Solving the Brain Puzzle

A Complete Layperson's Guide to Achieving Brain Health

— Bill Code M.D. —

◆ FriesenPress

Suite 300 - 990 Fort St
Victoria, BC, V8V 3K2
Canada

www.friesenpress.com

This book contains advice and information relating to healthcare. It is not intended
to replace medical advice and should be used to supplement rather than replace
regular care by your doctor. It is recommended that you seek your physician's advice
before embarking on any medical program for treatment. All efforts have been
made to assure the accuracy of the information contained in this book as of the
date of publication. The publisher and the author disclaim liability for any medical
outcomes that may occur as a result of applying the methods suggested in this book.

Lucinda Sykes M.D., Contributing Author
Denise Code MSc Nutrition, Contributing Author
Teri Jaklin ND, Contributing Author
Karen D. Johnson M.D., Contributing Author

For bulk purchases by groups or educational facilities, or for audiobook and other
languages, contact info@drbillcode.com

ISBN
978-1-5255-2724-1 (Hardcover)
978-1-5255-2725-8 (Paperback)
978-1-5255-2726-5 (eBook)

1. MEDICAL, ALTERNATIVE MEDICINE

Distributed to the trade by The Ingram Book Company

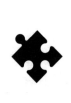

Contents

Section Five — Diagnoses

Section Six Interventions

Preface

I wrote my first personal book, *Who's In Control of Your Multiple Sclerosis?* (2005), because I was living with this diagnosis. The subtitle was "Pieces of the MS Puzzle." The answer to the question that the title poses is still the same: you are! In my ten-year journey since my last book, I have continued to search out pieces of the puzzle. I completed a two-year fellowship program in integrative medicine at the University of Arizona under Drs. Andrew Weil and Tierona Low Dog. I have attended multiple functional medicine courses and five conferences on integrative medicine for mental health. This includes being a guest lecturer at three of these on solutions for MS.

In conjunction with Dr. William Shaw, PhD, of Great Plains Laboratories (GPL) in Kansas, I have studied MS patients. We conducted a broad series of urine and blood tests, giving us a great deal of information about micronutrients, fatty acids, heavy trace metals, and gut flora. In addition, I have spent countless hours reading scientific literature, articles, and books in my quest for new solutions.

I have applied many of the solutions to my own situation and to a considerable number of clients. My credo is twofold: first, "Do no harm" and second, "Leave no stone unturned." Yes, I am fortunate to be able to understand most of these ideas or concepts due to my anesthesiology and intensive care specialty and, more recently, my background in integrative medicine.

I understand now how important it is to empower an individual on his or her journey. Indeed, if a person simply sits down and says, "Fix me, Doc," and is not invested in the process, I am handcuffed, because diet and lifestyle changes are what initiate and maintain one's health and improvement.

The other thing I have learned is that you can only take some people so far so fast. This is one reason for this book. Hopefully, it will help people progress at their own speed. Also, it will allow them to incorporate the choices they are currently capable of incorporating. I realize that geography, economics, and interaction with our loved ones must all be factored into our personal health journey.

Finally, I write this book primarily for the layperson, not the health care professional, although many new or different ideas in this book may help health care professionals. Most importantly, this book may assist you personally, your loved ones, or your clients in their journey to optimal health. If this book helps you as an individual or as a caregiver, then I will be grateful and feel rewarded.

How to Use this Book

This book is based on my forty years of medical experience. Included is a four-year stint in rural family practice, a specialty in anesthesiology, with board certification in Canada and the United States, six years in academic neuroscience research in anesthesia and stroke, twenty-two years of living with my own multiple sclerosis diagnosis and thirty-five years of migraine headaches.

I wrote this book to assist others with their own brain well-being. Brain transplants are not an option! Thus, what are our best alternatives? Like it or not, your best bet for brain health is in your hands. I initially used the phrase "Pieces of the Brain Recovery Puzzle" on the cover of this book to demonstrate how a number of small to modest incremental interventions can help you toward your goal of brain recovery/health. The subtitled changed, but the concept of puzzle pieces did not. Guides toward brain recovery are scarce, but bright spots (articles and books) exist. My goal is to provide these puzzle pieces to you in general groupings and individual chapters.

In this journey, you can choose each puzzle piece at your own speed. One benefit of chronic illness is time. You get to determine your own degree of urgency!

We are all a composite of our environment (air, water, and food intake) and our genetics. The good news is that we can modify genetics and environment, and by so doing, we can assist ourselves in general health and brain recovery. Our genetics can be assisted by epigenetics, which means turning good genes on and not-so-good genes off. Three major ways to do this are vitamin D, increased oxygen, and improved microbiota. Environmental improvement is a gradual, stepwise consideration of reducing our intake of toxins and assisting our body in getting rid of the toxins that we have accumulated to date. Most of us who are chronically ill are "canaries in the coal mine," because we become or stay ill while those around us do not.

Health Interventions Within Our Grasp

I have divided this book into six sections. Some people will read it in order. Others will pick and choose where they want to begin. Either approach is fine. The first section is on detoxification. This includes chapters on how to minimize toxins for prevention and how to remove them. The second section is on nutrition and supplements, including a chapter on energy and mitochondria. The third section is on anatomy and physiology. My hope is to give you enough information to understand how arterial, venous, and lymph circulation can be improved. This circulation is critical in the delivery of oxygen and the removal of toxins, which include by-products of energy, ATP, production. Oxygen is a critical component in our survival and has been missed as an intervention in our brain recovery. This error can now end with the information I provide. Finally, the previously unrecognized but vital component of our anatomy and physiology is the microbiome.

The next section is on pharmacology. This allows me to comment on many drugs that can help us. Some of these have a high cost/benefit ratio and so must either be avoided or used in a limited fashion. Other "drugs" include cannabis, which has a major chapter and references partly because of the controversy and unreasonable fear from its recent past, especially in the 1930s.

I have also included a list of diagnoses, because most of us are used to starting there in our recovery journey. This naming of illnesses has come at a cost, because the label or diagnosis has superseded our individuality. An example is the pain of a Crohn's disease patient, which can casually be left at "pain of Crohn's," while a lethal cancer of the rectum develops. Similarly, an MS patient with fatigue can have their hypothyroidism diagnosis delayed or missed altogether.

Finally, I discuss interventions toward brain recovery. There will be overlap, seeing as I touch on these subjects within earlier chapters. However, I list these, because they are recent enough to need some description for most readers. Cannabis is not listed in this group, but it certainly could be. Oxygen therapy is listed here, because it is too useful and critical not to be emphasized again and again. Photobiomodulation therapy (PBMT) and Gut Flora Transplant,GFT, or its earlier name, Fecal Microbiota Transplant (FMT) therapies are the new "kids on the block." I have also included additional practitioners who can guide you in this journey through integrative medicine, functional medicine, or other approaches.

Admittedly, there is a wide diversity of topics, because there are many pieces of the puzzle. These range from dental care, reducing electromagnetic smog, sleep issues, exercise, air quality, and cellular issues, especially energy and optimal mitochondrial function. Each chapter explains the specific concern and offers suggestions you can implement. Please, do not take these lightly, because the power of healing is dramatic and within your grasp.

Happily, you can initiate and individualize your own journey. Access to "technical" solutions, such as oxygen therapy, portable neuro stimulation (PoNS), photobiomodulation therapy (PBMT), and Gut Flora Transplant,GFT, also called fecal microbial transplant (FMT) is possible, because these are mostly private or outside the medical system at this time in most of the world. If you need assistance in your personal journey, read chapter 27 to find a list of experts to help you.

I have used all the therapies I discuss, as have hundreds of my clients. They are safe and follow the important medical diction in Latin, *"primum non nocere,"* which translates to "First, do no harm." This is one of the principle precepts of bioethics that all health care students are taught. Some practitioners have forgotten this sensible concept, but I have not. Therefore, you are safe to proceed with all the non-surgical interventions I discuss in this book. The only surgery I suggest, in select cases, is venous balloon angioplasty and only with a skilled and well-informed interventional radiologist, such as Dr. Salvatore Sclafani.

Section One
Toxification Issues

1: Detoxify and Live Better

My goal with this chapter is to convince you that detoxification is necessary for achieving optimal health and for recovery from illness. I've changed my thinking considerably since my early days as a general practitioner in my late twenties. At that time, I thought there was a drug solution for nearly every diagnosis. I was wrong and naïve. Detoxification has several components, and for this to occur, consider it a long-term detoxification lifestyle. In this chapter, I address the concept of reducing toxic exposure, better personal detoxification, and the importance of clean water, air, food, and your immediate environment.

Detoxification is a critical task of every single cell in your body. Without a good detoxification plan, we get sick earlier and die younger. Coupled with this will be the reduced function of your brain, including memory problems and even dementia. The detoxification process involves mobilization and biological transformation and elimination of toxins within (by-products of energy production) and without (enter the body from the food, water, and air we breathe). Much of this discussion is from a superb article by my friend, John Cline, MD, BSc, IFMCP (Functional Medicine) (Cline 2013). His article, "Nutritional Aspects of Detoxification in Clinical Practice," was published in *Alternative Therapies Journal*. He also wrote an excellent book in 2008 called *Detoxify and Live* (Cline 2008). It is still popular and valid. If you are looking for more detail, then his book is an excellent place to start. If you want more in-depth information, I suggest Sherry A. Rogers' book, *Detoxify or Die* (Rogers 2002).

In Dr. Cline's article, he outlines that patients often request a detoxification program and are actually surprised to learn it is *not* a program. Instead, people need to adopt a *detoxification lifestyle*. Components of this lifestyle include:

1. Avoidance of environmental toxicants, such as heavy metals, persistent organic pollutants (including glyphosate, a.k.a. Roundup), and electromagnetic radiation
2. Mobilization or elimination of toxicants by a loss of excessive fat and use of saunas, chelation therapy, and exercise
3. Optimal gastrointestinal health
4. Excellent nutrition and hydration
5. Attention to stress and resilience to relational health (improved relationships)
6. Adequate sleep and relaxation

Healthcare practitioners should model this detoxification lifestyle. This encourages patients to adopt similar health practices.

The most important recommendation is to reduce your toxin intake. Breathe the cleanest air possible. If you choose to live in one of the toxic localities or cities where you can "see" the air, then you should put a HEPA filter in your home and office heating or air system. This applies to a large number of people, including those living in most major cities, such as the industrial belt of all nations. In Canada, this includes all of southern Ontario. In the USA, this includes the entire Northeast, at least as far west as Chicago.

Be aware of all the toxins that originate outside the body. These include drugs, both pharmaceutical and recreational, heavy metals, chemical herbicides and insecticides, food contaminants and additives, household cleaners, and makeup and body care products, to name a few. Our skin is a good protector, but it is not infallible. Whatever is applied to the skin or worn close to the skin may be absorbed through the skin. Examples of these are body care products, cosmetics, and laundry soap. I recommend that you get rid of your lawn fertilizers and sprays. I have a client who insists he must use two major weed sprays to maintain acceptability to his neighbours in a gated community. Meanwhile, his MS continues to progress. This is so wrong! Perhaps he needs to move or advocate change in his community. Fortunately, many healthy and non-toxic products that benefit you and the environment are available.

In addition, do not drink tap water just because you've been told it is safe. Your drinking water will probably benefit from an inexpensive under-the-counter reverse-osmosis system. Our bodies are more than 70 percent water, and we need a significant amount every day. Remember the following concept: "Dilution is the solution to pollution." Drink plenty of pure water daily to flush toxins from your body. Finally, be aware of the origin of all your food and drink. Eat organic whole foods whenever possible.

The body's detoxification involves multiple steps within the cells. These steps are needed to change the mainly non-polar, lipid-soluble toxicants into polar, water-soluble compounds. Then these water-soluble compounds can readily be eliminated in the bile, feces, urine, and sweat.

The body has two major paths for detoxification. These are referred to as phase 1 detoxification and phase 2 detoxification.

Phase I Detoxification

Phase 1 detoxification occurs mainly in the liver and the gut cells, including our microbiota (gut bacteria). The liver is critically important in this process. A sign of this is its ability to regenerate over several months. Significant detoxification and biotransformation also occur in the brain, lungs, kidneys, and skin. This phase 1 system is made up of at least 57 pathways, called the cytochrome P450 (CYP) enzyme family of mixed function oxidases. The term "P450" is derived from the spectrophotometric peak at the light wavelength of the absorption maximum of the enzyme (450 nanometers, i.e., nm) when it is in the reduced state and complexed with carbon monoxide. These CYP enzymes have been identified in all kingdoms of life, including animals, plants, and fungi. Cytochrome P450 enzymes are present in most body tissues. They play important roles in hormone synthesis and breakdown, including estrogen and testosterone synthesis and metabolism, cholesterol synthesis, and vitamin D metabolism. Cytochrome P450 enzymes come from the light frequency of 450 nm, at which these enzymes have maximum effect.

The nine most common CYP enzymes are 1A1, 1B1, 2A6, 2B6, 2C9, 2C19, 2-D6, 2E1, and 3A4. I mention these specifically, because they are the ones most commonly featured in genetic testing to see you if you have a reduced ability to use one of these pathways. This is predicated on your genetic makeup. However, before you rush out and spend a lot of money on this, remember that you can often adapt the genes you have by optimizing your genetics. This is done with wise food choices and supplements that have an epigenetic effect. "Epigenetic" means foods and other substances are able to turn genes on and off. One of the most significant of these is vitamin D. Also, a careful history of your life and exposure and responses to medications, environmental toxins, and even makeup may give some major clues to the experienced clinician in environmental toxicology. A good functional medicine physician or integrative physician will either have this skill set or know someone who does. If this clinician suggests genetic testing, and you can afford it, then go ahead. But remember, you have control over what goes into your body, so if you are not willing to change what you do, then why bother testing?

Almost all of us ignore our detoxification issues and eat, drink, and breathe almost anything, until we get sick. Then wise people wake up and shift their paradigm. Those who do not wake up and change their ways do so at their own peril. It took me more than a year or so to wake up after my diagnosis of MS in 1996. I could have chosen to let the neurologist direct my life and start on disease-modifying drugs. Similarly, most neurologists say dietary changes are useless and that there is no support for this in the literature. They are incorrect. I soon realized their direction was misleading and skewed by pharmaceutical choice. Most of the disease-modifying drugs for MS are quite toxic. In addition, the last twenty years has revealed they have virtually no value in reducing long-term disability. Several long-term literature reviews have confirmed this, including one by neurologist Dr. Ebers of Oxford (see MS Hope.) In contrast to the drug path, we can embark safely on our own personal diet and lifestyle changes.

Before proceeding, I would like to emphasize that all drug products, whether prescription or over-the-counter, have major effects on our many detoxification pathways. This includes all painkillers, such as ibuprofen and acetaminophen, opiates, gabapentin, and antiseizure medication. If you must take these, then you should be extra careful with all the other toxins that you take in, because you are already having to adapt to the effects of the drug on your detoxification pathways. Similarly, if you still have mercury amalgam fillings in your mouth, you should have them removed. Once you get ill, you need to make many small changes to your health. Rarely are there single silver bullets for us to get well again. If you are fortunate and are not yet ill, you can typically make fewer corrections. If you make these optimal changes, you will move toward improved health. Dementia and other chronic illnesses start twenty to thirty years prior to the diagnosis. So, if fear motivates you, use it. For more details, see chapter 23 on Alzheimers.

For the P450 pathway phase 1 detoxification enzymes to work effectively, we must eat high-quality bioavailable protein and a host of nutrients, botanicals, minerals, fats, and carbohydrates. All body tissues can use healthy saturated fats as a source of energy. This includes the brain and the heart. The benefit of these fats is that they burn cleaner than carbohydrates. Consequently, by using fat as our major source of energy, we reduce the toxic metabolic by-products that are producing energy within our cells by some 30-40 percent. This is particularly well described in Dr. Joseph Mercola's recent book, *Fat for Fuel* (Mercola 2017).

Once the toxins have gone through the phase 1 detoxification process, the changed molecules are often more toxic than the parent compound. These intermediate metabolites can cause cellular damage. The body protects itself while waiting for the phase 2 detoxification process to occur. This is where antioxidants are your best friend. Antioxidants quench the free radicals created by the toxic intermediate metabolites and stop them from creating havoc within the cell. These antioxidants include a large number of plant derivatives, vitamins, and minerals. Any time you eat these foods or foods containing these components, you are improving your detoxification and cleaning your body.

Antioxidants from Food

Carotenoids:	lycopene, beta-carotene
Carotene:	lutein, zeaxanthin, astaxanthin
Vitamins:	C, E (mixed tocopherols)
Minerals:	copper, selenium, zinc, manganese
Other antioxidants:	Coenzyme Q10 Alpha lipoic acid
Glutathione boosters:	Cysteine from quality whey protein N-acetylcysteine from supplements (NAC)
Thiols:	garlic, onions, cruciferous vegetables
Bioflavonoids:	silymarin,Quercetin:broccoli,citrus and red and yellow onions
Polyphenols:	pomegranates, green tea, raspberries, grapes
Anthocyanins:	blueberries,blackberries,cherry,Concord or Muscadine grapes
Other pigments:	Curcumin,Red beet root,Chlorophyll

Phase 2 Detoxification

The majority of the intermediate metabolites produced from phase 1 progress onto the phase 2 conjugation pathways. These compounds are joined to other molecules, such as glucuronide sulphate, glutathione, various amino acids, such as taurine, glycine, arginine, glutamine, serine, proline, and other small carbon formations (methyl and ethyl groups). Glutathione is especially important as it is the body's most significant antioxidant and detoxifying agent. One way to enhance this is with NAC i.e., N-acetylcysteine, which supplies the most needed of three amino acids, namely cysteine. This is well described in an excellent review, "N-acetylcysteine (NAC) in neurological disorders: mechanisms of action and therapeutic opportunities" (Shahripour 2014). Undenatured whey protein is another source of this key building block of glutathione (Bounous 1988). I discuss my use of whey protein later. Following this phase 2 reaction, most compounds are water soluble. They can be excreted by bile and feces or the serum plasma with perspiration, sweating, or lung exhalation or, the most common method, through the kidneys and urine. For example, the gas anaesthetic, halothane, is excreted in the skin, lungs, and the liver. Evidence in animal models shows that an algae, Chlorella, may inhibit the reabsorption of heavy metals and some organic pollutants. This, of course, would help the process of detoxification.

"Let food be thy medicine and thy medicine be food." — Hippocrates, the father of medicine, 431 BC.

Your best path to safe, healthy detoxification is from the dozens of protective nutrients in many different fruits and vegetables. Aim for fifty different foods per week. This is the same as my recommendation for optimal microbiota. I hope repetition burns this into your brain. A broad spectrum of fruits and vegetables and other plants will positively modify the expression of your good signalling and help cell-to-cell signalling within the body as well.

Chelation

I would be remiss if I did not comment on this valuable tool. The Chlorella mentioned above is a form of oral chelation. So is the fibre you eat daily, so keep up your fibre intake! Also, oral DMSA (dimercaptosuccinic acid) or citrus fruit pectin are other types of oral chelation. I realize some people think of the more dramatic intravenous chelation. Yes, this can be dramatic for severe heavy metal toxicity. It must be dramatic, as one episode of the TV series *House* used intravenous chelation in their intensive care unit as a lifesaving event. It is an option, but most of us would be best guided by a health care practitioner who is knowledgeable in this arena. I rely on my nearby colleague, Dr. John Cline, because he is much better in this field than I am. A huge study on chelation, done by the National Institutes of Health (NIH) in the USA, validated the potential value of intravenous chelation "JAMA" (Lamas 2013). They studied the use of disodium EDTA chelation regimen on cardiovascular events in patients with previous myocardial infarction. When compared with a placebo, they found the disodium EDTA modestly reduced the risk of adverse cardiovascular outcomes.

This use of intravenous disodium EDTA chelation was particularly helpful in the subset of patients with diabetes mellitus and a prior myocardial infarction. A detailed study on this was reported in the journal *Circulation* (Escolar 2013). They describe a 41 percent reduction of combined cardiovascular mortality, nonfatal stroke, or nonfatal MI (myocardial infarction). There was a 52 percent reduction in recurrent myocardial infarction and a 43 percent reduction in death from any cause. The authors recommended further study, but there were more than 300 patients in each group. Therefore, I feel comfortable in recommending this as a possibility, particularly in the diabetes mellitus group, as this is often one of the poorest respondents to other interventions. In addition, for individuals unwilling, or unable, to be adequately compliant with diet and lifestyle changes, intravenous disodium EDTA chelation is another possibility.

Glymphatics: The Brain Lymph System

A final important detoxification method is the glymphatic system within the brain and spinal cord. Recent evidence from universities in the USA and Finland have confirmed that we have a lymphatic "drainage" or cleaning system within the brain and spinal cord (Xie 2013). This fluid link between the cerebrospinal fluid, CSF , and the lymphatic system is called the glymphatic system, which is a blend of the words "glial" and "lymphatic." Glial cells are also called astrocytes and are as numerous and important as neurons in brain support and function.

In descriptive terms, a flushing occurs with CSF along glial cells and in between brain cells. This flushing removes many of the by-products or "exhaust" of energy production by the brain cells' mitochondria. In addition, this "brainwashing" removes many toxins, such as heavy metals and herbicides, which, if not removed, further injure brain cells. We know this glymphatic brain wash, described earlier (Cook 2007), occurs best and almost completely during sleep. Therefore, be sure and read chapter 13 to learn how sleep can help optimize the glymphatic detoxification body function. We also now know EMF,more in Chapter 3, interferes with cellular detoxification processes. Therefore any time you further reduce your EMF exposure you help your detoxification.

2: Dental Care

This subject has several components. These are bruxism (grinding teeth at night), gum disease, dental extractions, and mercury amalgam fillings.

In my forties, my dentist told me I must be clenching my jaw during the day. This was a possible trigger of my headaches. Also, my teeth were wearing down, consistent with night clenching and grinding. My dentist gave me a night guard to minimize this problem. A few years later, after my MS diagnosis and after changing my mercury molar fillings with non-amalgams topped with gold crowns, my bite was much improved. It also seemed to help align my jaw, so I clenched less and quit grinding my teeth at night.

Another therapy that helped my jaw and clenching came from a NUCCA (National Upper Cervical Chiropractic Association) procedure. NUCCA chiropractors perform a precise, non-invasive, gentle touch to realign the neck and upper spine. I learned from my chiropractor that optimal positioning of the C1 to C2 vertebrae reduced jaw spasms. This same chiropractor also helped me conquer the terrible pterygopalatine (back of the molars) muscle spasms that I had after my wisdom teeth were extracted by an excellent oral surgeon.

Gum disease has been an ongoing problem for me despite good oral care. Now I recognize two contributing factors. One was the anti-depressant tricyclic Imipramine, begun in 1982 and taken for nearly twenty years. It has major anti-cholinergic (drying) side effects, with much-reduced saliva. The second contributing factor was my CCSVI (chronic cerebrospinal venous insufficiency), which I talk about in chapter 9. Four of our five salivary glands—mainly two under the tongue, the submental, and maxillary salivary glands on each side— drain to the internal jugular vein. In my case, this drainage occurred above my constricted internal jugular vein valve. Once this valve was ballooned at the narrowed site, my saliva has maintained better than ever. A further case of this was one of my young clients who, at age thirty-three, also had treatment for CCSVI for neurological issues. Before treatment, he had minimal saliva flow and significant gum disease despite excellent dental care. After his venous angioplasty, ballooning of his relatively stenosed internal jugular vein valves, his saliva and dental health improved dramatically. This was confirmed by his dentist, who initially diagnosed the problem as "dry socket," although it was actually due to inflammation-triggered muscle spasms. Another helpful treatment was my chiropractor massaging the inner jaw area behind my molars with a gloved hand. After two to three weeks of grief and pain, I realized again "too soon old and too late smart." However, I was grateful for the chiropractic treatments, which eased my jaw pain.

I am sure my personal journey with mercury began with molar cavities in early elementary school, even though I only had candy on allowance day (Saturday) and Halloween. Perhaps my dental health was also negatively impacted by the reduced saliva from my neck vein problem. It's hard to tell. However, by the time I was twelve, I had a mouth full of amalgams.

My other habit of chewing food thoroughly probably heightened the amount of mercury vapour I inhaled. Inorganic mercury (mercury vapour) is exceedingly toxic to the brain and spinal cord. Another common source of mercury is fish, which was rare in my youth, being a Protestant lad growing up on the prairies. Hence, methylmercury from fish was a small issue for me until 1992, when we moved to the west coast of Canada, where I had greater access to fresh fish.

It is probably worth mentioning that I had all my vaccinations, which all contained mercury as either an immune adjuvant (to enhance the immune response to the vaccine), a preservative, or both. This mercury is ethyl mercury, which is taken rapidly to the brain and quickly transforms into inorganic mercury, the most toxic form. This mercury can take months or years to be removed from the brain. As a medical student, I received all possible vaccines, including the first available hepatitis B vaccine in 1981. This particular vaccine may have been the tipping point for me. Also, one French study suggests this vaccine seems to precipitate MS.

I met a naturopath in the spring of 1997 who suggested a urine challenge with DMPS (sodium 2, 3-dimercapto) to evaluate my heavy metals. He found that both mercury and lead were very high, so he gave me ten rounds of intravenous EDTA (ethylene diamond tetra-acetic acid) chelation. Curiously, my light touch returned for several weeks after the DMPS challenge test but disappeared again four months later. It is still absent today. A further DMPS urine challenge in 2011 revealed that mercury and lead were still relatively high, but my consultant admitted EDTA was not very good at removing mercury. By then it was thirteen years since my amalgams had been removed. Then, in 2013, I had a hair analysis for heavy metals, which revealed mercury and lead were still quite high. I know now that hair mercury is almost all methyl mercury and is not indicative of how much circulating inorganic mercury is in the body. This knowledge was assisted by Dr. Chris Slade of Quicksilver Scientific. Mercury has a significant effect on the entire cardiovascular system (Houston 2011). This is critical in brain blood flow and oxygen supply, so be sure to read chapter 20, "The New MS," further on.

Imagine yourself in a canoe or rowboat that springs a leak. All is fine until you take a considerable amount of water on board. Once that happens, you must do something, or you will drown. Mercury is much the same. Returning to the boat analogy, the bigger the hole, the sooner the toxic level is reached. If it starts raining hard, that adds to your problem. Dental amalgams constantly release mercury vapour, which you swallow and breathe in. Every time you chew, it "rains" harder. The other factor that increases the speed of absorption is a vaccination containing mercury. You can switch the rain off by having the amalgams removed. This should be done by a skilled and, if possible, biologic dentist. These dentists are particularly concerned with the consequences on our general health secondary to foreign metals placed on our teeth or gums. It is best to have a rubber dam in your mouth to protect you from breathing in the mercury vapour while the drilling is being done. In addition, they should have the suction running the entire time to minimize your contact as well as the dentist's and his assistant's contact with mercury. It is also best to take a significant number of antioxidants in preparation for and during the procedure. This includes at least vitamin C, vitamin E, coenzyme Q-10, alpha lipoic acid, and glutathione, or at least its precursors. For these precursors, see chapter 6, especially my comments on whey protein.

The solution is to use a bailing can to remove the water from the boat. If you have a large amount of mercury in your body, you are an individual with slow metabolic removal, i.e., you have a small bailing can. If, however, you improve your body's removal by enhancing the critical amount of glutathione and the four detoxifying minerals (selenium, zinc, copper, and molybdenum), then you can dramatically increase the size of your bailing can and thus remove your mercury load.

The final variable you can improve is the active transport system in your kidneys, which sends mercury out in the urine. These are particularly injured by cadmium, arsenic, lead, and NSAIDs (nonsteroidal anti-inflammatory drugs—see chapter 14). By lowering these elements, you improve the health of the active transport cells in your kidneys.

I want to give you a few more details about methylmercury, the type that is derived mainly from fish. Some of us are limited in our ability to remove mercury and should avoid fish. This can be determined through laboratory testing, such as that available from Quicksilver Scientific. It is also recommended that pregnant or breastfeeding mothers minimize their fish intake. We also know that large predators or bottom-dwelling fish, such as swordfish and halibut, have considerably more mercury. Although salmon tends to be lower in mercury, some choices in this group are better than others. It is better to eat sockeye salmon, a plankton feeder, than a large Chinook or King salmon, as these two are predators and accumulate more mercury during their lifespan. Size matters too. If a salmon or tuna is more than ten pounds (4.5 kilograms), then they have considerably more mercury. In other words, know where your fish comes from.

The FDA (Food and Drug Administration) and the EPA (Environmental Protection Agency) in the United States have issued guidelines for fish and seafood consumption with respect to mercury. These guidelines are also applicable to women who are planning a pregnancy or who are already pregnant. These guidelines are as follows.

1. Do not eat shark, swordfish, king mackerel, or tilefish.
2. Eat twelve oz (360 grams) or two meals per week of lower-mercury fish and seafood. This includes shrimp, canned light tuna, salmon, pollock, and catfish.

Albacore tuna is higher in mercury and should be limited to six oz (180 grams) per week.

3. If eating fish from contaminated local waters (rivers and lakes), limit intake to six oz (180 grams) per week.

Another factor in how well we are able to eliminate mercury is the particular strains of abnormal bacteria that may be in the gut. Some of these bacteria make us quite susceptible to methyl mercury. Methyl mercury absorption is also an issue if we have "leaky gut," which can arise from damage by gluten, casein, antibiotic use, chemotherapy, NSAIDs, and, over time, excess heavy metals (see chapter 11).

Looking back at my life, I had several complicating factors that made mercury a problem. First, I had reduced saliva flow due to reduced venous blood drainage, probably since birth. Next, I had a large number of amalgam fillings at an early age. Then, at age twenty-eight, I was put on a mouth-drying antidepressant, reducing my saliva, which resulted in more amalgam fillings and consequent gum disease. As I note in chapter 11, I also had a lot of antibiotics as a child. Though born vaginally, I was raised on formula. By age twenty-nine, I was advised I had irritable bowel syndrome, and I eventually determined that I was gluten sensitive. Hence, this would have compounded mercury toxicity in my body. Fortunately, when I started on a large amount (50–60 grams per day) of a quality whey protein isolate, I boosted my glutathione. Glutathione is made up of three amino acids, the rate-limiting one being cysteine. Cysteine is readily available in whey protein that has not been overheated or put through a high-speed blender. This boost in glutathione dramatically assisted my body in removing heavy metals, particularly mercury. Finally, the total removal of all amalgam mercury fillings by age forty-four was an excellent assist.

Optimal dental care is a critical part of health. Healthy teeth can add up to eight years of life. The only individual item that is as striking as this is stopping smoking. It is beyond my expertise to cover dentistry well, so find a quality dentist. If this individual does not accept the concern about mercury, then find a different dentist. Healthy teeth and gums permit optimal chewing, which is a keystone in the absorption of nutrients from the food you eat. Your microbiota begins with your teeth.

3: Dirty Electricity, Electromagnetic Fields (EMF), and Your Brain

By Dr. Teri Jaklin, ND

Just about everyone today carries some sort of Wi-Fi device on their body. Despite research warning us against it, nobody seems to be all that worried about it. Cell towers loom in our communities, and most homes, businesses, schools, and even cars are Wi-Fi enabled. This is not a good thing.

Dirty electricity, such as electromagnetic fields (EMF) emitted from Wi-Fi devices, has become an unavoidable pollutant. It is everywhere, and to make things worse, it is invisible. It flows along anything metallic, like household pipes and wires, and radiates from them into your home. Your exposure to dirty electricity is compounded by wireless routers and wireless devices like game consoles, computers, cell phones, plasma TVs, baby monitors, (yes, baby monitors), cordless phones that use DECT (digitally enhanced cell technology), "smart" meters installed by hydro companies (with and without your permission), compact fluorescent lightbulbs, and even neighbors who are close enough to share *their* dirty electricity load. Now look out your window. The telecom giants have sneaky ways of concealing cell towers. I have seen them camouflaged as flagpoles outside workplaces and retirement residences. They are often found on top of condo and apartment buildings, and then there is the towering inferno—the classic, ugly old cell tower. The most ironic thing I have ever seen was at a church, whose decorative cross, which stood a good 100 feet (30 meters) had been turned into a cell tower. Ironically, the base of that cross/tower was a sign for their pre-school, which went by the name "Small Fry."

Dirty electricity cannot be seen, felt, heard, or tasted. Therefore, you have no idea you are even being exposed. Basically, you are smothered daily by a blanket of electromagnetic smog. This smog has a scientific basis for its ill effects on your health, and there is precious little you can do about it. In fact, the previous American administration made a commitment to connectivity everywhere in the nation. You know what that means: more cell towers, more exposure, and more cellular damage . . . for everyone.

Many people do not do well with exposure. Many more do not even know it could be a contributing factor to their ill health. The World Health Organization (WHO) has classified symptoms arising from this exposure as electrohypersensitivity (EHS) or idiopathic environmental intolerance. Still, a body of scientists says if it doesn't physically burn you (Health Canada Safety Code 6 standards), there is no basis for thinking it harmful. My guess is that they work for the telecom industry, because if you look, there is an abundance of quality research expressing concern.

In 2009, I came across the Bioinitiative Report, a collection of research gathered by a group of scientists, researchers, and public health policy professionals calling for "biologically-based exposure standards for low intensity electromagnetic radiation," such as that emitted by the wireless devices mentioned above.[1] In 2012, the Bioinitiative Report was updated

---

[1]   Read the entire report here: www.bioinitiative.com.

to include 1,800 of the most current scientific articles on the subject. These scientific articles demonstrate "the bioeffects (effects on the body) of EMF are clearly established and occur at very low levels of exposure." These effects can occur within minutes of regular cell or cordless phone use or whole-body exposure to cell towers, Wi-Fi, and wireless smart meters. The report goes on to state "chronic levels of this exposure can result in illness."That is probably not what you wanted to hear, but it begs the question: what are these bio-effects? To summarize directly from the Bioinitiative Report (Carpenter 2012), the DNA is impacted in many ways, leading to direct DNA damage with the loss of DNA repair capacity in human stem cells,[2] the protective function of free-radical scavengers—particularly melatonin—is reduced,[3] neurotoxicity in humans and animals,[4] carcinogenicity in humans,[5] effects on offspring behavior,[6] and effects on brain and cranial bone development in the offspring of animals that are exposed to cell phone radiation during pregnancy.[7] Too much information? This is only a snapshot of the evidence presented.What is the bottom line? Electrosmog causes physiological stress in the body. When the body can't keep up with its attempts to repair the damage, disease symptoms begin. Mechanisms of action include heat shock proteins, which damage the DNA, changes in blood-brain barrier permeability, and increased free radical damage.

When I dug deeper, I discovered that the concept of dirty electricity and its ill effects is not new. Dr. Samuel Milham, MD, MPH, connected the introduction of electricity to

---

[2]   Sections 5, 6, 7, and 15

[3]   Sections 5, 9, 13, 14, 15, 16, and 17

[4]   Section 9

[5]   Sections 11, 12, 13, 14, 15, 16, and 17

[6]   Sections 18, 19, and 20

[7]   Sections 5 and 18

America with a notable increase in death from most diseases (Milham 2010). His data was ignored for almost a century. By the time a study began on how electromagnetic fields (EMFs) affect the human body, in 1979, the entire American population had been exposed to EMFs. There was no longer a pure control group, as required for scientific studies. Canada's own Dr. Magda Havas, PhD, is one of the foremost researchers and world educators on the subject of EMR. She is also a leader in the field of dirty electricity, a topic that, until recently, has been largely ignored by the scientific community.

I have had the privilege of connecting with Dr. Havas on two occasions. The first meeting was when the community I live in fought a major carrier's attempt to locate a monstrous cell tower in the heart of our small hamlet. More recently, I did an interview with her for this chapter. I encourage you to go to her YouTube channel and learn from her yourself (Havas 2016). She is a tireless advocate for your health in the face of EMF. While you are there, check out Dr. Milham (Milham 2010) and the Bioinitiative Report (Carpenter 2012) as well.

Now, let's get specific on the role of electromagnetic fields and its impact on the brain. The fact is, few studies directly connect EMF and individual brain conditions, but it is just a matter of time, since brain health is a hot topic. Some work has been done with ALS (amyotrophic lateral sclerosis, a.k.a. "Lou Gehrig's disease"). Dr. Havas herself has worked with people with MS and found that dirty electricity can exacerbate their symptoms.

Dr. Havas agrees it is hard to prove in MS, because the measurement is so subjective. Having said that, her research shows that once dirty electricity is reduced, the health of people with MS improves. The inspiration for her study was a high school principal in Wisconsin who has MS. The school suffered from dirty electricity, and the principal was set to retire, because her symptoms had become so bad. Once the school cleaned up the dirty electricity, she recovered. However, when she was exposed to dirty electricity in other aspects of her life, she relapsed. In the recently published results of this study, the improvement in individuals with MS occurred in as quickly as two to six weeks after the dirty electricity in their environment was cleaned up. Dr. Havas concludes, "electrosmog can be an irritant for people with MS" (Havas 2006). It affects the central and autonomic nervous systems as well as the immune system, not to mention the free radical damage and consequential physiological stress.

What about the brain in general? What about traumatic brain injury, Alzheimer's, Parkinson's, ALS, and even conditions like depression, migraines, and ADD/ADHD? The research is growing in these areas as well (check the Bioinitiative Report). But bear in mind we are in a time where the understanding of the mechanisms of action is far ahead of the proof for EMF in each individual condition. So, let's look at the big picture: the blood-brain barrier (BBB).

A healthy brain is maintained by the blood-brain barrier. The BBB protects the sensitive brain tissue from toxins present in blood and lymphatic circulation. This ensures a pristine environment for the sensitive brain tissue and its executive functions.

Many things can cause increased permeability of the BBB, leading to neuro-inflammation and damaged neurons. Dirty electricity, including cell phone radiofrequency radiation (RFR), is one of them. Many studies show that low-intensity exposure to RFR can affect the BBB. The Bioinitiative Report sums up the research, stating,

> it is more probable than unlikely that non-thermal EMF from cell phones and base stations do have effects upon biology. A single two hour exposure to cell phone radiation can result in increased leakage

of the BBB, and fifty days after exposure, neuronal damage can be seen. The levels of RFR needed to affect the BBB have been shown to be less than holding a mobile phone at arm's length and BBB effects occur at about 1000 times lower RFR exposure levels than the US and ICNIRP (International Commission on Non-Ionizing Radiation Protection) limits allow.

Essentially, no safety legislation is in place in Canada or the USA, to protect consumers from the health hazards specific to this radiofrequency communications electrosmog. The most frightening thing of all is that this happens twice as fast in people who start using a cell phone before age twenty (Hardell 2008). Do you know anyone younger than twenty who uses a cell phone?

In 2009, when I was interviewing people for our cause, I spoke to a gentleman who had worked for one of the major telecom carriers just as the cell phone explosion began. He had clocked 3,000 cell minutes per month for three years, long before we started thinking about headsets and hands-free. He was in his late thirties and had a clearly visible flash of white in his otherwise brown hair just above his right ear, his cell phone ear. He confirmed that this flash of white occurred two years into his cell phone-focused work. He went on to explain that, since then, five years after he left that company, if he held a cell phone to that ear, it triggered a terrible headache.

Are you asking the same question I am? If the BBB can be damaged at such low exposure, and neuroinflammation is indicated in brain injury in general, how could it possibly *not* affect whatever process is at work in any disease that plays itself out in the brain? And with the current statistic of one in nine people over age sixty-five with Alzheimer's disease, what does that mean for future generations, who have been exposed to EMF since conception? Beyond the BBB, I cannot help but think about the impact on other delicate structures, like the microbiome, whose health is already connected directly to the brain.

Recently developed metering and filtering equipment provides scientists with the tools to measure and reduce dirty electricity. Graham/Stetzer (GS) filters have been installed in schools with "sick building syndrome," and the health and energy levels of staff and students have improved. Individuals diagnosed with MS have better balance and fewer tremors. Those requiring a cane walked unassisted within a few days or weeks after GS filters were installed in their home. The number of students needing inhalers for asthma was reduced in one school, and student behavior associated with ADD/ADHD improved in another school. Blood sugar levels for some diabetics respond to the amount of dirty electricity in their environment. Type 1 diabetics require less insulin, and type 2 diabetics have lower blood sugar levels in an electromagnetically clean environment. Scientists like Dr. Havas, retired Washington State University biochemistry professor Martin Pall, who has proposed a biological mechanism for EHS, and Harvard neurology professor Martha Herbert, who has suggested there could be links between EMFs and autism, all have scientific evidence of a connection between electromagnetic pollution and health conditions (Carpenter 2012). This connection needs to be investigated on a wider scale, so we can determine the true story behind the number of people sensitive to this form of energy, how it is impacting their health, and what it means to other unexplored areas, such as brain health.

How many people with MS or any other brain injury are electrohypersensitive? What role does electrosmog play in neurodegeneration? Skeptics say the science is not there. Advocates tell a tale of urgency. We live in a revolutionary time in the history of medicine, where science is changing faster than the evidence base can keep up.

You may not have control of the blistering rate that cell towers and cell sites are going up around you, but you have the freedom to make choices. When that cell tower was scheduled to go up in our community, my husband and I began making arrangements to sell our house and move. It was that important to us. About 5 km (3 miles) south of my home is a busy intersection that I avoid as much as possible. I call it "dirty corners." Not only is the air dirty from the volume of traffic, there are also three cell towers and a high-voltage power line passing through it. I feel strongly enough about EMF exposure to stay away!

At times, it can get overwhelming. It seems that free Wi-Fi is a basic human right, not an option or, heaven forbid, a health hazard. It seems everything from baby monitors to guitars are wireless. I know young people who have never known safer options, like a landline, much less a rotary phone! But you can put some electro-boundaries in place to protect yourself and your family.

Whether you are convinced or not, you can still take some simple steps to reduce dirty electricity in your home, or at the least set some healthy boundaries around connectivity. If you have children, I recommend implementing these now. Let the science prove us wrong, which I am fairly confident it will not. Some of these may make you wince or even squirm a bit. That's okay. Once they are in place, you'll find it hard to believe you ever did it any other way.

Creating a Protection Plan

1. Use your cell phone as little as possible. Use airplane mode whenever you can, and turn it off when you go

to bed. Leave it as far away from your body as possible while you are sleeping, preferably in another room. One of the worst-case scenarios is charging your phone on the bedside table while you sleep. Do that on the kitchen counter, where it is not directly adjacent to your treasured brain. I have a number of patients who collect all the household phones at night, turn them off, and return them in the morning, so the family is not pathologically connected to the phone overnight. Night and sleep are preciously rejuvenating for the brain and body, not a time for texting or social media.

2. Explore the settings on your wireless router. Routers are getting increasingly powerful, emitting more and more EMF. You can decrease the transmitter's power to the point where it meets your needs. Most router software has a timer, so use it! Set the timer to shut the Wi-Fi down at a specific time, so you and your family are not exposed for the eight hours you sleep each night. In our house, the router shuts down at 10:00 p.m. and comes back on at 7:30 a.m.

3. You can also install a demand switch, so you can turn the router on and off, and it is only on when you require an internet connection. If you really want to get way from Wi-Fi, install an ethernet cable in your home office or to your TV.

4. Some general household tips include not using compact fluorescent bulbs, heating pads/blankets, or waterbeds and removing anything that is plugged into a wall socket close to the head of your bed (e.g., clock radios, lamps). Keep them at least two meters from your bed.

5. Remove all cordless phones that use DECT. The base station on a DECT phone is constantly communicating with the handsets, which means you do not have to be on a call for the device to be in transmit mode. This

means it is constantly spewing electrosmog. When I first began learning about the health hazards of EMF, we had just purchased a new, fancy cordless phone set. The gentleman I was interviewing at the time told me not to worry so much about my cell phone. He said if I had a DECT base station, it was like having a cell tower in my living room! Needless to say, I returned it the same day.

If you want to take it a step further, you can install GS filters in your home to reduce dirty electricity. Depending on how impacted you are by electrosmog, a number of other shielding products, from paints to fabrics, are now readily available. In 2009, as part of my learning curve, I had our home tested for dirty electricity and EMF exposure and took measures to correct them. It did not involve GS filters, but I feel now is a good time for them. Even without the cell tower, I know our exposure has gone up. When we moved into our current home fifteen years ago, there was just one point in the entire home where we could get cell coverage. Now we can even use our cellphone in the basement. Like so many others, we had our hydro meter replaced with a (not so) smart meter, despite a sign forbidding them to do so. We also have a router, cell phones, iPads, and multiple computers in the house. It is definitely time to revisit our electrosmog situation.

It is said that EMF is the "new tobacco" or "asbestos," where the industries engaged the top researchers and stopped funding others who were finding evidence of harm. Clearly, the wireless industry will not support the needed research and will most likely stay silent rather than take the lead. No one wants to admit that something so lucrative and so essential could possibly cause illness. As a result, damning research is silenced until the detrimental health effect can no longer be ignored, and the research can no longer be denied. This cycle has repeated itself through history.

If the "new tobacco" theory and the findings of scientists outlined not just here but all over the world are even partially true, we are in big trouble. The explosive growth of everyday devices emitting EMF has been called a twentieth-century epidemic. Are we paving the way to a twenty-first century epidemic of disease and death caused by a silent yet formidable foe?

As overwhelming as this sounds, do what you can. Continue to educate yourself, and make decisions on equipment that might minimize EMF exposure. Turn off and relocate devices. While it is naïve to think we can create an EMF-free world at this point, work to minimize your electro-toxic exposure.

Dr. Code's Comments

I usually give patients an outline or summary of what they can do. To begin, I suggest that the healthy, tolerable amount of electromagnetic smog is about 100 units per day. When we have Wi-Fi within our house, it puts out 30,000 units whenever it is on. Similarly, the hands-free phones that many people use within their house put out 50,000 units. These issues are much more dramatic than the smart meters that everyone talks about from the hydroelectric power industry. I suggest you consider using only corded phones and get rid of your hands-free units.

If you are going to use Wi-Fi, at least turn it off at night, giving a rest to the brain when it needs it most during sleep. Similarly, when using a smart phone, tablet, or computer try not to have it plugged in and charging while you are using it. This dramatically reduces your exposure. Ideally, you should only use your smart phone on speakerphone or through Bluetooth to minimize the immediate exposure to the brain.

Finally, if you live close to a cell phone tower, you might consider the Swedish concept of a silver fibre enclosure around the top and outside four regions of a four-poster bed for protection while you sleep. These are certainly available and recommended for anyone with a significant neurodegenerative brain health challenge. These include MS, stroke, traumatic brain injury, Parkinson's, or Alzheimer's.

EMF (Dirty Electricity)

Is grounding/earthing good for you? When we are outdoors, especially among trees and soil, we are connected to the earth's electromagnetic frequency. This is called the Schumann Resonance, which is exactly 7.83 hertz. Contact with these healthy ions is part of what feels so good about being out in nature. To learn more, watch the excellent film *Resonance—Beings of Frequency* (Russell 2013).

In our homes are obvious components, such as W-Fi routers, cordless phones, and major appliances. Perhaps even more significant are the frequencies of your home's electrical wiring. These frequencies are called electromagnetic interference or "dirty electricity." Ideally, your electrician should have installed shielded wiring, such as MC cable or EMT conduit, but this is recent and rare. Unfortunately, earthing or grounding mats do not guarantee your well-being either. EMF professionals do not recommend these products. So, save your money. Instead, I suggest the following.
1. Disconnect the bedroom circuit breaker at night.
2. Spend at least thirty minutes outdoors daily, ideally barefoot on the seashore or lakeshore or in damp grass.

3. Get rid of cordless phones, and use your cell phone on speaker or Bluetooth and sparingly. Text rather than speak.
4. Hardwire more of your computer and attachments, such as keyboards, printers, and tablets.
5. Turn your Wi-Fi off at night.
6. If you live near a cell tower, purchase a Silver Shield (woven mesh over your bed, which acts like a Faraday cage). See photo below.

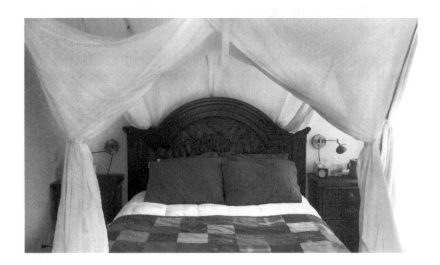

Section Two
Nutrition and Supplements

4: Healthy Eating

By Denise Code, MSc Nutrition, spouse of Dr. Bill Code

Then and now . . . how things have changed in our world. This certainly applies to our food supply and our health. While we have had many good changes that have improved our lives, other changes have not. Today, as compared to years ago, we are threatened by toxins in the environment. Our food is being produced on depleted soils and has lower levels of some nutrients. Thanks to big industry, we have over 30,000 foods to choose from in our grocery stores, but are we better off?

Compared to decades ago, we have soaring rates of obesity, diabetes, cancer, and heart disease. In North America, 69 percent of adults are overweight and obese. Eleven million Canadians and twenty-nine million Americans are diabetic. Autoimmune diseases and brain disorders (Parkinson's, Alzheimer's, dementia, and autism spectrum disorder) have also become more common. The next generation of children will not live as long or as healthfully as their parents. For the first time in years, the United States has reported a decline in lifespan for men and women. What is at the root of our changing health and decline in longevity? It may be as simple as what we put in our mouths. Yes, nutrition may be at the root of our health challenges.

As a health care professional, I bought into the nutrition teachings during the 1970s and into the 2000s. As health professionals, we were instructed by "evidence-based" science, our government bodies, and our professional organizations to communicate this health information to our patients and society in general, information such as:

- Fat is bad. Reducing fat is the solution to heart disease and cancer.
- Don't eat eggs. The cholesterol in them is bad for your heart.
- Carbohydrates are good. Eat at least six to eight servings of grain products a day.
- No need for vitamin/mineral supplements. A healthy diet is sufficient.
- Don't eat butter. Margarine is better for your heart.
- All foods are part of a healthy diet.
- Don't worry about the additives and preservatives in food. Your liver and kidneys will deal with them to pass them out via urine and stool.
- If you are diabetic, use artificial sweeteners instead of sugar.

We have been led astray by the organizations that are supposed to protect us and our health. I am angry at the way we have been manipulated by big pharma, big industry, and big food companies. Perhaps in the beginning, their goal was noble, to produce medicine to cure diseases, chemicals for better crop yields, and packaged food for quick, easy meals. But now we know that the medicines, our environment, and our food are all working together to make us sick, not healthy.

With greater maturity and understanding, I've peeked behind the curtain. Through reading books by authors like Michael Pollan (2016), Joel Salatin (2007), Dr. Michael Doidge (2015), Dr. Terry Wahls (2015), Dr. David Perlmutter (2015), Dr. Joseph Mercola (2017), and others, I have a completely different view when it comes to nutrition. This view also came about because of my experiences working in health care and through the experience of my husband achieving control of his MS symptoms through intensive nutritional therapy. For those naysayers who say there is no evidence for these shifts in the nutritional view, I challenge them. The evidence is in the scientific literature, if one approaches with an open, inquiring mind.

As a young student studying nutrition, food was promoted as providing calories, protein, fat, carbohydrates, vitamins, minerals, and fibre. This is true. Now we know that food is composed of thousands of other nutrients. These nutrients and the other components from food act on our genes. Nutrients can communicate with our genes to turn them on and off. That means food has a profound influence on how our genes express health and/or disease. Food also affects the bacteria in our gut. These bacteria or microbiome protect us from disease. When "bad" bacteria dominate in our gut, illness results. Thus, food is information for our body. Food is the source of our physical and our mental health.

We have lost common sense when it comes to our food, including how it is grown and processed. Perhaps this book will help you to gain perspective and help you understand how important it is to get back to basics, how important it is to eliminate some foods and focus on eating other foods. Good food choices will work with your genes and with the gut bacteria to produce a healthier, more vibrant you.

The Challenge of Eating Healthy

Eating a healthy diet can be quite a challenge today. There is so much choice in food—over 300,000 foods and beverages are available. Food is everywhere—at gas stations, leisure centres, offices, mini-marts, and large grocery chains. Supermarkets carry 30,000–40,000 food products. The average consumer is confused about what to buy. Make grocery shopping easy. Shop in the outer rim of the store. That is where you will find fresh meat, fish, poultry, dairy products, and fresh fruits and vegetables. The messages we receive regarding health and food are confusing and contradictory. The result: people feel like they are in a constant "food fight," stressed out over food and unable to enjoy the pleasures of eating.

What Is Healthy Eating?

Healthy eating is choosing to eat the most nutritious foods most of the time in amounts that allows you maintain a healthy weight. Which foods are the most nutritious? Those that are closest to their original form in nature. These foods are often called *whole foods*. Another way to think of them is as *real foods* (unprocessed foods).

Less-healthy foods generally come in packages; that is, they have been processed. Processed foods are often high in sugar, manipulated fat, salt, and chemical preservatives. Some added chemicals do not need to be listed on the table of ingredients if they are added for ease of processing or preservation.

For example, a whole apple is very nutritious. It contains vitamin C, natural fruit sugar, fibre, phytonutrients, antioxidants, and water. A Fruit Roll-Up made from apple contains little nutrition from that apple. Other ingredients, including sugar, have been added to make the snack.

Healthy Eating for a Better Brain

The following is meant to help you with your food choices for better brain health. Keep in mind, that which improves brain health will also improve total body health. It is never too late to make dietary changes. Your body is constantly shedding dead cells and making new ones. Indeed, it is reckoned that all the body cells turn over in seven years. This shows that your body has a tremendous ability to heal itself. It just needs the right ingredients. Given the right ingredients, it will produce healthy cells.

Vegetables and Fruits

Countless studies link consumption of vegetables and fruit to good health. They are nutrition superstars. They provide vitamin C, folate, beta-carotene, fibre, minerals, and thousands of phytonutrients. Plants manufacture phytonutrients (phytochemicals) to protect them from diseases and pests. These same phytochemicals protect us from disease. Studies show that phytochemicals:
- Stimulate the immune system
- Block substances we eat, drink, and breathe from causing cancer
- Reduce inflammation
- Prevent DNA damage and help DNA repair
- Reduce damage from free radicals, which lead to diseases and aging
- Slow cancer cell growth
- Trigger the death of damaged cells
- Regulate hormones
- Protect the brain and enhance memory and learning

Thus, phytochemicals are protective throughout the body, and their effects are felt in the brain too. Examples of this for brain health are many. Flavonoids, such as citrus tangeretin, improve memory and learning. Sulforaphanes from broccoli and cruciferous vegetables protect neurons from oxidative stress. Polyphenols from apple, grape, and citrus fruit juices offer stronger protection of brain neurons than antioxidant vitamins.

Apigenin, a flavone found in celery, parsley, oranges, and other plants, has anti-cancer activity. It also acts on the brain to reduce inflammation, decrease anxiety, and stimulate new neuron cell production.

These are just a few examples of the power of phytochemicals in fruits and vegetables. We need to eat a variety and an abundance of fruits and vegetables each day to protect our health and promote healing. Over 8,000 phytochemicals exist. Although much is known now, scientists continue to discover how these plant chemicals help us. Furthermore, it has also been shown that these phytochemicals have an additive and synergistic effect. That is, we need a variety of plants to provide a variety of these compounds, so that, like an orchestra, they work better together.

A great example of this phytochemical synergy is an apple. A 100-gram apple contains nearly 5 mg of vitamin C. However, when we eat an entire apple, the phytonutrients in it provide the equivalent body protection of 1,500 mg of vitamin C. In addition, apple juice has been shown to halt brain decline and boost brain hormones in Alzheimer's patients. Studies in rats showed that feeding apple juice concentrate protected their brains from free radical damage and cognitive decline and also helped to maintain healthy brain neurotransmitter levels. That is the power of only one food. Consider adding broccoli, kale, carrots, beets, onions, and berries—a symphony of foods, with countless phytonutrients as well as vitamins, minerals, and fibre.

Choose Organic Fruits and Vegetables

Organically grown produce should be your first choice. More than 600 chemicals are registered for agricultural use. These pesticides, which include herbicides and insecticides, contaminate produce. Although some can be washed off, others enter the plant through the roots and invade the edible parts. When we eat pesticides, they accumulate over the years and increase our "body burden." Even at low doses, pesticides increase our risk of cancers (e.g., leukemia, lymphoma, brain tumors, breast cancer, prostate cancer). Pesticide use is also linked to an increased risk of Alzheimer's disease, Parkinson's disease, depression, and respiratory problems. Farm workers, children, and pregnant women are most at risk for health problems from pesticide exposure.

The Environmental Working Group (EWG) in the United States publishes the "Dirty Dozen" list. This lists produce that should be avoided because of pesticide residues. For example, in the testing of strawberries, seventeen different pesticides were detected, and in the testing of grapes and sweet peppers, fifteen different pesticides were found. It's best to avoid the Dirty Dozen and buy them organically. The EWG also has a "Plus" category for the Dirty Dozen list. This is for leafy greens (kale and collard) and hot peppers, which should also be avoided. Buy these organically grown. Fifty-one pesticides were detected on the leafy greens. The hot peppers had particularly toxic insecticide residues, which are extremely harmful to the nervous system.

The EWG also publishes the "Clean 15." This is a list of produce with low levels of pesticide residues. Because of this, you can choose these conventionally grown fruits and vegetables rather than the organic ones. The Dirty Dozen and the Clean 15 are listed below:

Environmental Working Group's Dirty Dozen

- Strawberries
- Grapes
- Cherry tomatoes
- Apples
- Nectarines
- Cucumbers
- Peaches
- Celery
- Spinach
- Tomatoes
- Cherries
- Sweet bell peppers

Environmental Working Group's Clean 15

- Avocados
- Onions
- Eggplant
- Sweet Corn
- Asparagus
- Honeydew melon
- Cabbage
- Pineapples
- Frozen sweet peas
- Kiwis
- Mangoes
- Papaya
- Grapefruit
- Cauliflower
- Cantaloupe

Organically grown produce may also contain pesticide residues. These are often due to pesticide drift from conventionally grown crops. However, it has been shown that the pesticide load is much smaller than that for conventionally grown produce.

A current debate is whether organically grown produce is more nutritious and healthier for us. Professional health organizations and government bodies say there is no difference between organic and non-organic produce. However, evidence exists that organically grown crops are higher in nutrients. A 2014 meta-analysis of over 300 studies showed that organic produce was higher in antioxidants. The organic produce had 50 percent more anthocyanins and flavonoids (phytonutrients known to be anti-inflammatory). In 2008, a study at the University of California, Davis, reported double the quercetin in organically grown tomatoes. Other reports have shown that organic produce has higher levels of essential minerals and vitamin C. Experts are skeptical if this will improve our health. However, we know two things: 1) phytonutrients have a positive impact on our health and 2) pesticides harm our health and the health of the soil. Thus, it makes sense to choose organic foods as often as possible. I believe that, over time, the evidence for the benefits of organic food will continue to accrue.

Dozens of studies confirm the health benefits of a diet high in fruits and vegetables. People who eat five or more servings of fruits and vegetables each day have half the risk of cancer compared to people who only eat two servings per day. High intake of fruits and vegetables is linked to decreased incidence of heart disease, stroke, high blood pressure, eye disease, obesity, and several cancers. Because a diet high in fruits and vegetable improves blood sugar control, there is a lower risk of type 2 diabetes.

What about brain health? Are fruits and vegetables important for brain health? Yes! Nutrients in fruits and vegetables impact brain health in several ways. Flavanols and polyphenols help the brain with learning and memory. Folate in foods, including spinach and orange juice, prevent cognitive decline. Alpha-lipoic acid, found in vegetables like spinach, broccoli, and potatoes, is important for memory and for reducing cognitive decline. Celery, peppers, and carrots have luteolin, which calms inflammation and helps to preserve memory. People who follow the Mediterranean Diet, which is high in fruits and vegetables, are 30 percent less likely to develop depression. In addition, researchers have found that:

1. Variety is as important as quantity. Different colours of fruits and vegetables offer different nutrients.
2. Diet + exercise + sleep = even more profound effects on brain health (Gomez-Pinilla 2002).

Phytochemicals are powerful antioxidants that protect us from disease. How do you know if your body has a good level of protection? One way is to measure the carotenoids. These phytonutrients are found in the yellow and red pigments in fruits and vegetables. There are 600 carotenoids in plants, but only 40 are found in our diet. A diet high in carotenoids reduces the risk for heart disease, diabetes, insulin resistance, metabolic syndrome, and some cancers. Studies have shown that in older adults, high levels of carotenoids in the blood protects against decline in walking speed and severe walking disability.

Fortunately, non-invasive technology exists. The Pharmanex company has developed a fast, easy, accurate way to determine the level of carotenoids in the body. By using a scanner, a light is shone onto the palm of the hand, and a carotenoid score is determined. This score has been correlated to overall body antioxidant levels. The greater the score, the greater the level of antioxidants and the lower the risk of disease and early death. The score is influenced by dietary intake of fruits and vegetables. A low score correlates with a low intake. Thus, it can be a great tool to determine if you are eating enough fruits and vegetables. Low scores can be boosted by increasing fruits and vegetables, by taking supplements, or by a combination of food and supplements. The score can be a great motivator toward improving dietary intake.

What to Choose and How Much to Eat for Health

Opinions vary as to how much fruits and vegetables one should eat. For optimal health, eight to twelve servings a day is recommended. A serving is typically 125–250 mL (1/2 cup to 1 cup) or a piece of fruit, such as an apple. Dr. Perlmutter recommends that two thirds of the dinner plate should be vegetables (Perlmutter 2015).

Other dietary guidelines suggest half of the dinner plate should be vegetables. Dr. Terry Wahls recommends three cups of green vegetables, three cups of coloured vegetables, and three cups of sulfur-containing vegetables (onions, broccoli, cauliflower) daily (Wahls 2015). Whatever guidelines you choose, when it comes to vegetables and fruit, more is better, and variety is important. Choose organically grown fruits and vegetables, and avoid those on the "Dirty Dozen" list. Avoid processed forms of fruits and vegetables, as they often contain added salt, sugar, and preservatives. Eat fruits and vegetables as close to their natural state as possible. You will reap the benefits of good health.

Carbohydrates: What You Need to Know

For years, dietary recommendations have focused on increasing whole grains. While it is true that whole grains are nutritious, they have downsides. Most often, people are not eating the natural, unprocessed whole grain. Instead they are eating processed foods in the form of breakfast cereals, granola bars, cakes, pies, cookies, breads, and crackers. These foods are attractively packaged and labelled, giving the impression they are good for us. But let's look at the dark side of carbohydrates.

Impact on Blood Sugar

When a whole grain is crushed to make flour, tiny particles of starch (carbohydrate) are formed. These particles are more easily digested and quickly act to raise blood sugar. High blood sugar is irritating to blood vessels and promotes inflammation. The body responds to the blood sugar by pumping out insulin to capture this blood sugar and use it for energy in the cells. Over time, high blood sugar levels and high insulin levels lead to a decline in the cells' response to insulin. A metabolic state of hyperinsulinemia (high blood insulin) and hyperglycemia (high blood sugar) results. The consequences are metabolic syndrome, increased body weight, diabetes, and damaging inflammation. Although whole grains alone can be healthy (i.e., brown rice, quinoa, whole wheat), they are pulverized and made into products laden with sugar, manipulated fats, salt, and preservatives. These ingredients can also have a negative effect on our health.

Allergies and Sensitivities to Grains

Allergies and sensitivity to grains is increasing. This is especially true for wheat, corn, and soy. These grains are present in 90 percent of our processed foods. Wheat, corn, and soy are what keep food prices low. The proteins in these grains have been changed through decades of traditional plant breeding and also by genetically modifying them. Genetically modified crops, such as soy, corn, and sugar beets, have been engineered to make them resistant to glyphosate (Roundup), and in the case of corn, to produce an insecticide, Bt toxin. Consequently, the protein in these foods has been altered. When our body meets a new protein, it mounts an allergic response through the immune system. This immune system response involves inflammation. That inflammation can be felt throughout the body, including the brain.

Gluten is the protein that is perhaps giving us the most problem. Gluten is found in wheat, rye, and barley. Thus, most cakes, cookies, granola bars, breakfast cereals, breads, crackers, baked products, and many processed foods contain wheat and sometimes barley or rye. Wheat tastes good and stimulates our appetite, so we eat more. This benefits the food companies but not our waistline. The health problems related to gluten are covered in chapter 5. Because gluten can be harmful to our body and to our nervous system (including the brain), it should be avoided.

Grains That Contain Gluten

Wheat, including Einkorn, Durum, Faro, Graham, Kamut, Semolina, and Spelt	Rye	Barley	Triticale

Foods/Products That May Contain Gluten

Beers (ales and lagers)	Nutritional supplements	Processed luncheon meats
Marinades		
Breading and coating mixes	Brown rice syrup	Croutons
	Pastas	Sauces
	Communion wafers	Gravies

Dressings	Soy sauce and Asian sauces	Thickeners
Self-basting poultry		Imitation bacon
Drugs and over-the-counter medications	Flour and cereal products	Vitamin and mineral supplements
Soup bases	Stuffings and dressings	Imitation seafood
Energy bars	Herbal supplements	Malt vinegar

Alternatives to Gluten

Rather than feeling deprived because you no longer eat foods containing gluten, embrace the variety and the flavours of gluten-free alternatives. A list of gluten-free options appears in the table below. These options include grains, seeds, legumes, and nuts, which can be important sources of vitamins, minerals, protein, healthy fats, fibre, and phytonutrients.

Gluten-free Grains, Flours, Seeds, and Nuts

Amaranth	Garbanzo, garfava (a flour from garbanzo beans and fava beans)	Quinoa
All seeds and nuts		Rice
Arrowroot	Millet	Sorghum
Beans and bean flour	Montana	Soy*
Buckwheat	Oats (certified to be gluten-free)	Tapioca
Corn*		Teff (a lovegrass native to Ethiopia and Eritrea)
Flax	Potato	

*Always buy these organic; conventional crops are genetically modified.

For people limiting carbohydrates in their diet, flours made from nuts, coconut meat, and legumes are low in carbohydrates. Flours from grains and seeds, such as quinoa, sorghum, brown rice, and buckwheat, are higher in carbohydrates. The highest amounts of carbohydrates are found in rice, arrowroot starch, potato starch, and tapioca starch.

In recent years, manufacturers have rushed to produce gluten-free products in response to the rise in gluten-free eating. Don't be misled. Even though these products are gluten-free, they are not necessarily healthy choices. The gluten-free flours, the sugar, and the other ingredients can be equally harmful, especially in causing blood sugar spikes and weight gain. Choose these products wisely, and use them only occasionally.

You can use gluten-free flours to make your own baked goods. Usually, a combination of two or more flours is needed for a successful product. Alternatively, you can buy gluten-free flours that can be substituted for equal amounts of wheat flour in your favourite recipes. Be aware that there will be differences in flavour and texture in gluten-free products. Thousands of recipes are available on the internet, along with information on gluten-free cooking. Some of my favourite cookbooks are from *Gluten-free Girl* (Ahern 2009), and Dr. William Davis' *Wheat Belly* (Davis 2012). Again, be cautious in how much of these carbohydrate sources you eat (Volek 2008).

Organic Matters

As with fruits and vegetables, your first choice should be organically grown gluten-free grains, seeds, nuts, and the flours and products made from them. These crops are not genetically engineered organisms (GMOs); however, when they are conventionally grown, they may be treated with pesticides. Some crops are sprayed with glyphosate to desiccate them or make them ripen within the same time frame for ease of harvest. This is a particular issue with wheat, potatoes, sweet potatoes, and sugarcane.

Protein

Protein is made up of smaller units called amino acids that are linked together in long chains. Humans need twenty different amino acids. Nine of these amino acids are considered essential and must be obtained from food. The other amino acids are considered non-essential, because our bodies can manufacture them.

Our bodies are 20 percent protein by weight. Protein is needed for growth, tissue repair, and immune function. Enzymes, hormones, and blood cells are all made from protein. In addition, protein is essential for brain health. Neurons communicate via neurotransmitters, which are made from protein. Protein helps to optimize brain function and is essential for getting nutrients to brain cells. Furthermore, during digestion, protein helps to slow down the process. This results in a more gradual release of digested carbohydrates and reduces blood sugar spikes. High blood sugars and subsequent release of insulin promote inflammation, which is harmful to all parts of the body, including the brain.

Guidelines vary as to how much protein is enough. A general guideline is 12-15 g per meal for women and 15-20 g per meal for men. More protein is needed for those who are physically active or recovering from an illness or injury. The minimum amount of protein needed daily for health is 0.8 grams per kilogram of body weight.

Protein can be obtained from many food sources, both animal and vegetable. If you choose to eat protein from animal sources, strive to eat meat from pastured, organically-fed animals (beef, lamb, pork, and poultry). This will reduce your intake of pesticides, herbicides, and, consequently, glyphospate. Bone broth made from chicken or beef is an excellent food choice. Bone broth is abundant in glycine, an amino acid that helps to heal the gut, form healthy joints, hair, and skin and has a calming effect. Bone broth is also rich in calcium, selenium, and magnesium, which are all important for brain health.

Seafood, besides being rich in protein, provides healthy fats—EPA and DHA. These are incorporated directly into the body's cellular and mitochondrial membranes. Best choices of seafood include wild salmon, wild-caught shrimp, oysters, clams, sardines, anchovies, mackerel, and herring. These fish will have less concentration of mercury and toxins than larger fish. As noted earlier, halibut, swordfish, king mackerel, white albacore tuna, sea bass, and farmed salmon contain significant amounts of mercury and should be limited, especially for pregnant women.

Eggs have been unfairly targeted as something to avoid. Eggs contain all essential amino acids. They also contain important vitamins, minerals, and antioxidants that protect our eyes and brain. Thus, eating eggs daily is a good habit. The cholesterol in eggs is *not* the problem that we have been led to believe. More than 80 percent of the cholesterol in our body is made by our own liver. Thus, dietary cholesterol is not the culprit in heart disease. Other risk factors, such as smoking and inactivity, are far more harmful. The best choice for eggs are from hens that are pastured, roaming free, and fed organically.

Dairy products are also excellent sources of protein. However, dairy is somewhat controversial, as those sensitive to gluten are often also intolerant of dairy. Butyrophilin and casein are two proteins which can be problematic. Casein is known to produce morphine-like substances in the body, and these can affect behaviour and mental clarity. Again, it is best to consume organic dairy products. Beware of many of the yoghurts and processed milk products, because they can contain a lot of sugars and additives.

All nuts and seeds are good sources of protein. They also supply healthy fat, vitamin E, B vitamins, minerals (magnesium, calcium, copper, and zinc), antioxidants, and fibre. Some people soak their nuts to minimize enzyme inhibitors. This is easily done by covering nuts in filtered water, adding one or two tablespoons of sea salt, and leaving them to soak overnight. Drain and rinse, then dry them in an oven at 37–65°C (100–150°F).

Vegetarians rely on nuts, seeds, and legumes for their protein needs. Legumes (beans and lentils) are rich in minerals, vitamins, and fibre. However, legumes contain lectins, proteins that bind to carbohydrates and are thought to be a natural defense mechanism for plants. Lectins are not digested and travel intact in the gastrointestinal tract. They can damage the intestinal wall and lead to leaky gut, inflammation, and possibly autoimmune conditions. Thus, some people cannot tolerate legumes and are best to avoid them. Lectins can be reduced by sprouting and fermenting. Also, soaking legumes and changing the soaking water two or three times can reduce the number of lectins. As with other foods, organic sources are best.

Fat

During the past fifty years, fat intake has been discouraged, and a host of low-fat or fat-free foods have been produced. It was believed that fat caused heart disease, cancer, and obesity and was responsible for our ill health. Indeed, certain fats are harmful and should be avoided. These are the processed fats and oils that have been manipulated at high heat. Consequently, these form trans fats, which are abnormal fats (Kummerow 2009). These abnormal fats are incorporated into cells and tissues, thus producing unhealthy cells and promoting inflammation. Trans fats and all industrially-processed fats are definitely to be avoided (Brandt 2017)!

Healthy fats provide fat-soluble vitamins, are a source of fuel for the body, promote satiety, and help absorb minerals. Fats fall into three categories, based on their structure: saturated (e.g., animal fat), monounsaturated (e.g., olive oil), and polyunsaturated fat (oils from nuts and seeds, such as corn, soybeans, safflowers, and sunflowers). Furthermore, fats are made up of smaller units called fatty acids. There are two families of essential fatty acids—omega-6 fatty acids and omega-3 fatty acids. Omega-6 fatty acids are transformed in the body into substances that promote inflammation. Therefore, excessive dietary omega-6 can be harmful. However, we do need some omega-6 for brain and immune function. The omega-3 family has the opposite effect on inflammation—they are anti-inflammatory. Because of the widespread use of seed oils, our diets have 16–20 times more omega-6 fatty acids, causing inflammation and ill health. Thus, we need to reduce the amount of omega-6 consumed and increase the amount of omega-3 fatty acids. A healthier ratio is one to one or five to one.

Omega-3 fatty acids are found in flaxseeds, hemp seeds, and walnuts. However, these fatty acids must be converted to EPA and DHA, the types of fatty acids that are then converted to anti-inflammatory substances. This conversion can be limited in some individuals, so omega-3 supplements of EPA and DHA can be beneficial. Grass-fed beef and pastured animals have fat higher in omega-3s than livestock fed cereal grains. Important sources of omega-3s are fish and fish oils. These contain omega-3s in the form of EPA and DHA, which are easily used in our body. Our brains are about 60 percent fat. DHA is found in cell membranes in the brain and allows the membranes to remain flexible and fluid and thus allow messages to flow between cells. DHA not only protects the mitochondria from damage but also promotes nerve transmission in the central nervous system. Omega-3s have been shown to help depression, mental disorders, and ADHD, as well as lower the risk of Alzheimer's, dementia, and heart disease. In addition, omega-3s are beneficial for eye health, bone and joint health, asthma in children, and sleep.

Because saturated fat affects cholesterol levels in the blood, they have been thought to be harmful. In the blood, cholesterol is carried along with protein, and these complexes are called lipoproteins. High-density lipoprotein (HDL) lowers the risk of heart disease, while low-density lipoprotein (LDL) is associated with a greater risk. There are different types of LDL when it comes to heart disease risk. The small, dense LDL particles are associated with a greater risk of heart disease. They penetrate the artery walls and lead to plaque formation. The larger, fluffy LD particles do not contribute to heart disease.

Saturated fat raises the larger LDL particles; thus, it is not as harmful as previously thought. Trans fats, refined carbohydrates, and sugar raise the small, dense LDL particles, providing one more reason to avoid processed trans fats, refined carbohydrates, and sugar. Indeed, people with high levels of the small LDL particles have triple the risk of heart disease. One saturated fat, butter, is a much healthier choice than vegetable oil margarines. When butter is clarified into ghee, the lactose and casein are removed. Ghee is a good source of butyrate, which is important for the gut's energy and cell health.

Thus, healthy fats support brain function, hormone production, and metabolism. Low-fat and fat-free diets should be avoided. We need a variety of fats from a variety of food sources. Saturated fat from organically grown meat, eggs, and dairy can be part of a healthy diet. Avocados and nuts provide healthy monounsaturated fat. So too does olive oil (extra virgin is best), and it has the added benefit of containing potent antioxidants. Coconut oil contains lauric acid, which is converted to a substance that is antiviral and antibacterial. It also contains MCT oil, which is a type of fat the does not require digestion and can be used directly by the brain for energy. MCT is also an excellent fuel for the mitochondria. All in all, healthy fat is not the enemy.

What is the bottom line when striving to eat healthfully? Choose organically produced foods as close to their natural state as possible. Aim for 50 different foods each week to feed your microbiome. Avoid processed, packaged, industrially produced foods full of additives and lacking in nutritional quality. Your body and brain will thank you.

5: Gluten

The Perils of Gluten

The information on the perils of wheat has exploded over the last ten years. Trust me; this is not a fad. It is a harsh reality. One of the factors increasing gluten intolerance is glyphosate, which aggravates the issue and is used to harvest 90 percent of wheat in North America (Samsel 2013). Gluten is a tenacious, elastic substance, especially from wheat flour, that gives cohesiveness to dough. It will interest you to learn that the word "gluten" comes from late Latin and means "to glue or paste." Unfortunately, this "glue" sticks open the openings between cells in our gut lining and causes and aggravates leaky gut. There are normally minimal openings, so-called "tight junctions," between gut cells, and these are ordinarily closed, hence the term "tight junctions," which are critical for long-term health.

This is a key protection mechanism to prevent toxins from our food and the environment from entering our bloodstream and body. This "glue" also triggers inflammation (swelling, heat, redness, and pain or loss of function) in our gut lining. Research by a group in New England in 2015 revealed that gluten triggered almost immediate gut inflammation in 100 percent of healthy subjects (reported to me in personal correspondence). This study was done with endoscopy, looking into the stomach and intestines with a fibreoptic scope before and after a gluten load. Meanwhile, the incidence of celiac disease is now present in at least 1 percent of all people, which is four times what it was 30 years ago. New data suggests this may now be as high as 2–3 percent of all people! Even more important is non-celiac gluten sensitivity (NCGS). Here the phrase "Gluten Sensitivity: Not Celiac and Not Certain" is a key discussion (Vanga 2013). NCGS is at least eight times as frequent as celiac disease. Almost all the problems related to NCGS are neurological. These include headaches, MS, epileptic seizures, cerebellar ataxia, depression, anxiety, ADHD, autism (Vojdani et al. 2004), and schizophrenia. I suspect gluten also will be implicated in Parkinson's and Alzheimer's, at least as an inflammatory trigger.

Gluten is a complex protein that humans are uniformly unable to digest. Gluten is a composite of proteins stored together in the seed's endosperm, which nourishes the embryonic plant during germination. This gluten complex accounts for 75–85 percent of total protein in bread wheat and slightly less in pasta or durum wheat. For more than forty years, we have rewarded wheat farmers for the amount of protein in their wheat. The world champion wheat is often from northern Alberta or Saskatchewan. Nature optimizes the gluten protein there to permit a "jump start" of rapid germination and growth in the spring because of the short growing season.

To use Dr. Tom O'Bryan's analogy: "If we think of a gluten protein as a one hundred pearl necklace, we are able to only digest it into ten or twelve pieces." Hence, we cannot break it down to its individual amino acids, which the body is programmed to absorb. Any or all of these pieces of gluten protein can trigger inflammation in the gut wall or microvilli interface. Normally, the cells in the intestine are tightly joined to prevent toxins and other unwanted particles from entering the bloodstream. When gluten particles cause inflammation in the gut, the tight junctions between the cells are disrupted. In essence, the tight junctions, which are the walls between the cells, become "glued" open, and the gut becomes leaky. The partial gluten proteins can then leak through the gut wall into the bloodstream. The body recognizes these proteins as foreign and mounts an immune response. There are now sixty-two different gluten proteins (and there may be thousands) that can trigger an immune response.

In Canada and the United States, the diagnosis of celiac disease is dependent upon a gastroenterologist's biopsy of the small intestine. This biopsy is then sent to pathology, where it is examined under a microscope to determine if it has qualities of grades 1, 2, 3, or 4. These grades determine the degree of the flattening of the brush border of the gut lining. Celiac is only diagnosed if grade 3 or 4 is present. This is when the gut lining is completely flattened. Long-term data suggests that many people do not recover from this severe damage. In Canada, it takes an average of six months to see a gastroenterologist and another six months to book an endoscopy and biopsy. Individuals must remain on gluten the entire time, despite sometimes agonizing symptoms. This is ludicrous. The only advantage to a diagnosis of celiac disease is the ability to deduct the extra cost of gluten-free foods from your federal tax return.

In Europe, no biopsies are done when gluten intolerance is suspected because of gastrointestinal symptoms. Instead, a number of antibodies against gluten are measured, and then all gluten is discontinued for three months. Whether or not the antibody test is positive, gluten is re-introduced. If the gluten challenge is positive for symptoms, then the patient is diagnosed as having celiac disease. This is a much more practical and economic approach and better for patients. I would suggest the Canadian and American model can no longer be afforded from the patients' perspective and from the cost to the medical care system, given its limited benefit.

Non-celiac gluten sensitivity does not usually require a gastroenterologist referral and biopsy in the absence of gut symptoms. Instead, the physician, hopefully a neurologist, has patients discontinue gluten for a three-month trial and notes any symptom changes. Individuals must be persuaded that complete removal of gluten is the only good way to test for non-celiac gluten sensitivity. If a patient is unwilling to do this, it does not help to confirm non-celiac gluten sensitivity. Perhaps stopping wheat will be enough (Carroccio 2013). Patients must feel empowered to implement dietary changes to recover their health. There are no shortcuts.

When the gluten protein leaks through the gut wall, the immune system attacks the foreign protein. This causes specialized cells, beta-lymphocytes, to create memory cells and antibodies, which bind to the proteins. These memory cells are identical to what happens when we have a vaccination as a child for measles, mumps, and rubella. A group of our immune cells, in the presence of a slight amount of the virus entering the body, mounts a major immune response to deal with the insult. This is why a 97-99 percent gluten-free diet will not be successful. Even a minute amount of gluten will trigger an immune response. It takes three to six months for this response to calm down again.

Eventually, the body mistakes these foreign gluten proteins for a particular body protein. This has been called autoimmune illness, as the body's immune system is now attacking body tissues that appear similar to the foreign protein. This is known as molecular mimicry. Frequent examples with gluten are the thyroid being attacked with the development of Hashimoto's thyroiditis (hypothyroidism). A second example is the immune system attacking the joint lining or synovium and the development of rheumatoid arthritis.

How About the Brain?

If you have leaky gut, you also have leaky blood-brain barrier. The blood-brain barrier is designed to protect the brain from products circulating in the bloodstream, such as bacteria, from entering the brain. However, if you have a leaky blood-brain barrier, the previously protected brain and spinal cord are now vulnerable. We have never found the "smoking gun," that is, antibodies to myelin, in MS despite searching for these antibodies for forty years! Yet, MS has been categorized by neurologists as an autoimmune disease.

Recent research published in *Nature* magazine in 2015 revealed that a small amount of blood in the brain initiates a major immune attack (Ryu 2015). This autoimmune attack is against the blood protein, fibrinogen. Fibrinogen is an important clotting protein that protects us from bleeding to death. This attack against fibrinogen may be the "smoking gun" for the autoimmune component of MS. At least 14 percent of MS patients have visible microbleeds on sophisticated MRI scans. This was seen in MS patients younger than fifty years of age. The normal population, younger than fifty years, has less than 1 percent of these microbleeds. Perhaps now neurologists can feel validated for their long-held theory that auto-immunity has been partly substantiated and move on to the question of why these microbleeds are present in the first place. A further suggestion I would make is that repeated traumatic brain injury or even a single episode can cause these microbleeds. This may help explain the severe damage in NFL players when they are eventually diagnosed with chronic traumatic encephalopathy (CTE). Time will tell.

Before leaving the topic of wheat, I need to mention wheat germ agglutinin. This is a component of wheat germ, a tiny portion from the wheat kernel. In the 1970s and early 1980s, wheat germ was believed to be healthy and, therefore, fashionable to add to foods. Now we know that wheat germ agglutinin is another powerful trigger of autoimmune diseases. Wheat germ is found in whole-grain flour and sprouted wheat products.

Now let's talk about a few of the brain diseases associated with wheat consumption. Research from Israel is quite definitive that at least 8 percent of MS patients are triggered by gluten alone (Shoenfeld 2013). I believe that most MS patients have their signs and symptoms aggravated by gluten. An example of this is bladder problems experienced by some people with MS that can be aggravated by eating wheat. The symptoms of chronic cystitis or bladder inflammation triggered by the gluten molecule can simulate a bladder infection. The patient notices pain with voiding, urgency, and frequency but will be unable to culture any bacteria in the urine. Often patients are given antibiotics in an attempt to control the symptoms. Now that we understand the negative impacts of antibiotics on the microbiota, this action will only make matters worse. I have one client who, before her early fifties, had more than 200 courses of antibiotics!

Epileptic seizures can be caused by wheat alone. These can even be full grand mal seizures. I have one client, now in his early seventies, who has had repeated seizures without any diagnosed reason on MRI scans. His physicians even started to disbelieve that he was having seizures until he had one in the emergency department. Typically, these gluten-triggered seizures are difficult to control with one, two, or even three anti-epileptic medications. However, being gluten-free can be the best way to become seizure-free.

Cerebellar ataxia of unknown origin (idiopathic) is another example of gluten's impact. In this illness, people walk on their heels, are unsteady, and appear drunk. If all other known causes are ruled out, including vitamin B12 deficiency, these are usually wheat triggered. The sooner the person discontinues gluten, the sooner brain recovery is likely.

Schizophrenia is often aggravated and sometimes triggered by gluten. This is a critical food problem that should be considered whenever someone is suffering from delusions and hallucinations. Why? Because these people are often treated aggressively with powerful anti-psychotic drugs. Once started on these or admitted to a psychiatric hospital, the rest of one's life story is written—badly. Options for education and employment become very limited, if not impossible. These options are even worse if admitted into the criminal justice system. Despite the efforts of Canadian psychiatrist Abram Hoffer and others, mental health diagnosis and treatment too often neglects the role of toxins, nutrition, and nutrient supplementation.

Anxiety and depression can also be triggered by gluten sensitivity. Some researchers report that 10-15 percent of people with gluten intolerance experience anxiety and depression. Other researchers have found that 30 percent of people with celiac disease suffer from depression. In retrospect, I believe my bouts of depression were aggravated by gluten. I look back to my last few months working in the operating room in 1996. My lunch was inevitably whole-wheat bread sandwiches eaten between cases. For the next sixty to ninety minutes, I had huge problems staying awake in the operating room. This is critical, as vigilance is the byword of the anesthesiologist. I have since learned that if you are drowsy after eating, one of the main triggers is food sensitivity.

Headaches are such a common problem with rarely an etiology or solution that they are often the bane of a neurologist. Gluten is a common trigger for migraines. I determined gluten is a trigger of my migraine headaches when my son brought home beer when he was visiting us from university. As a typical student, he would buy wheat beer with 7 percent alcohol, because it was the same price as lower-alcohol beer. If I drank one of them, I would get a headache. Meanwhile, I could have two of the 5 percent non-wheat beer, made with barley and with less gluten, and not get a headache. The penny finally dropped: wheat was causing my headaches. Headaches are seen in up to 50 percent of celiac disease and up to 70 percent of MS patients.

Now that I can look back, I realize I developed several diagnostic suggestions for gluten sensitivity. Severe migraine headaches by age twenty-six was one of them. Depression, diagnosed at age twenty-eight, was another. I was diagnosed with mild osteopenia (thinning of the bones) at age forty-one. After a major ankle fracture, brought on by minimal injury, I should have thought about osteoporosis. However, I did not. It was only two years later, after lifting a 120-pound emu onto a truck, with subsequent severe back pain, that I started to get sorted out. I was referred to an endocrinologist who specialized in osteoporosis. She ordered an X-ray of my spine and carefully measured my height. The X-ray revealed a L-2 lumbar full compression fracture. My height was five feet 10 inches (175 cm). In high school, I was six feet tall (180 cm). It is normal to lose one inch (2.5 cm) of height by age 50. If one loses two inches, it is due to vertebral compression fracture. My diagnosis was "upgraded" to severe osteoporosis.

Other clues of osteoporosis secondary to gluten sensitivity are height within a family. I have two brothers living who are 6 feet 3.5 inches and 6 feet 5.5 inches, respectively. My other brother, who passed away in 1994, was 5 feet 11 inches. I have three sisters, one whom is 5 feet 10 inches, one 5 feet 9 inches, and one 5 feet 2.5 inches. The shortest sister was told at age forty that she had the bones of an eighty-year-old, secondary to severe osteoporosis. We now know that one of the causes of osteoporosis is untreated celiac disease or gluten sensitivity. The damage by gluten in the gut impairs absorption of critical nutrients needed for bone formation and density. We also know that reduced height is one of the signs of gluten sensitivity.

Irritable bowel syndrome (IBS) and similar gut issues are frequently worsened with the intake of gluten. My first diagnosis of IBS was at age thirty, twelve years before my MS diagnosis. My IBS has persisted but is almost better if I remain gluten and casein free. Yes, 80 percent of people sensitive to gluten have a cross-sensitivity to casein, the major protein in cow's milk. My great weakness is ice cream, but if I'm smart, I choose coconut ice cream. True dairy sensitivity is almost always due to casein. Parts of the casein molecule are similar to the gluten molecule.

Lactose, on the other hand, is a sugar found in milk. It is poorly tolerated by some people, because they lack the enzyme to digest it. Virtually all sensitivities and allergies are protein-based. The casein in cow's milk is particularly allergenic and somewhat less so in goat and sheep milk. Meanwhile, the whey in milk from all three species is almost always tolerated, because it is almost identical to the whey protein in human breast milk.

Corn is the third protein one might consider if one is sensitive to gluten and casein. Wheat, corn, and other grains are interesting, as their lectin proteins are bitter and evolved to protect these grains from being eaten. Yes, ideally the animal feels unwell when they eat these grains, so they avoid them. We also know the most common food sensitivity in any society will be the grain that dominates their diet. Thus, in North America, wheat is number one, and in Japan and most of Asia, rice is number one. I suspect number one in Mexico is corn in some regions. You are getting glimpses of the reasoning behind the Paleolithic Diet or Dr. Wahls' Diet (Wahls 2015).

The final issue with most grains occurs when we pulverize them into flour. This dust-like substance has a high surface area, allowing the starches to be nearly instantly absorbed in the gut. Then they are quickly converted into sugar. This sugar or glucose spike results in an insulin spike and subsequently an inflammatory spike. Hence, all highly processed grains (flours) have this same downside. Similarly, all processed foods compound this further, with the addition of sugar or high-fructose corn sweetener. As a consequence, modern North Americans are becoming more and more obese and suffer more and more excess inflammation. Suffice it to say that almost all brain diseases, including MS and Alzheimer's, become worse or progress faster if an individual is obese. Finally, a possible solution to help some gluten sensitivity is fermentation (Biesiekierski 2013). This is why sourdough is often tolerated better. Almost all fermented foods are better for you, because they support our microbiota.

6: Supplements

To supplement or not? That is the question. The answer is a definite "yes." I answer as an integrative physician and as a patient with MS, IBS, and severe osteoporosis. Eating healthy organic food is, and will always be, critical for me. It should be for you too.

In this chapter, I suggest:

1. Critical supplements for specific problems
2. General, all-around supplements important for everyone
3. Supplements that can optimize our genetics
4. Supplements that can detoxify our body from previous and ongoing mistakes

To begin, allow me to address a healthy blood sugar level. Many of us currently have type 2 diabetes or early warning signals thereof. We need to minimize our sugar spikes, because these provoke insulin spikes, which provoke inflammatory spikes. Excess inflammation triggers or aggravates a multitude of unwanted illnesses, such as heart disease, arthritis, depression, anxiety, Alzheimer's, Parkinson's, MS, and others. Almost all blood sugar spikes come from carbohydrates and alcohol. Yes, even alcohol has its price. When you combine that fact with the principle that alcohol is virtually empty of most nutrients, as is soda pop, I hope you understand the consequences.

Once you eat a healthy, mostly organic, mostly whole-food diet of 50 foods per week, you will have obtained most of your nutrients. However, a few key ones should be included daily. I will list these for you. My baseline trio to recommend is 1) Vitamin D-3, 4,000 IU (international units) per day, 2) Fish or krill oil source of 2,000–3,000 mg per day of EPA and DHA combined, and 3) a multivitamin/multimineral without iron, unless you are a woman having menstrual periods. If you already have a health challenge, such as my MS and osteoporosis, you will need nutritional supplements to return to baseline. Some may need four to five times as much of some nutrients to achieve this. For example, in chapter 7, I suggest three months of those listed items as a minimum trial period. Similarly, three months is a good length of time to see if a supplement is benefitting you.

Magnesium

To begin, let's talk about magnesium. Magnesium deficiency is widespread and present in 50–80 percent of people. Magnesium has been described as the "cheapest ounce of prevention." Magnesium deficiency can be at the root of many pathologies or health problems. Treating magnesium deficiency for pennies a day may produce an incredible decrease in illness and pain. If you focus on getting your magnesium just right, you may achieve significant results. I use 500 mg of slow-release magnesium at bedtime for my muscle spasms and sleep problems. Magnesium is our least abundant serum electrolyte. Yet, it is extremely important for the metabolism of calcium, potassium, phosphorus, zinc, iron, sodium, lead cadmium, hydrochloric acid, acetylcholine, and nitric oxide. Magnesium is also critical for more than 300 enzymes, stability within the cells, and for the activation of thiamine, which alters a wide variety of body functions.

Magnesium absorption requires a large number of green leafy vegetables in our diet and the cofactors selenium, parathyroid hormone, and vitamins B6 and D. Magnesium concentrations are depleted by alcohol, salt, phosphoric acid (sodas), coffee intake, profuse sweating, severe and prolonged stress, heavy menstrual periods, diuretics (fluid pills), and some parasites, such as pinworms.

Magnesium deficiency contributes to a large number of illnesses. These include increased blood pressure, cardiovascular disease, liver disease, kidney disease, peroxynitrite injury (with resulting aggravated migraine), MS, glaucoma, and Alzheimer's disease. In addition, recurrent bacterial infection can occur due to this lowered nitric oxide in all body areas, including the sinuses, vagina, middle ear, lungs, and throat. Furthermore, deficiency increases the risk of fungal infection and thiamine dysfunction, which includes low gastric acid, behavioural disorders, and PMS (premenstrual tension syndrome).

Other mineral deficiencies, such as calcium deficiency, can contribute to osteoporosis and hypertension, mood swings, dental cavities, hearing loss, type 2 diabetes, cramps, muscle weakness, PMS, impotence, aggression, and fibromas. Potassium deficiency can precipitate heart arrhythmias, hypertension, and some cancers.

Most of us will benefit from some magnesium supplementation. However, calcium supplementation is no longer indicated for most people. If you want to read an excellent discussion of magnesium, go to *Medical Hypothesis* by S. Johnson (2001). An interesting side note is that the intake and circulation of magnesium is inversely proportional to cardio-vascular disease. The Weston A. Price Foundation states,

> magnesium shines brightest in cardiovascular health. It alone can fulfill the role of many common cardiac medications; magnesium inhibits blood clots (like Aspirin), thins the blood, blocks calcium uptake (like calcium channel-blocking drugs) and relaxes blood vessels (like ACE inhibitors, common blood pressure lowering drugs). Where else could you potentially replace many drugs including blood pressure control? Finally, magnesium is an excellent nutrient to reduce your C-reactive protein, which is a very good indicator of lowering your inflammation (Czapp 2010).

How much magnesium do you need to supplement each day? The RDA is 310–420 mg per day; however, some people need 600–900 mg daily for optimal health. I suggest you start at 200 mg of oral magnesium citrate and gradually increase until you develop slightly loose stools. Dr. Carolyn Dean's book, *The Magnesium Miracle* (Dean 2017), is a great resource. Alternatively, you can read her blog post, "Gauging Magnesium Deficiency Symptoms."[8]

Iron

Iron is also critical for a host of reasons. Iron deficiency is still the most common cause of anemia in children and women

---

[8] https://drcarolyndean.com/2010/06/gauging-magnesium-deficiency -symptoms/

of childbearing age. Once women reach menopause, they join men in requiring much less iron. The best and easiest iron to absorb is when it is attached to the heme molecule, as found in meat. This is the same form of heme that is found in your red blood cells. If you are vegan or vegetarian, ensure that you have vitamin C in your meal when you eat foods containing iron.

Excessive iron is an important concern for many of us with the possibility of hemochromatosis. This is genetic and is especially common in people of Irish descent, like me. Postmenopausal women and men should avoid multivitamin/multimineral supplements with iron, as it is not needed. Monitoring your hemoglobin and serum ferritin are important lifelong concerns. Normal ferritin in women is listed up to 200 nanograms/ml and in men up to 300 nanograms/ml. Ideal maintenance for both is 25-75 nanograms/ml. If your ferritin is greater than this 200-300 nanogram/ml guideline, you need lab evaluation of your fasting serum iron and total iron binding capacity. If these are awry, you need to see a specialist in hemochromatosis, who will include genetic testing. Patient complaints may include weakness, fatigue, lethargy, apathy, and weight loss. Consider excessive iron if you experience arthritis, especially of the finger joints, diabetes, menstrual periods stopping suddenly, loss of libido, impotence, congestive heart failure, and arrhythmias. Iron excess can even lead to encephalopathy (brain swelling and confusion). For further discussion regarding excess iron, refer to the chapter on the thyroid.

Copper

Copper deficiency is rare. However, it is still possible, and occasionally, copper can be in excess (Wilson's Disease), which can be quite harmful. Copper and zinc are in a teeter-totter balancing act within the body. If you have excess copper, you are usually deficient in zinc. Copper is important in the synthesis of two neurotransmitters: norepinephrine (noradrenaline) and dopamine. Clinical indications of copper deficiency include rheumatoid arthritis, abdominal aortic aneurisms, osteoporosis, and peptic ulcer disease. An excess of copper can produce rapid thought patterns, insomnia, depression, memory loss, hallucinations, paranoia, and even obsessive-compulsive disorder. The diagnosis of excess copper is best done via a hair sample analysis. Some patients with schizophrenia, depression, autism, tardive dyskinesia, or memory loss have elevated copper. The initial treatment is to increase zinc intake. There is usually enough copper within a multimineral, providing 1-4 mg daily. Measurement of serum copper and ceruloplasmin can help assessment.

Zinc

Zinc is involved in many biochemical pathways, including DNA and protein synthesis. Zinc plays a key role in visual function, hearing, and taste. Furthermore, zinc stabilizes cell membranes and has an anti-inflammatory effect and antiviral activity, especially against herpes simplex (cold sores). Deficiency can trigger anorexia, pica, depression, impaired mental concentration, intention tremor (a tremor that occurs when you begin a motion), and a host of other non-brain functions. Zinc deficiency is more common in malabsorption, liver cirrhosis, sickle cell disease, chronic kidney disease, alcoholism, and the elderly. Regular lab tests are not that useful. Many drugs interfere with zinc; hence, more supplementation may be needed. These include aspirin, protein pump inhibitors, ACE inhibitors, diuretics, steroids, tetracyclines, fluoroquinolone antibiotics, and penicillamine. Iron and zinc compete as well. It should be noted that almost anyone with a mental disorder needs zinc replacement. This may need to be substantial, with as much as 50 mg three times per day for two to three months. Most commonly, 30 mg per day of elemental zinc will be sufficient. This is probably the suggested amount unless under the care of a health care practitioner. Zinc is best tolerated in the citrate or picolinate form. Of course, lower doses are needed in children.

Selenium

Selenium is a co-factor in glutathione pathways and an antioxidant, and enhances immune function and has antiviral action. Selenium plays a key role in converting thyroid hormone T4 into T3. Significant brain issues can be related to an impairment of conversion of T4 into T3. This should be considered if hypothyroid symptoms persist with administration of T4 alone. Excessive selenium is toxic. Symptoms include peripheral neuropathies, pain, depression, fatigue, and even convulsions and paralysis. Most adults will tolerate a supplement of 200 micrograms per day, and this is quite safe. Hair analysis is a good assessment tool.

Manganese

Manganese is a cofactor in cartilage synthesis and bone formation, and manganese deficiency impacts these structures. Critical is excess manganese, which can occur in miners but also from drinking well water containing excess manganese. Several areas, even on Vancouver Island, have wells high in manganese. Bottled water or the use of reverse-osmosis filters is a solution to well water high in manganese.

Adverse effects of manganese excess include psychosis and neurological symptoms resembling Parkinson's disease. Clinicians vary in their acceptance of this possibility. I suggest well-water testing if high levels of manganese are found in trace mineral hair analysis. Multivitamin/multimineral supplements providing a dose of 2-7 mg per day are adequate. Occasionally, clinicians prescribe 10-60 mg per day. Calcium interferes with manganese absorption, so if one is on high doses of calcium (which I do not recommend), a multivitamin/multimineral supplement containing manganese should be taken.

Other Trace Minerals of Clinical Importance:

Lithium

This as a drug used for bipolar illness or depression control. That dose is in the 600-900 mg per day range. I am talking about 5-20 mg per day as a brain calming and boosting of BDNF (brain-derived neurotropic factor).

In a hair analysis study with Great Plains Labs on twelve MS patients, we found almost all were low in lithium. This group lived on Canada's wet west coast, where heavy rains wash away trace minerals. This certainly happens with selenium. Meanwhile, most of my prairie and Ontario clients have normal lithium. I have routinely taken 10 mg per day to assist with my calmness and BDNF for my brain. Excellent discussions on lithium abound.

Molybdenum

This mineral is key in four body pathways and is also measured in the GPL hair analysis for metals and trace minerals test. At Great Plains Laboratory (GPL), we found four of the twelve MS patients low in this mineral. One of the important pathways is the formation of uric acid—yes, the gout indicator. There is almost no gout in MS patients, and if their uric acid is below one half of normal or mid-range, I suggest the supplement molybdenum, available at health food stores, until the uric acid normalizes. Uric acid is one of our key antioxidants and is especially key in humans, because we cannot make vitamin C the way most mammals can. Uric acid is about ten times as potent an antioxidant as vitamin C.

Methylation: B6, B12, and Folate

William Walsh, PhD, author of *Nutrient Power: Heal Your Biochemistry and Heal Your Brain* (Walsh 2012), specializes in nutrient-based psychiatry and nutritional medicine. He asked why some people become violent. Could it be something in their brain or body chemistry? Dr. Walsh went on to work with Dr. Carl Pfeiffer, who was studying heavy metals and schizophrenia. They found that levels of metals, including copper, zinc, and manganese, were all abnormal in criminals compared to the general population. One of the effects of this was pyrrole disorder, which includes severe zinc deficiency and undermethylation. People with pyrrole disorder have extremely low levels of B6 and zinc, which seriously affects brain function. B6 deficiency is quite common among children with ADHD.

In Pfeiffer and Walsh's studies, they found six or seven nutrient factors that dominated everything. These nutrient factors are either involved in the synthesis of a neurotransmitter or the functioning of a neurotransmitter. In their massive database of ADHD and autism, they found 70 percent of humans in the USA have normal methylation, 22 percent are undermethylated, and 8 percent are over-methylated. About 70 percent of all people with a metabolic disorder have one of these methylation disorders. Similarly, almost all these people are deficient in zinc and improve with supplemental zinc.

Methylation in Mental Health, Especially Autism

The number one cause of undermethylation is single-nucleotide polymorphism (SNP) or mutations for the one carbon methylation cycle. The main factor is the enzyme MTHFR (methylenetetrahydrofolate reductase). Everyone has thousands of these SNPs. Some have the more serious MTHFR SNPs of C677T and A1298C. However, if a person has the homozygous of the C66T, the "worst" form, they may not be undermethylated. The reason for these people not necessarily being undermethylated is epigenetics (the area of science that studies turning off and on certain genes). For example, vitamin D can have epigenetic effects on more than 2,000 genes. Oxygen affects over 8,000 genes. You may need individual help with your epigenetics. If you study your personal genetics with 23 and Me (www.23andme.com) and have concerns with your methylation genetics, you should seek some expert advice.

In my practice, I test for homocysteine at a local lab. High levels of this protein are harmful to the endothelium (lining of the blood vessel), so you are at increased risk for endothelial injury, blood vessel dysfunction (Schalinske 2012). This dramatically accelerates your risk of atherosclerosis and neurodegenerative diseases such as Alzheimer's. Treatment of elevated homocysteine is supplemental B6, B12, and folate, all in their methylated form. Ideally, a homocysteine level less than 7 mcmol (micromoles)/L is best, not the normal value listed at 12 or 13 mcmol/L. If you need a more individualized approach, then I strongly recommend "Your Expert Resource on MTHFR Gene Mutations" at www.drbenlynch.com. He is an expert in this area.

Dr. Walsh now trains physicians in his approach, because he believes this can help change mainstream psychiatry. He has spoken to the USA Surgeon General's office, the US Senate, and the National Institutes of Health. He has also spoken to the American Psychiatric Association. He speaks from his huge chemical database about how depression is comprised of at least five completely different disorders. Through his description of these biotypes, along with some inexpensive blood and urine testing, he can individualize the best treatment protocol. He determines which patients would be ideal candidates for antidepressant medications (SSRIs) or benzodiazepines, or better yet, those who can be helped with nutrients.

A more recent area in mental health is that of over-methylation, which occurs in many persons who suffer from anxiety and depression. This results in excessive activity at dopamine, norepinephrine, and serotonin receptors. These people exhibit many symptoms, such as chemical and food sensitivities, sleep disorders, underachievement, upper-body pain, and an adverse reaction to serotonin-enhancing substances (e.g., Prozac, Paxil, Zoloft, St. John's Wort). Because of their genetic tendency to be deficient in folates and other B vitamins, treatment focuses on replenishing these nutrients. This results in a reduced activity of dopamine and norepinephrine.

An important side note here is why SSRIs induce violence. Over-methylated individuals are intolerant to SSRIs. Evidence suggests this genetic intolerance is a factor in violence. Apparently, forty-two of the fifty major school shootings in the USA since 1990 were done by teens or young adults taking an SSRI (Brogan 2017). The package insert of SSRIs, like Paxil and Prozac, warn that they may make some prone to suicidal or homicidal behaviour. It behooves us to learn about this risk before we or a loved one start on these medications. For more details, visit www.walshinstitute.org.

Omega-3s: EPA and DHA

Omega-3 fats are anti-inflammatory and omega-6 fats are pro-inflammatory. Also, oils high in omega-6 will keep on the store shelves for years, while omega-3 fats degrade over weeks. They will smell badly and probably do more harm than good in the body. Omega-3 fats are best fresh or freshly frozen, encapsulated or sealed in a dark bottle.

Almost all the omega-3 clinical research has been done with fish oils that contain DHA and EPA. Krill oil and DHA from fungi are other possibilities, especially for vegetarians and vegans. However, there is not much confirmation in the literature that these are equivalent to fish oils (Alexander et al. 2017). Men and post-menopausal women have difficulty converting the type of omega-3 (ALA) in flax, hemp, or walnuts to EPA. Thus, these people need omega-3 in the form of EPA and DHA. Small fish, like herring, anchovies, and sardines, are excellent sources of omega-3s. These fish are lower on the fish food chain and, as a result, have lower levels of mercury and dioxins, which are prevalent in our oceans today. The best omega-3 oils are those that have had the toxins removed by carbon dioxide extraction. Salmon oil is rarely treated by this extraction method; hence, I do not recommend it.

Studies abound on the value of omega-3 oils. They decrease the risk of sudden cardiac death, an electrical phenomenon, by half. Similarly, they also diminish epilepsy. We know the brain is 70–80 percent fat, almost all in the form of omega-3s, EPA, and DHA. These molecules are called essential fatty acids (EFAs), because the human body cannot produce them. The other EFA is omega-6, but this is rarely insufficient in the North American or European diet. Why? Omega-6 is prevalent in most nuts, seeds, and vegetable oils. The optimal ratio of omega-6 to omega-3 in the Paleolithic or Stone Age diet 10,000 years ago was 1:1. We are much the same genetically today, yet our ratio of omega-6 to omega-3 is 20:1 or 10:1. We need less omega-6 and more omega-3 for health. We can make omega-9, which is found in olive oil. The Mediterranean Diet is still my favourite. It contains a lot of omega-9 oleic acid, which is a monounsaturated fat. Another valuable consideration is Dr. Mercola's book *Fat for Fuel* (2017). If you are diabetic and obese, you might go further to a ketogenic diet (Dashti et al. 2007). Saturated fats have been vindicated (Feinman 2010) and simple carbohydrates implicated (Feinman et al. 2015; Siri-Tarino 2010).

Many studies confirm the value of omega-3 supplements (Alexander 2017). They help depression, anxiety, and even

ADHD. All brain challenges have a major excess of inflammation. The most obvious choice for curbing inflammation is omega-3 fats. Omega-3s are so important in brain building that the unborn fetus steals these from the mother's brain. This is why pregnant women should be on omega-3 supplements. Lack of omega-3s is a major factor in postpartum depression. Indeed, postpartum depression increases after multiple pregnancies, because subsequent fetuses each steal a little more of the mother's omega-3 fatty acids.

If you get heartburn from taking omega-3 supplements, try them with food. Alternatively, take a digestive enzyme containing lipase when you take your omega-3. If still unsuccessful, try freezing your capsules. If you swallow them frozen, they are further down the digestive tract when they thaw out. Fat, including omega-3, can help open the lower esophageal sphincter. If this valve at the bottom of the esophagus is open, acid from the stomach can splash up and cause heartburn. I recommend 1,000–1,500 mg per day of DHA and an equal amount or more of EPA. For simplicity, I suggest a supplement of 3,000 mg of EPA and DHA combined.

Vitamin D

I have left this till last, because this has been my favourite nutrient of the last twenty years. Vitamin D is closer to a hormone than a vitamin. Also, we are able to make our own, on our skin, from sunshine. Hence, this de-classifies it as a true vitamin. This is a brief summary related to brain optimization and well-being.Vitamin D is given in International Units,IU,or micrograms (1000 micrograms = 1 mg).4,000 IU = 100 micrograms, 400 IU = 10 micrograms,1000 IU = 25 micrograms.

Lack of vitamin D often starts in the womb. Pregnant women should take 4,000 IU of vitamin D per day, or at least 2,000 IU. At least 2,000 IU is needed if one lives in the northern part of the continent or at a latitude of 35 degrees or higher. I live about the 49th parallel, so I am at risk of insufficient vitamin D from sunshine. In fact, fertility is enhanced by adequate vitamin D. If women do not receive enough vitamin D during pregnancy, babies are more prone to type 1 diabetes, MS, and childhood cancers. Newborns are best on vitamin D in breast milk, providing the mother is on vitamin D supplementation. However, if concerns exist, then a supplement of 800 IU per day can be given to the baby. For decades now, children in Finland have been given 2,000 IU per day, beginning at one year of age. I also suggest this routinely in Canada.

Vitamin D is one of our most favourable epigenetic agents. It turns on up to 2,000 good genes and turns off hundreds of bad genes. This reduces inflammation throughout the body and brain, enhances the well-being of the microbiome, and prevents up to 50 percent of 18 types of cancer, including bowel, breast, uterus, ovarian, and prostate cancers. This is secondarily important, as cancer chemotherapy ravages the brain. "Chemo brain" and depression are very real phenomena.

New research confirms adequate vitamin D levels reduce the risk of Alzheimer's (Sommer 2017). Years of research have demonstrated adequate vitamin D concentration (25-OH) in the blood as being a key component in diminishing MS attacks and the severity of attacks. I have taken a considerable amount of vitamin D for years upon the advice of my colleague, Dr. Ashton Embry of Direct-MS.org. My goal, and yours, should be a blood vitamin D level of 40–60 nanogram/ml or in SI units of Canada and Europe, 100–150 nmol (nanomoles)/L. (The conversion ratio is 2.5, so 60 ng/ml equals 150 nmol/L.) Please know which measurement you are reading.

For years, I needed 12,000 IU per day to maintain a blood value greater than 100 nmol/L, likely because of malabsorption from my IBS. Once I quit gluten, I was able to reduce my vitamin D supplement to 7,000 IU per day. Nowadays, we are more aware of absorption issues with vitamin D, so if we measure lower vitamin D than we would expect from a particular intake, then malabsorption should be diagnosed and the appropriate intervention implemented (i.e., avoid gluten and possibly dairy).

Food cannot provide enough vitamin D to meet your needs. Fluid milk and some dairy products are fortified with vitamin D, but levels are regulated by government agencies. For example, a cup of milk or yoghurt may contain 100 IU of vitamin D. Salmon and mackerel contain about 400 IU of vitamin D per 4 ounces. Other foods only have small amounts of vitamin D. Sunlight is an excellent way to get vitamin D, but this is not foolproof. Sunscreens, such as 30 percent SPF, block 99 percent of the sun's rays, which make vitamin D in the skin. Also, the ability to make vitamin D on our skin declines with age. Thus, the best way to ensure adequate vitamin D is to take a supplement.

In conclusion, I suggest 1,000 IU per day in the first year of life and 2,000 IU per day at year one until age 30 or so. Then 4,000 IU per day or enough to achieve a blood level of 100–150 nmol/L (which is 40–60 ng/ml in the USA). If your physician won't measure your vitamin D, then get it measured privately. Your brain and optimal well-being depend on it.

In this chapter, I outlined some of the key supplements you must consider for brain health. This is not an exhaustive list. In addition, the mitochondrial/energy suggestion list in the following chapter should be considered, especially if brain recovery is sought. Remember, you are in control!

7: Fatigue, Low Energy, and the Mitochondria

"I'm too tired." Have you ever uttered this phrase? Perhaps you have said it to yourself rather than out loud, recognizing that people do not really want to hear it. Dr. Terry Wahls' first book, *Minding Your Mitochondria* (2010), comes to mind. Happily, our understanding of mitochondria as our energy source has continued to progress dramatically since she wrote that book nearly ten years ago. Despite many chronic illnesses having fatigue as one of their core components (e.g., rheumatoid arthritis (RA), systemic lupus erythematosis (SLE), fibromyalgia (FM), myalgic enephalitis (ME), chronic fatigue syndrome (CFS), and even MS), this description of fatigue is usually given short shrift or is ignored medically. Meanwhile, the science has caught up and moved past this inaction. I suggest it is time physicians listened and acted on this complaint. However, in the short-term, it is in your power to change most of these resolvable items. Mitochondria rely on a food source, such as glucose or fatty acids, and the oxygen that we breathe. In the presence of these two components, our mitochondria are able to make adenosine triphosphate (ATP), the currency of cellular metabolism, very efficiently. In this chapter, I outline the other critical components that may be awry, even if adequate oxygen and food sources are available.

In short, the mitochondria are in every living cell of our body, including the microbiota, gut flora. These organelles are critical for supplying energy for almost all cell functions. These energy powerhouses use oxygen by separating the high-energy bond between the two oxygen atoms in a controlled "explosion." This oxygen combustion helps to break up food and convert it to the energy packets of ATP. If enough oxygen is present, then mitochondria can produce thirty-four molecules of ATP per molecule of oxygen. However, if there is insufficient oxygen (hypoxia), then the anaerobic or lactic acid pathway produces only two molecules of ATP. An average human cell has 2,500 mitochondria. The exception is the red blood cell, which has no mitochondria. In addition, the mitochondria have their own DNA, from the maternal line, called mitochondrial DNA (mDNA). When healthy, the mito-chondria are able to control or quench almost all the reactive oxygen species created from oxygen breakdown. If unhealthy, then mitochondria are susceptible to damage due to the proximity to the explosion of the tightly bound oxygen molecules. Consequently, mitochondrial damage and dysfunction occur.

The causes of mitochondrial damage are well outlined in Dr. Dean Raffelock's chapter in James M. Greenblatt and Kelly Brogan's book, *Integrative Therapies for Depression* (Greenblatt 2016). These include: 1) oxidative stress, 2) radiation exposure, 3) environmental toxins, 4) some infections, including Epstein-Barr virus and hepatitis viruses, 5) hormone deficiencies, most notably hypothyroidism, 6) genetic mitochondrial disease, and, 7) pharmaceutical agents (drugs). Oxidative stress is a significant component of neurodegenerative diseases, so antioxidants matter (Uttara 2009).

It is critical for your own health and energy to know this list and how to compensate with supplements if you and your physician decide you need to stay on one of these agents, particularly the pharmaceutical drugs. These include simple ones, such as Aspirin, acetaminophen (paracetamol), and nonsteroidal anti-inflammatory drugs (NSAIDs), as well as more complex drugs, especially antipsychotics, statins, benzodiazepines, and metformin (commonly used in type 2 diabetes mellitus). All the above drugs are known to have tough side effects. All cause mitochondrial damage and dysfunction. Small wonder many of us say, "I'm too tired." Most clinicians learn the Krebs or citric acid cycle in medical school but not the important mitochondrial nutritional cofactors. By learning more about these, you will open a new doorway to optimize your brain's healing and function.

Important Mitochondrial Nutrition Cofactors

How does food in the form of fatty acids, amino acids, and carbohydrates get into the mitochondria? First, it is absorbed through the gut lining into the bloodstream. Then it travels to the liver, where some processing occurs, and then to the heart, the lungs, and on to the entire body, including the brain. In the brain, glucose and free fatty acids are able to cross the blood-brain barrier (BBB). Once they cross the BBB, they can enter the brain cells, including neurons, if conditions are correct. However, it should be noted that in Alzheimer's disease, this pathway is often broken. This is why one of the nicknames for Alzheimer's is type 3 diabetes mellitus. Many of these patients are resistant to insulin, so the glucose does not enter the neuron. Low energy levels in the cell and poor-quality thinking are the consequences. It is also why some of these patients respond well to free fatty acids in the form of medium-chain triglycerides (MCTs). The best known of these is coconut oil as an alternative fuel source to blood sugar (glucose).

Each of the nutrients named above needs to be converted into acetyl-CoA, which can then be used in aerobic energy production. L-carnitine, actually acetyl carnitine in the brain, is needed to move free fatty acids into the inner mitochondria to be used as energy. This is a critical step. A large number of nutrients are needed for this transformation to occur. These include the amino acids lysine, methionine, and serine. Other cofactors that are critical for this are vitamin B6, vitamin B12, folate, trimethyl glycine, vitamin C, vitamin D3, biotin, and iron. Glucose needs vitamin B1, vitamin D3, vitamin B5, and biotin. Take heart, because at the end of this chapter, I include a summary list that will allow you to try three months of these supplements to see if you can reverse your low-energy problem.

Once inside the mitochondria, within the citric acid cycle and the electron transport chain, other nutrients are needed. Both of these pathways require coenzyme Q10 (CoQ10), magnesium, zinc, and vitamins C, K, and B3 to produce and recycle the much-desired ATP energy packets. These steps require vitamin B1 (thiamine), vitamin B2 (riboflavin), vitamin B3 (niacin, as NADH), vitamin B6 (pyridoxine), alpha lipoic acid, magnesium, sulphur, iron, and phosphorous. When each of these nutrients are combined with twelve individual amino acids, they help form eight organic acids that are needed in the process of the second energy-producing pathway within the mitochondria, called the electron transport chain. It is critically important that all the components are present to produce the much-required ATP. In fact, this is like rechargeable batteries, but the ATP molecule needs to be recharged nearly 1,000 times a day!

Protecting Your Mitochondria from Harm

The three key antioxidant molecules that protect against free radicals, or reactive oxygen species (ROS), are glutathione (GSH), coenzyme Q10, and alpha lipoic acid (ALA). GSH is the major free-radical scavenger in the brain. Fortunately, early in my recovery journey, I learned how to raise my cellular GSH. I was able to do this by ingesting increased amounts of the usually rate-limiting amino acid of the three amino acids that make up GSH. This critical amino acid is cysteine. To do this, I began taking a quality whey protein isolate, prepared at lower temperatures to protect this vulnerable cysteine molecule. At that time, I used the whey protein isolate from Immunotec Research Limited in Quebec. I travelled around Canada, the United States, and Mexico as one of their speakers for five years. Needless to say, I am well versed on this topic.

I was impressed by the McGill research work of Drs. Bounous and Kongshavn (1988). They first confirmed the power of quality whey protein and published these concepts. Today, I recommend whey from New Zealand, because their cows are grass fed, and it is prepared in the important low-temperature technique. It is easy to look back and realize a major part of the significant GSH benefit is improved cellular function. Much of this improvement is due to more energy, secondary to improved mitochondrial function. European Union whey is no longer useful for this, because it has been pasteurized at too high a temperature to conform with EU regulations. Unfortunately, this destroys (denatures) this critical cysteine molecule. Similarly, whey products targeted to the physically active—like bodybuilders and athletes— are often produced without the low-temperature technique, because it is more expensive. Finally, I choose New Zealand whey, because it has less glyphosate and other herbicides, less abnormal proteins (GMOs), and less bovine growth hormone.

Therefore, even though many types of whey protein products help with muscle recovery, they do not contain much of the critical undenatured cysteine. An important reminder is that when you purchase a quality undenatured whey protein, you should not put it in a blender or into an extremely hot liquid, because this will damage the important cysteine molecule.

Think of how an egg white turns white in the frying pan or egg-poaching unit. This protein, egg white, is now denatured. It will no longer have the valuable undenatured cysteine in it. I cannot recommend raw eggs because of the risk of salmonella. Therefore, a quality whey protein is a decent alternative. Fortunately, the whey protein from cows is reasonably close to the whey protein from human breast milk. Consequently, only about 1 in 10,000 people will be sensitive to it. It is the casein (cheese protein) within milk that humans usually respond to in a negative fashion. Of course, lactose can also be a problem for many. I took 50 g of quality whey protein daily for over fifteen years in my own personal recovery journey. I believe it dramatically helped my mitochondria recover, because my energy returned considerably. As a side note, it is important to look at the detoxifications chapter (chapter 1), because GSH is critical here too. You must also reduce the offending toxins to be successful!

The other two key antioxidants mentioned above are CoQ10 and ALA. CoQ10 is high in organ meats, such as liver. This is one of the major reasons that Dr. Terry Wahls recommends organ meats (Wahls 2015). Personally, I've had more success with suggesting supplements than trying to convince people to eat organ meats. With CoQ10, I suggest 200 mg three times a day. The original and cheaper ubiquinone will usually be adequate, if you are less than forty. If you are over 40 you may need to take the more expensive ubiquinol. Alpha-lipoic acid (ALA), the third mitochondrial protector, is also present in the organ meats (heart, liver, and kidneys). However, it is also available in supplements and in vegetables, such as broccoli, spinach, tomatoes, brussel sprouts, rice bran, and some peas.

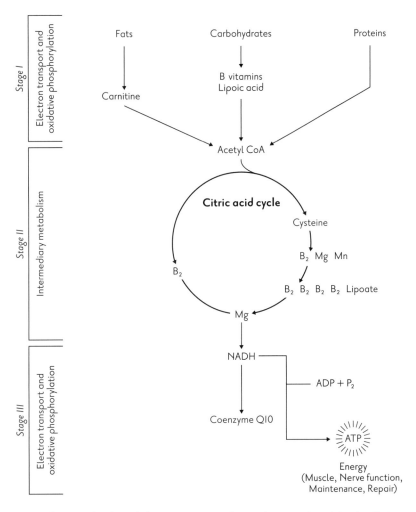

Figure: Citric acid cycle and electron transport chain with required nutritional cofactors

Nutritional Modulators of Mitochondrial Oxidative Phosphorylation

Nutritional Agent	Daily Range	Influence
Ascorbate (Vitamin C)	500-6000 mg	Part of glutathione-lipoic acid antioxidants
Catechin	50-1000 mg	Hydroxyl radical and peroxynitrite quencher
Copper (Cu)	1-3 mg	Necessary for ZN-Cu superoxide dismutase Superoxide dismutase (SOD): major anti-oxidant calming oxygen and nitric oxide free radicals
Manganese (Mn)	2-5 mg	Necessary for MnSOD
Zinc (Zn)	10-50 mg	Necessary for ZnCuSOD
CoQ10 (ubiquinone)	20-1000 mg	Maintenance of electron transport chain function
D-ribose	5 gm twice per day	Can improve energy reserves especially in heart Failure and chronic fatigue
Glutathione	100-1000 mg	Antioxidant and Phase II glutathione formation
Lipoic acid	50-1000 mg	Multiple roles in mitochondrial protection
Magnesium	50-1000 mg	Mitochondrial Krebs cycle activator
Omega-3 fatty acid	500-3000 mg	EPA/DHA protect mitochondrial membrane and block action of cytokines

Nutritional Agent	Daily Range	Influence
N-acetyl-carnitine	50-1000 mg	Fatty acid transport into the mitochondrion
N-acetyl-cysteine (NAC)	50-1500 mg	Stimulates mitochondrial glutathione synthesis
Niacin (Vitamin B3)	10-50 mg	NADH and NADPH production in energy creation
Niacinamide (Vitamin B3)	200-2000 mg	NADH and NADPH production in energy creation
Riboflavin (Vitamin B2)	10-200 mg	Coenzyme for producing energy from carbohydrates, fats and protein
Selenium	100-500 mcg	Activator of glutathione peroxidase
Thiamine (Vitamin B1)	10-200 mg	Transketolase activator for hexose monophosphate shunt
Vitamin E (tocopherols)	100-1000 mg	Mitochondrial membrane protection
Vitamin K	100-1000 mcg	Electron transport chain protector

Consequences of Insufficient Antioxidants GSH, CoQ10, and ALA

Excessive oxidative stress creates mitochondrial dysfunction. The brain cannot create the large amount of energy needed if the mitochondria are not functioning properly. As a consequence, many of the neurons become "idling neurons." This means they are alive but not functioning. If enough brain neurons are not functioning, this can masquerade as depression, cognitive challenge, memory loss, or loss of executive function. I have had all these at one time or another and would rather not experience them again. The consequence of oxidative damage from lack of optimal amounts of antioxidants is premature cellular aging and disease. This is nowhere more obvious than in the "energy hog" of the brain.

In her report, "Micronutrient Deficiencies and Mitochondrial Dysfunction," C. Marrs states, "the mitochondria also regulate inflammatory cascades, steroidal genesis, neurotransmission, nerve degeneration, ion homeostasis (calcium, sodium, potassium, and magnesium), heme synthesis, reactive oxygen species production and detoxification, and, ultimately, cell death" (Marrs in Greenblatt 2016).

Women in particular are more at risk for hormone dysregulation. This hormonal dysregulation represents some of the least-recognized signs of mitochondrial dysfunction. When a patient presents with an almost unending complex of unrelated symptoms, there is a good chance it is a mitochondrial problem of nutrient deficiency. The solution to this mitochondrial problem might be solved without pharmacologic drugs (Velarde 2014; Reddy 2008).

Environmental Factors of Mitochondrial Health

Nutrient deficiency in our food is present in all societies. This includes wealthy Western nations. In fact, the situation may be much worse in Canada and the United States. Modern industrial farming methods have depleted crop nutrients in the harvested foods, and everyone suffers secondary to this. Poor nutrition is not just present in overweight, sedentary people but also in fit-looking and highly active people, including athletes. Organic and nutrient-dense whole foods circumvent part of this. When you add environmental pollutants and prescription drug use to the lack of nutrients, the potential injury to our mitochondria goes up astronomically. Some of my main pet peeves, because they can be huge contributors to the problem, include protein pump inhibitors, statin drugs, and glyphosate.

We have cultivated out 95 percent of the genetic variation from different food crops. This reduces to almost nothing the greater than 200,000 plant components that provide subtle nutrition for us (Daniel 2012).

Eighty to 90 percent of the dry weight of modern fruits, vegetables, and grains bred specially for high production come from carbohydrates. Secondary to this, they have far fewer key phytonutrients. These key phytonutrients are nature's molecules, which can keep us healthy or restore our health. In Canada and the United States, almost 85 percent of the topsoil has been depleted in the last 100 years, resulting in a depletion in the nutritional content of our food. In fact, topsoil depletion is worse than this, because that number was reported only until 1992. Europe and South America have experienced a 72 percent and 76 percent reduction in topsoil, respectively. Consider this if wondering whether to take a daily multivitamin/multimineral. The short answer is, yes!

Drug and Environmental Exposure

Medicines, vaccines, and environmental toxicants induce mitochondrial damage. One of the key triggers of this damage is vitamin B1 and thiamine depletion, which occur from the use of antibiotics, metformin, loop and thiazide diuretics, estrogens in hormone-replacement therapy, and oral contraceptives. Vaccines do the same. Statins deplete CoQ10 dramatically. All types of psychotropic (brain-altering) drugs directly trigger mitochondrial damage. This includes antidepressants, antipsychotics, anti-anxiety drugs, and sleeping pills. Even NSAIDs, such as ibuprofen, naproxen, diclofenac (Voltaren), ASA, and acetaminophen do this.[9] If you believe the FDA (Federal Drug Administration) and Health Canada will protect you from the above crisis, then you are mistaken. The impact of drugs on mitochondrial function is only a recent understanding. As a result, there is no requirement for mitochondrial injury or nutrient impact to be researched or mentioned with a new drug. Therefore, this useful warning is not present on any of our current established drugs.

Now for the Brain Matter. Yes, the Brain Matters!

Despite the lack of acceptance and knowledge of poorly functioning mitochondria in neurology, primary care, and psychiatry, this problem is a huge component of illness. Remember, the brain has the highest number of mitochondria per cell, with greater than 2,500. When this is coupled with the fact that brain cells need more energy per unit of mass than any other organ, then you can understand the significance of the problem.

---

[9]   Linus Pauling Institute: Micronutrient Information Center. Available at: http://lpi.oregonstate.edu/infocenter/. University of Maryland Medical Center: Vitamins. Available at: http://umm.ede/health/medical/reports/articles/vitamins.

Nerve function and communication require a lot of energy. Some of the activities that require large amounts of energy include ion channel transfer, receptors, neurotransmitter vesicle release, and neurotransmitter recycling. Lack of energy aggravates nerve-to-nerve communication problems. In addition, the maintenance of cell well-being, homeostasis, becomes problematic. This precipitates many neuropsychiatric conditions, including some of the relatively irreversible neurodegenerative problems, such as Alzheimer's, Parkinson's, and ALS (Kidd 2005; Swash 2016).

Compensation for Brain Mitochondrial Dysfunction

Our body has brilliant backup methods that allow it to cope when the mitochondria are not functioning properly. The three following body processes help the brain manage energy for a time:

I. Orexin/Hypocretin Neurons

These neurons need five to six times as much energy as regular neurons. This allows them to sense and monitor brain energy resources early. Hence, they are an "early warning system" for us and our brain.

Whenever orexin/hypocretin neurons have insufficient stores of ATP, they stop firing. This permits the brain to do a relocation of energy. An analogy of this is an electrical company moving power from one station to another. When orexin/hypocretin neurons are firing, wakefulness is induced, and we have a maintenance of arousal and eating. If orexin/

hypocretin neurons are turned off, melatonin is increased, which induces sleep (Sakurai 2007).

Orexin/hypocretin neurons originate in the lateral hypothalamus (just above the pituitary or master gland). Their neurons reach throughout the entire central nervous system and into the peripheral nervous system. Their innervation extends to the adrenals, testicles, and ovaries, and they even have receptors in the kidneys and small intestine.

Sleepiness, fatigue, malaise, and anorexia in most illnesses and mitochondrial distress are a consequence of resource allocation by the orexin/hypocretin system. These same neurons also modify pain receptors and digestion (via neuropeptide galanin), and can trigger depolarization of neurons found in migraines and epilepsy. In fact, low cerebrospinal fluid concentrations of orexin/hypocretin are found in major depression and suicide (Takahashi 2006).

In summary, wakefulness and feeding are key components of healthy optimal mitochondria. When energy resources are low, and you see a new-onset sleep disorder, such as excess sleep or narcolepsy, think of this orexin/hypocretin system. Why are migraines and seizures generated? It may be the brain's effort to compensate for changing brain ion homeostasis. Therefore, consider mitochondrial dysfunction for this group of symptoms. If you experience a new and recent onset of fatigue or migraines, consider toxins that may have triggered it. (Picard 2014). This may be a new medication, vaccine, reduced thyroid function, or new exposure to an environmental toxin, even a food sensitivity. Food sensitivities that trigger migraines for me include wheat, dairy, and sometimes wine and chocolate, much to my chagrin!

2. Lactate Production as a Marker for Mitochondrial Dysfunction

Most of us have heard of lactate production or lactic acid. We know it happens during prolonged exercise, especially if we are not used to the repeated exercise of our muscles. In addition, lactate production is a signal that we are nearing our limit of exercise. Why? Because the making of ATP, energy packets, with oxygen in aerobic exercise makes thirty-four molecules of ATP. However, without adequate oxygen, lactate production increases, and the mitochondria make only two molecules of ATP. We know that brain lactate formation occurs when we are short of oxygen. This occurs not only during exercise but also with other major stressors. Therefore, increased brain lactate production also signals a shift from aerobic to anaerobic metabolism. Evidence suggests the brain can also convert lactate to ATP.

A great deal of lactate production results from brain trauma. This is a huge stressor, and oxygen and glucose are depleted rapidly. We can now measure, through specialized brain imaging, the brain shift toward anaerobic metabolism and excess lactate production. When this occurs during rest and minimal exertion, it indicates mitochondrial distress. This is more prevalent in mitochondrial abnormalities, such as myalgic encephalitis, chronic fatigue syndrome, and MS (Cruz 2012; Shungu 2012; Narayana 2005).

More recently, magnetic resonance spectroscopy can be used to identify lactate doublets in diseased brain mitochondria. These abnormal "lactate doublets" have been found in acquired mitochondrial dysfunction. People with acquired mitochondrial dysfunction include those with autism and bipolar disorder, and those who are aging prematurely. Clinical indications are reported as fatigue, muscle pain, and weakness. Another name, "hitting the wall," applies to athletes who have reached this threshold of exertion (as in a marathon). An acute onset of energy depletion in the brain signifies trauma or brain injury. This gives a whole new approach to assessing mild concussions. When someone sustains a blow to the head and feels tired, we should realize this is secondary to energy depletion and prescribe rest. Research on bipolar disorder has suggested disrupted mitochondrial energy was secondary to neurochemical imbalance. Finally, lactate production can initiate and/or maintain inflammatory cascades. Neuro-inflammation is associated with every brain illness I know of, both neurological and psychiatric.

3. Vitamins and Brain Inflammation

Mitochondria are a large component of the possible mechanisms of triggering inflammation. Not surprisingly, some of the same nutrient deficiencies that injure mitochondria also initiate or trigger inflammatory cascades and activate neurotoxic chemicals. An example of this is vitamin B6, which is needed in over 100 enzymes, including the making of Coenzyme Q10 and the amino acid tryptophan. Tryptophan is needed for the synthesis of serotonin and melatonin. Hence, lack of vitamin B6 disturbs neurotransmitters. It can also lead to cell death in brain areas, such as the hippocampus, basal ganglia, and cerebellum. Is this part of the early stages of Parkinson's or other movement disorders?

Furthermore, when vitamin B6 is deficient, the incomplete breakdown of tryptophan produces the metabolite quinolinic acid. I learned from Dr. Bill Shaw, PhD, of Great Plains Laboratory that quinolinic acid is a potent and self-perpetuating neurotoxin in the brain. It produces reactive oxygen species and over-activates NMDA (n-methyl-d-aspartate) glutamate receptors, which injures cells, even to the point of cell death. At the same time, quinolinic acid inhibits the brain's astrocytes from cleaning up excess glutamate, which is a further neurotoxin. This ensures continued brain inflammation and damage.

The point of the above somewhat complex discussion is that vitamin B6 deficiency can have profound brain influence. Today, this quinolinic acid pathway can be evaluated with the extremely valuable organic acid test on the urine. This was pioneered and optimized by Dr. Bill Shaw, initially at the CDC (Center for Disease Control) and now in his own lab for the past twenty years. Defects in vitamin B6 metabolism are linked to seizures, which are often drug resistant. In addition, vitamin B6 reduces brain atrophy in Alzheimer's patients, tardive dyskinesia (automaton-like walking), schizophrenia, and diabetics with depression. Low vitamin B6 likely aggravates Huntington's disease.

Vitamin B1, also called thiamine, is every bit as critical to mitochondria and brain health. One study found that 75 percent of both type 2 and type 3 diabetics were thiamine deficient. Obesity worsens this problem, as does being postoperative from bariatric surgery. It is interesting that the use of yeast in vaccines for HPV (human papilloma virus) and HBV (hepatitis B) aggravates this vitamin B1 deficiency as well (Lương 2013).

Regular consumption of some foods high in thiaminase, the enzyme that breaks down thiamine, worsens vitamin B1 deficiency. These include coffee, tea, and other foods. Medications depleting vitamin B1 include all antibiotics and protein pump inhibitors (e.g., Nexium). In addition to absorption problems, these drugs aggravate the same deficiencies. I accept that I am at high risk for this because of my longstanding irritable bowel syndrome. This is also true for any inflammatory bowel disease, including Crohn's, ulcerative colitis, and celiac disease.

We need thiamine badly, because without it, the entire mitochondrial engine grinds to a halt. White matter abnormalities in the brain, such as MS, are common with mitochondrial disorders. Early or mild mitochondrial insults will trigger orexin/hypocretin slowing. Certainly, sleepiness, anorexia, fatigue, depressed mood, and apathy are cardinal symptoms of MS. Sufferers may also experience pins and needles, numbness, tingling, muscle pain, dizziness, and brain fog or fuzzy thinking (cognitive dysfunction).

Once moderate- or longer-duration thiamine deficiency occurs, we may see gastrointestinal issues. These include prolonged gastric emptying, excessive vomiting, diarrhea, and irritable bowel syndrome. In addition, we may see neuropathic pain, ataxia, tremors, and even fainting. In some patients, we see abdominal or chest pain, sleepwalking/talking, insomnia, night terrors or panic, night sweats, and anorexia. Some people will change quickly with high or low blood pressure, tic-like movements around the eyes, and even diminished knee reflexes. Extreme cases of deficiency may include heart palpitations, low blood pressure, slow resting heart rate, high, fast heart rate with uneven beats, and even balance problems. Finally, if this deficiency persists, people can develop delusions, hallucinations, and disorientation to time, place, or even people. Happily, these quickly respond to thiamine supplementation. Fortunately, this is extremely safe, so it may be worth a trial of replacement or supplementation.

Fatigue and Depression

Common symptoms in those suffering from depression include loss of energy, loss of motivation, severe fatigue with or without muscle weakness, and excess sleep. These people may be diagnosed as depressed and occasionally as having an undertreated hypothyroid condition. Medically unexplained symptoms such as the above can be seen in anywhere from 25-75 percent of patients in outpatient care. If you happen to be one of these patients, now you know that you have more options!

Autonomic Dysregulation

It surprises me how often I see this in patients simply by asking. I routinely inquire about the problem of cold hands and cold feet, sudden light-headedness when getting up quickly, and intermittent diarrhea or constipation. This may be due to the autonomic nervous system being especially sensitive to mitochondrial dysfunction and lack of energy. The autonomic nervous system is a combination of the sympathetic and parasympathetic systems. The sympathetic tends to be our adrenaline side, with the fight-or-flight response. Meanwhile, the parasympathetic tends to be our calming side but occasionally with nausea and even vomiting due to overactivity of the vagus nerve.

Autonomic dysregulation is a common problem in nearly 70 million people worldwide. This translates to 3 million Americans or approximately 1 percent of all people. The most common symptoms are temperature dysregulation, increased or decreased heart rate relative to the changes from sitting to standing, blood pooling in the legs, fainting, dizziness, seizures, blurred vision or changes in vision, significant noise and light sensitivity, intense salt and water cravings, nausea and vomiting, irritable bowel syndrome symptoms, mood lability, fatigue, inertia, and severe anxiety attacks. At times, I thought I was over these symptoms, but I still have irritable bowel syndrome. I am happy to have most of the rest of these symptoms behind me. Maybe you can too. Autonomic dysregulation is not psychosomatic but is instead a sign of mitochondrial distress. Consider that each episode is triggered by stress that exceeds the energy resources at the moment in these very sensitive neurons. This problem can be improved dramatically without medication. More energy is provided from optimal mitochondrial nutrients, food, and more oxygen—simple to say and not that complicated to do.

Cerebellar Dysregulation and Ataxia

Cerebellar ataxia is commonly caused from mitochondrial disease and damage (Greenblatt 2016). These can present from subtle to gross gait and balance changes. However, they can progress to the stage where a person is barely able to stand or walk. Patients may collapse to the floor, losing muscle strength intermittently. Even seizures have been documented to occur after certain medications or vaccine reactions. I always ask and listen for timing and triggering factors. Patients often know this but need a few open-ended questions to jog their memory.

Cerebellar dysregulation can incorrectly be diagnosed as depression. Ideally an MRI rules out cerebellar injury. In addition, comprehensive lab testing of thyroid function should be done. If all these are normal, you should consider mitochondrial distress. Sometimes, vitamin B1 deficiency, CoQ10 deficiency, or both can be the cause (Artuch 2006).

Psychiatric and Cognitive Disturbances

Both of these are common signs of mitochondrial distress. Early on in a mild phase, it may simply be a loss of energy or motivation. Later, when it is more moderate, it can be seen as mood swings, anxiety, personality changes, and even psychosis. Cognitive troubles may be secondary to a medication/vaccine adverse reaction. Symptoms can include difficulty finding words, naming and fluency, understanding written text, reduced attention span, and visual and verbal memory deficits. It may simply be described as an overall decline in cognitive ability.

Myopathy and Myalgias

Muscles need a lot of energy to perform, so a drug or nutrient depletion can induce muscle pain and weakness. Symptoms can include pain, inflammation, cramping, and tendinopathies. Low CoQ10, which disturbs the electron transport enzyme, is often to blame. The ones I love to hate here are the statin drugs. Statins block the formation of CoQ10, and all these drugs when sold have an insert suggesting that patients should be put on CoQ10 whenever a statin is started. However, this is rarely done. Antibiotics, especially fluoroquinolones, cause increased mitochondrial reactive oxygen species and deplete magnesium and thiamine. Trials with CoQ10, alpha lipoic acid, vitamin B1, and creatine may reduce muscle pain and weakness. They are safe, relatively inexpensive, and well worth a try.

Gastrointestinal Dysmotility

This condition is common and present in up to 15 percent of patients with mitochondrial disease. Consider mitochondrial dysfunction if there is unexplained abdominal pain, chronic constipation, cyclic vomiting, and diarrhea. Depression, migraine, and gastrointestinal dysfunction can be clustered together. Watch for this unhappy triad.

Anorexia (remember orexin/hypocretin neurons), slow-emptying stomach, and pseudo-bowel obstruction are other signs of mitochondrial dysfunction. Occasionally, there is profound weight loss as well. The symptoms are not psychogenic but likely secondary to regular and diminished supply of energy to the nerves. Inflammation is often a core or critical piece, because managing the inflammation taxes the mitochondria energy supplies even further. Once again, the use of CoQ10 and l-carnitine can often be dramatic in their solution of the above (Finsterer 2016).

Mitochondrial Support

There are frequent literature reports of mitochondrial cocktails of vitamins, minerals, and other nutrients (Tarnopolsky 2008). Below are my suggestions for an affordable three-month trial to help you resolve your lack of energy (Greenblatt 2016). If you don't see an improvement in those three months consider consultation with an integrative/functional medicine professional.

- B 100 complex twice a day (best choice would contain methylfolate)
- Vitamin C, 1 g twice a day
- Vitamin E, 400 mg of mixed tocopherols once a day
- Magnesium, 500 mg at bedtime and 250 mg in the morning, if still needed for muscle spasms
- Alpha lipoic acid 200 mg twice a day or three times a day if peripheral neuropathy
- l-carnitine 500 mg three times a day or acetyl carnitine (crosses BBB) for cognitive problems
- CoQ10 200 mg three times a day
- Zinc 30 mg per day
- Iron supplementation, but only if the labs indicate this is needed
- GSH (glutathione) supplementation via whey, NAC, or liposomal GSH
- Essential fatty acids, especially omega-3 in the form of 2,000 mg of EPA plus DHA in combination, e.g., clean fish oil
- Occasionally in women, 500 mg of omega-6 as evening primrose oil, borage oil, or hemp oil

"I'm too tired." This is the phrase that I talked about in my first paragraph in this chapter. I've attempted to outline some of the treatable causes of this lack of energy. My suggestions do not contain any pharmacologic drugs, because none of them really work to solve this problem. Instead, it is a critical feature of nutrition components that can be initiated in the form of supplements. However, it is also critical to remove the offending or triggering agents that are causing the mitochondrial dysfunction. This is more of an individual story that each of us must determine on our own. Fortunately, a group of physicians and other health care professionals are trained in integrative and/or functional medicine. If you are experiencing fatigue/lack of energy, and you need help in your own journey, I suggest you consult with one of them.

8: Let's Get Growing a Garden

Gardening for the health of it! When I spoke to others about my next book, several suggested that I should include a chapter about gardening. One of these people was Joan Beal, who was the force behind bringing Dr. Paolo Zamboni's vein treatment to North America. As you recall, Dr. Zamboni pioneered the use of intravenous balloon angioplasty to treat blocked veins in the neck to improve blood drainage from the brain. This has become known as CCSVI (chronic cerebrospinal venous insufficiency). Joan is a visionary; thus, when she suggests something, I listen.

My wife, Denise, and I have been operating a certified organic fruit and vegetable farm on Vancouver Island for seven years. For the three years before certification, we worked within wholly organic guidelines. In fact, for the fifteen years prior, we had used no chemicals. We had been raising emus for their production of oil and meat, right from egg incubation to adulthood. I realized almost ten years ago that I would often mention the value of organic food in my talks and my writing. I decided if I was going to "talk the talk," then I had better be prepared to "walk the walk." In addition, I now appreciate the parallel or overlap between healthy soil and a healthy microbiota within humans.

In more recent years I have become aware of an even more critical reason to garden. The act of organic gardening is incredibly healthful for the individual doing it. It doesn't just get you out in the sunshine and fresh air; the exposure to soil and the healthy microbiota within it are the biggest reason. We know now that regular exposure to soil and soil organisms work as a fabulous probiotic for our gut flora. Any healthy and successful gardener or farmer will tell you that their success is completely tied to the general health and well-being of their soil. Healthy soil can hold up to 100,000 organisms within a single gram. Normal soil will average about 3,000 organisms per gram. If the soil is optimal for diversity and type of microbiota, then the plant root systems penetrate deeper and are much more diverse and have many more tiny root hairs. This allows the plant to be resistant to infection, drought, excess moisture, and pesky insects. You may recognize that these are many of the things that we want to be resistant to as humans as well. A negative input into the health of our soil, such as salt exposure, herbicides, pesticides, artificial fertilizers, and antibiotics will all reduce the health and diversity of the soil organisms. This is why organic soil and gardening is so important. This is an exact parallel to the health of our personal gut microbiome.

A second reason to talk about the health of gardening is its value as a hobby. It is the number one activity and the fastest-growing hobby on the west coast of Canada. Perhaps even more important to the chronically sick is the role of economics: growing some of your own organic food saves money, though I am not trying to put organic farmers out of work. Far from it! I know how little farmers earn. Organic farmers farm and garden as a lifestyle choice, not an economic one. It might interest you that 54 percent of Canadians buy some organic food weekly. Also, organic food demand is increasing by 16 percent annually.

By growing your own fruits and vegetables, you achieve several important pieces for your health. By this I mean recovery from chronic illness or preventing chronic illness. First, you completely control the inputs. Hence, you can avoid chemical fertilizers, poisoned water, weed and insecticide sprays, glyphosate, heavy metals, and even road dust. Road dust can be high in cadmium and even arsenic if you live within a twenty-five-mile radius of a coal-fired power plant.

Second, you can choose what to grow. These days, that can be a wonderful adventure with a seed catalogue or a visit to an honest nursery. You are best to avoid large chain stores with tomato plants: your purchase may not be fully mature or have had some unmentionable spray or nutrient in its short life. Such places are driven primarily by profit. This is what has turned wise people away from mega-supermarkets in the first place.

Third, you get enjoyment from the process. Watching something grow is a magical experience for almost any human being. Similarly, harvest or plant death is part of the lifecycle. All of us need to appreciate and accept the lifecycle. Those around children know there is no better learning venue than the lifecycle, whether it be planting a seed and watching it grow or incubating an egg and watching it hatch. What a gift to watch and/or teach a child to do this.

Fourth, inputs and costs are minimal; you can control your personal venture. A good example of this is "square foot" gardening, a method developed by Mel Bartholomew. For the metric people among us, this is "30 cm square" gardening. In his book, Squa*re Foot Gardening: A New Way to Garden in Less Space with Less Work* (1981), he shows that a four-by-eight-foot area (120 x 240 cm) can produce enough vegetables for a family of four for the entire growing season. Perhaps the best way to start this is to construct a 6 inch (15 cm) high wooden frame that is four by four feet (120 x 120 cm). This so-called raised bed permits you to add soil, whether you are growing on hard clay or even concrete. This raised bed permits an 80 percent reduction in the space required for row gardening. Also, it uses up to 90 percent less water. If you want to put this raised bed overtop of grass, I suggest you put down several layers of newspaper first. Fortunately, newspapers today are printed with canola oil ink. Also, almost all newsprint is whitened with ozone rather than chlorine bleach. It is best to water this raised bed with sun-warmed water that has sat out at least overnight to allow the chlorine to gas off and protect the plants. It is best to situate this raised bed in a part of your yard that gets at least six hours of sunshine in midsummer. Your summer will vary depending on whether you are in the northern or southern hemisphere. I mention this in deference to my good friend, Don Parker, in Melbourne, Australia. Aussies hate being forgotten, and I don't blame them. Remember, our summer is their winter and vice versa.

The fifth feature is the benefit of handling and even eating soil. Include some root crops, such as beet or beetroot, carrots, potatoes, onions, sweet potatoes, and leeks. We know how important healthy soil is for plants and for us. Some of the bacteria in soil are especially healthy for our own gut microbiota. Therefore, it's okay to get covered in a little soil or even eat some soil. I suggest you do some of your gardening with your bare hands. This is true whether you are a small child or even honouring the child within you. So, pull out the occasional carrot, shake off the dirt, and eat it. The benefits are many. The soil itself is nutritious, and the vitamins are optimal, as they are not depleted by storage or cooking. Also, you will learn to eat "ugly" vegetables. These are the less-than-perfect, non-symmetrical ones, such as a carrot with one long and one shorter tip. I assure you that farmers or farm workers always eat these first, because they are less marketable. If you buy this type of vegetable, you can often purchase more for less money. Ugly or wonky vegetables have become incredibly popular in the UK recently as they sell for less than premium price. Certainly, ugly or wonky vegetables are equally healthy for you and also helps you confirm it is real. Some of our tomatoes that are bred for long travel and storage no longer taste real or have the same optimal nutrients.

Sixth, grow some heritage or heirloom seeds for variety. Frequently, these taste better. A further benefit is that you can save seed from them, and it will grow true to form next time as well. You also have the advantage over market gardeners in that you can pick and eat your products when they are at their peak. One helpful hint: if you do not know where to get some of the seed for things like garlic or potatoes, then buy certified organic produce at your grocery store and use them. Then you can be assured that these seeds, bulbs, or tubers have not been irradiated or treated to minimize or eliminate sprouting. This is all done in the name of profit, not health. We have purchased certified organic produce for sweet potatoes, turmeric, and ginger to grow in experiments for ourselves.

To determine how much sun you have in the location you have chosen, simply keep track of how long the sun hits the ground or surface between the hours of 10:00 a.m. and 6:00 p.m. on a midsummer day. If you have light shade, which is two to three hours of the above timeframe without sun, then you can grow root vegetables, such as turnips, radishes, carrots, and beets. If you have partial shade, which is four to five hours without direct sun within that eight-hour window, you can still grow leafy vegetables such as arugula, radicchio, kale, spinach, mustard greens, chard, and scallions. If your climate permits, or you are gardening indoors, then you can readily do two plantings per year. A further suggestion is not to plant vegetables that grow to a large size near smaller vegetables. This is a practical way to avoid the smaller plants being overshadowed by the larger ones.

If you have a balcony, and you have your apartment super-visor's or condo strata's approval, then this is a wonderful place to grow food. By combining PVC pipe and putting plastic sheeting over it, you can develop a small greenhouse. An even smaller greenhouse involves taking a 2–4 Litre pop or milk bottle and cutting it 15 cm from the bottom. You should also make tiny holes in the bottom for drainage and then put in 10 cm of soil. Once the seeds are planted, replace the lid you created and tape it on. Now you have a miniature greenhouse, but remember to use a thermometer so the heat inside it is no more than 25°C (80°F). If the temperature rises above this, you must either take off the lid or move it to a cooler place, or you will cook your plants. An even simpler variation is to use a small pot and put four short bamboo sticks around it and invert a small clear plastic bag over it and secure it with an elastic or tape. Once again, ensure it does not get overheated. Another option is using a discarded aquarium or ice chest or even an inexpensive storage container. These can have soil inside them, and the above principles apply. It is a good idea before you put the soil in the old aquarium to put 2 in (5 cm) of small pumice stone or non-toxic peanut foam under the soil. This will help drainage.

You may be uncertain as to what to use for soil. I suggest the simple formula developed by inventor Mel Bartholomew, which is a combination of one third peat moss, one third weed-free compost, and one third vermiculite. Alternatively, you can use one half peat moss and one half compost. Over the growing season, if you can, refresh the top of the soil with compost three to six times. If you are planting in one of the four-by-four-foot squares, once you have placed the soil, put a grid over the soil with squares that are 1 inch by 1 inch (2.5 by 2.5 cm). Within each grid, you will plant seeds. If the par-ticular plant requires 30 cm spacing, you will be putting one in each square. If it requires 15 cm spacing, you will have four per square. If the plant is best at 10 cm spacing, then you will have nine per square. Finally, if it is best with a 5-cm spacing, then you would have 16 in each designated square. Another helpful hint is to plant root crops beside root crops and water almost daily. Deeply rooted plants, such as tomatoes and squash, may need water only once or twice a week. If you are ready to get more sophisticated, you can use drip irrigation and even a timer. However, if you simply have a small limited garden, I suggest you do almost everything by hand.

If you have space and access to a shelf, whether it is metal or plastic, you can put containers of plants on the shelves and then cover it with clear plastic, which is taped on. In Canada, we often talk about the value of duct tape, and it is incredible what it can help you to do.

A final comment is how deep to plant your seeds. A good suggestion is to plant the seed at a depth of one or two or at most three seeds' thickness. In his first attempt at gardening, a friend of mine planted his seeds 15–20 cm deep. Not surprisingly, nothing grew.

If space is a concern, then simplify and be creative. Put in some houseplants that may not be edible. These alone will detoxify the environment in your flat, condo, or house. This is well stated by psychiatrist Dr. Kelly Brogan in her recent and fabulous book, *A Mind of Your Own* (Brogan 2017), in which she says, "Keep as many plants in your home as possible, as they naturally detoxify the environment. Spider plants, aloe vera, chrysanthemums, Gerbera daisies, Boston ferns, English ivies, and philodendrons are good choices." She suggests eight to ten per 1,000 square feet of floor space. Some of these can be on the ceiling or around windows. No windows? Get a full-spectrum light bulb, as it is healthier for you too.

Now you know at least enough to have fun and get started. Everyone learns from his or her mistakes. In fact, it is difficult to progress within gardening without making multiple and repeated mistakes. Just when you think you have it all figured out, usually a few parameters, such as the weather, change. Gardening is not only humbling it is also very healthful! If you become totally enthused, then look at Eliot Coleman's book, *Four-Season Harvest* (Coleman 1999).

Section Three
Anatomy and Physiology

9: Circulation – Arteries, Veins, CCSVI, and Lymph

The topic of circulation in the body may seem like old news. Fortunately, many of the concepts that we have learned over the last forty years regarding cardiovascular health can now be applied to the brain. There is one major difference in that the brain requires a huge amount of oxygen to function optimally. Although the brain is only 2-3 percent of the body mass, it requires more than 20 percent of the oxygen the heart delivers. The primary job of the circulation system is to deliver oxygen and energy, in the form of glucose and free fatty acids, and to remove the waste products of metabolism. The brain's high requirements for energy result in its high density of blood vessels within its microcirculation, 5-100 microns (100 microns = 0.1 mm).

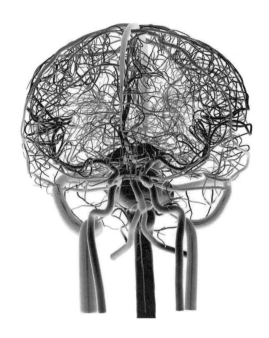

Metabolism is the combining of oxygen with glucose or free fatty acids within the mitochondria to make energy packets in the form of ATP (adenosine triphosphate). If enough oxygen is available, the major by-product is carbon dioxide. If there is not enough oxygen, then lactic acid is produced (just like after major muscle use). If this metabolism process is occurring optimally in the neurons, they function effectively, and we can see well and think clearly. However, as mentioned, if these same neurons have inadequate energy to function optimally but enough to stay alive, then we call them "idling neurons." Two factors determine if cells make enough energy: 1) blood flow and 2) the amount of oxygen dissolved in the blood when it reaches the tissues. This chapter discusses the factors involved in blood flow. The topic of oxygen and hypoxia (lack of oxygen) will be reviewed in a different chapter.

Blood flow to the brain or any other part of the body is equal to blood pressure divided by the resistance. If stated correctly, this is called Ohm's law (V=IR, or I= V/R, where I=amps or flow, V=volts or pressure, and R=resistance). In our youth, our blood vessels are usually flexible and elastic. As we age, with the ever-increasing atherosclerosis (hardening of the arteries and veins), they become much stiffer. This increased resistance must be overcome by increased pressure to maintain the same flow. The brain definitely requires the same flow, so blood pressure rises. It may seem a mystery to you why we treat blood pressure as aggressively in an eighty- or ninety-year-old person as we do in a sixty-year-old person. It mystifies me as well. I believe we must have some flexibility and compensation for this, or we make our elderly people less able to think, balance, and walk.

Hence, as we age, the body can compensate to some degree for the narrow pipes. Where is the narrowing of blood vessels most dramatic secondary to atherosclerosis? This commonly occurs where the carotid blood vessel in the neck splits or bifurcates into the internal and external carotid. This narrowing frequently occurs in a place of flow turbulence. Whenever a tube splits into two, turbulence occurs at the site where flow changes from laminar flow, or optimal, to turbulent and more chaotic flow. Here also is where atherosclerosis or wall-thickening plaque build-up and injured blood vessels occur.

We know this atherosclerosis can be reversed with sufficient and persistent change of diet and lifestyle (Ornish 1990). Avoidance of trans fats should be a priority. In fact, if diet and lifestyle are not altered, then almost all angioplasty and/or vein bypass grafts, as in coronary artery bypass grafting, are occluded within six to twelve months. This has been well documented for the last thirty or more years and occurs whether you have one, two, or seven different bypass grafts. This same blockage occurs in cardiac stents. So, while you may buy some time with the assistance of your cardiologist or cardiovascular surgeon, it is up to you what happens thereafter. Furthermore, your microbiome health matters, too. A recent paper by Menni et al. "Gut microbial diversity is associated with lower arterial stiffness in women" (Menni 2018). Therefore, more microbiome diversity literally slows "hardening of the arteries" or atherosclerosis. I am suggesting by increasing your food diversity you increase your microbiome diversity which can improve your blood vessel health. This may slow and even reverse your atherosclerosis.

This same example of cardiac health is repeated abundantly within the brain. However, in the brain, we are mostly unsuccessful at either bypasses or stents. Therefore, in brain health and recovery, the onus is on you, the individual, to reverse the narrowing blood vessels (Ornish 1990). The two methods for enhancing brain blood flow occur in the neck. First it is the surgery or stent placement within the carotid artery to prevent strokes. Second is venous balloon angioplasty of the jugular veins, which is almost always at the valve region. (I will talk more about my personal experience with this later.) Happily, all the diet and lifestyle changes that help reverse this vascular disease are also anti-inflammatory and, hence, to a great degree slow or even reverse the aging process. So, listen up!

So far, I have talked mostly about arteries. It will interest you that there are nine cases in the published literature where a confirmed diagnosis of MS was caused by abnormal arteries. Each of these were unusual and, therefore, documented and involved an abnormal vertebral artery anatomy. In each case, the path of the vertebral artery was through the neck muscles. Hence, certain activities and movements compromised blood flow. In turn, this compromised oxygen supply and caused neuron and oligodendrocyte injury. This led to the pathology of MS. I hope this discussion alone helps you understand chapter 20, "The New MS."

If you review Dr. Schelling's book about MS, *Multiple Sclerosis—The Image and its Message,* you will note that lack of oxygen to certain brain areas causes injury consistent with

MS. Hence, in many ways, MS is like a stroke or cerebrovascular accident. The above examples of vertebral artery abnormality are the closest examples of how MS is like a stroke. Dr. Schelling describes how venous blockage or "hypertension" can and does cause brain injury (Schelling 2018). If you look carefully at the stroke literature, you will find that approximately three percent of strokes occur due to a blockage to the venous system.

Drainage of the blood from the brain via the veins is also a key component of adequate brain oxygen and nutrient supply. You will understand this best if I use a traffic analogy. If you block the superhighway leaving a city (I choose leaving the city to mimic the blood leaving the brain through the venous system) from four to one or two lanes, you dramatically reduce traffic flow. This occurs even if all the smaller highways parallel to the superhighway are open. The traffic is hugely delayed until the superhighway is restored. I'm suggesting that the same occurs when there is relative blockage of the superhighway of venous drainage from the brain. This blockage occurs primarily in the internal jugular veins but also to some degree in the azygos and vertebral venous system.

The above traffic analogy is certainly mimicked in the body's response to a partially or completely blocked jugular vein. The body develops collaterals, alternate pathways, that are never as big and, even though there are a number of them, never achieve the same rate of flow. Poiseuille's Law is a scientific description of the above highway analogy. It states that the flow through a tube is related to the fourth power of the radius. This means if you reduce the radius of a tube by half, you reduce the flow to one sixteenth. So, if your neurologist says the collaterals do the same job, I suggest he or she does not understand Poiseuille's Law.

The venous system cannot increase the flow by increasing the pressure, because it is downstream to the extremely low resistance area of the capillaries. Instead, the fresh blood from the heart tends to bypass the regions of the brain that have a relative obstruction of the outflow component. In my traffic analogy, the drivers of the cars know about the relative accident ahead, so they take an alternate or collateral route. Our arterial blood flow does the same thing, so the newly oxygenated blood bypasses the regions drained by the veins that are relatively blocked. In a nutshell, this describes CCSVI (chronic cerebrospinal venous insufficiency) and why these people's brains do not function as well. The same brain regions are more hypoxic until the relative obstruction is relieved by balloon venous angioplasty.

The most common restriction of venous brain drainage is the valve in the internal jugular vein. Yes, just as your leg veins have valves, so do your jugular veins. This is a common area of turbulent flow. Turbulent flow begets vessel injury (i.e., atherosclerosis), and this worsens over time. A few of us have a small variation in the internal jugular vein valve, even from birth. The medical term for this is "congenital." Over time, this abnormality can worsen, further obstructing flow. The jugular vein valve is usually just above where the internal jugular vein joins the brachiocephalic vein. This term "brachiocephalic" denotes the flow to the arm (brachio) and the head (cephalic). If you look at the vein from surface anatomy, it is just above the level of the sixth and seventh vertebra or just above the collarbone or clavicle.

There is a superb clinical example of hypertension of the veins and subsequent injury to the jugular vein valves in kidney failure patients once they have an arteriovenous shunt placed in their wrist vessels to facilitate dialysis. Subsequent to this, they require a venous balloon angioplasty of their jugular vein valves two to four times a year to maintain optimal brain function. It is unfortunate that many specialties within medicine do not talk to each other about clinical parallels of patients.

If the interventional radiologists or vascular surgeons spoke with the neurologist about this, then perhaps the neurologist would be less mystified with the concept of CCSVI.

I would now like to tell you of a clinical example of a woman with MS in Canada who had her partially blocked jugular vein valves treated within the Medicare system. The woman was in a severe car accident and spent time in a coma. She proceeded to have kidney failure in the intensive care unit. Next, she had an arteriovenous shunt placed in her wrist. The vascular surgeon noted she already had some blockage at her jugular vein valves. He did the standard procedure of balloon venous angioplasty on her jugular vein valves. When she woke up from her coma, she was delighted that her MS was considerably better. Usually, the stress of the accident and time in hospital would have worsened her MS. She related her story to others with MS in Canada on social media. Therefore, I suggest she is the first and only individual with MS to have her treatment paid for by the Medicare system in Canada.

We still have this major roadblock in Canada of people with MS being denied venous angioplasty. In fact, I have several friends who have been refused consultation by a vascular surgeon, even though they had a consult request from a family doctor, because they have MS. One vascular surgeon stated that MS patients must have a consult instead from an MS neurologist. I suggest this is simply a power game on behalf of the neurologists, and I find it irritating and unfair. I have a dream that one day MS patients will be treated the same as everyone else. I suspect this will not happen until the current generation of neurologists leave medical practice. In the meantime, MS patients will have to leave Canada for this balloon venous angioplasty if they have these partially blocked jugular vein valves. These patients now have an additional option of home oxygen. You can read more about this in chapters 30 and 31.

In October 2015, I was lucky enough to spend four days in Austria with Dr. Franz Schelling. For more than thirty years, he has studied anatomy and the literature on brain diseases and their causes. This journey, long and arduous, even cost him his career as a medical doctor. This is despite confirmation of his concepts in the standard medical literature. He wrote about his findings and published his book online (2018). This book is a detailed discussion about MS. This chapter is for those who can, and want to, understand in detail the true pathology and physiology of MS. I have outlined my understanding of his work in an effort to help you understand how your own brain health can be impacted.

Dr. Schelling is something of a modern-day Sherlock Holmes. I like detective mysteries and Sherlock Holmes, so that spurs me on in understanding the early findings about the pathology of MS. The first recorded pertinent information was Dr. Robert Carswell's testimony in 1830 (see www. ms-info.net) about two different cases of the same unknown kind of lesion. This discovery became public a few years later as Carswell became chair of pathological anatomy in London. These lesions were described "as a peculiar diseased state" with a special form of scarring (think sclerosis, as this is what it means). In his plain drawings, he drew these pathological changes so clearly, they could hardly be mistaken for anything else. He noted "points" punched in the pons of the brain. However, he focused especially on "patches" in the spinal cord. His entire picture is of major significance and first held the key to understanding the process of spinal MS.

Then, from 1839 to 1841, leading Parisian pathologist Jean Cruveilhier drew two new spinal cord specimens from his patient's autopsy. These two were marked by scars unmistakably identical to Robert Carswell's "patches." Cruveilhier's drawings showed how these lesions lined up preferentially along the spinal cord's posterior midline.

In 1865, Dr. J.M. Charcot, described as the father of neurology, drew another such specimen while working as a pathologist in Paris. Admittedly, he included it only as a footnote. This footnote seems to constitute the sole historical advance. This original anatomically substantiated understanding of spinal MS showed how the lesions were along both sides of the spinal column. He made this intuitive leap when he combined his observations with those of Carswell's and Cruveilhier's identical findings. Now, 150 years later, there has been no substantial advance in the gross characterization of the spinal "patches" of MS. Only now, with advanced magnetic resonance imaging (MRI), are we able to diagnose and describe these MS lesions in the spinal cord with live patients as opposed to post mortem.

Detection of distinctive brain lesions is also possible with MRI. However, in early pathology, one of Carswell's and both of Cruveilhier's archetypal MS specimens also had lesions in the pons region of the brain. Both pathologists felt these were related pathologically to the spinal lesions. Then, in 1867, in a thirty-five-year-old victim of MS, Charcot also found both spinal cord and brain lesions. This is well described in Dr. Schelling's quote, "truly revolutionary, however, was Charcot's masterly depiction of the lesion quite simply described as a sclerotic plaque affecting the wall of a lateral ventricle elsewhere characterized as grey sclerotic plaque like scars, in the walls of the ventricles, to a thickness of 1 cm. The lesion embeds prominent veins, coursing within distinct, eccentrically widened perivascular spaces" (Schelling 2018). What this means is that even Charcot, in the earliest days of understanding MS, noted that these scars were always formed around veins and that this area was usually around the ventricles of the brain. Hence, Charcot had it correct in the beginning, but this was lost over time and had to be rediscovered.

Charcot's contributions may well be his most momentous achievement, perhaps missed by many until now, because these key illustrations were part of the thesis of his little-known pupil, Leopold Ordenstein. Ordenstein, however, focused mostly on living patients with MS. Hence, Charcot's important pathology contribution has been missed until recently.

The next contribution in describing this brain injury came from Dr. J.W. Dawson, pathologist. In 1916, Dawson wrote, "in the extensive areas of sclerosis immediately contiguous with the brain's ventricles, some large collecting veins running immediately underneath the ventricular lining, so-called subependymal, are directly outlined by zones of gelatinous tissue. The involved vein walls appear to be partly homogenized, blocking their normal structural differentiation, and are encompassed by distinctly widened perivenous spaces in which residues minor hemorrhages are to be found" (Schelling 2018). This is the first mention of minor hemorrhages or small bleeds in MS in the brain. I now appreciate how important this is due to David Utriainen's talk at the 2016 ISNVD meeting in New York. Studies by Utriainen and Haacke have shown that tiny microbleeds can trigger major inflammation in the brain consistent with the pathology of MS. At least 14 percent of MS patients have had these microbleeds. Similarly, microbleeds occur in concussion/traumatic brain injury (Zivadinov et al. 2016).

In 1937, Tracey J. Putnam, an American neurologist, and Alexandra Adler, an Austrian neurologist, illustrated for the first time "that cerebral plaques characteristically spread in a rather odd, specific relationship to large epi-ventricular veins and, further, to bizarrely altered affluents of these vessels" (Schelling 2018). Their drawing of lesions from the patient demonstrates a ventricle-based cone-shaped lesion, otherwise known as a Dawson finger, as per Dawson above.

In 1965, Torben Fog, a Danish neurologist, found that distinctive MS plaques were almost always around vein segments, i.e., perivenular. In 1970, an American, Charles E. Lumsden, observed that MS-specific plaques in the brain stem consistently originate in veins. Then, the results of Colin W. Adams effectively confirmed that, "the early stage of periventricular plaque is the formation of the lesion around a subependymal vein" (Schelling 2018). These veins, separate from arteries, run underneath the cerebral ventricular lining. Even though MS lesions appear to arise on the edges of the cerebrospinal fluid-filled ventricles, this fluid-filled area does not play any direct role in their formation. Instead, it is these critical veins, as they are at the end of the longest distance from the heart. Therefore, their flow and dissolved oxygen concentration is the lowest. This is incredibly important in the start of MS.

There, we have the story in a nutshell! That is, for 150 years, we have recognized that the lesions or brain scars of MS surround veins in the areas around the cerebrospinal fluid-filled ventricles. This is the part of the brain that neurologists search for typical MS lesions or UBOs (unidentified bright objects) when they look at MRIs. Until MRIs came along in the 1970s, we could only look at the brains of dead people with pathology. Happily, MRI has solved this problem. Also, I have learned from MRI experts that we should ideally take more pictures in the quiet four to five minutes after injecting the contrast gadolinium. This permits us to see the arterial brain flow and then the venous blood flow. Unfortunately, this is rarely done. Well-documented protocols for this are described by Dr. M. Haacke of Wayne State University (Haacke 2012).

This "additional free" information is rarely ordered for a patient known to have MS or suspected to have MS. Instead, neurologists do not request it and tend to concentrate on only the T2 information for UBOs, or, to MS patients, "white spots." These, too, are lesions that form around small veins, just as Charcot, Dawson, and Putnam (see below) described from pathology investigations. What I am suggesting is that when these patients have an MRI, the study should include data collection of the arterial blood supply and the venous blood draining the brain. This timing component is possible when the patient has a pulse oximeter device on his or her finger. This times photos of MRI with the pulse, permitting blood-flow calculation. Then we can better understand an individual's anatomy and flow or physiology of the circulation. This is probably one of the significant components in the onset and progress of MS.

Now that I have attempted to describe some of the mysteries about how MS lesions form, I would like to summarize some of the important things that happen at the microscopic level. The medical term for this is histology. Early descriptions of MS lesions in the spinal cord were very accurate, in that they talked about dense fibre-filled lesions. We now understand that when astrocyte cells sustain an injury (probably hypoxia), they frequently create many small fibrils (think pieces of string) within. Once these multiple fibrils are formed nearby each other, they frequently contract together, forming a tightened web that we visualize as a scar. When these early changes are occurring in astrocytes and neurons, only minimal lymphocytes and immune cells are present. In fact, there are no more lymphocytes or other immune cells present in a new MS lesion than there are in a new stroke. Neurologists do not use autoimmune drugs in stroke treatment. Why do they use them in the treatment of MS? I firmly believe they need to re-examine the history and information from pathology and MRI scans when planning therapy.

In the foregoing paragraphs, I have attempted to describe the gross pathology and histology of MS lesions. These lesions, easiest seen in the brain, occur around a vein centre. My hope is that this allows us to talk about the features that create this venous injury in the first place. This is an important consideration, because these lesions are one of the major features within MS. Similarly, it is also a significant feature in the cause of Parkinson's disease and early Alzheimer's. I am not suggesting that all these diseases are caused by vein problems, but many of them are initiated at least in part by this venous problem. Certainly, each has a vascular component that precipitates the development of the disease.

Now that we have reviewed some of the history, let us begin with venous injury from another perspective. This perspective is that of Dr. Paolo Zamboni of Ferrara, Italy. He researched venous injury in varicose veins and stasis of the veins in the legs for most of his career as a vascular surgeon. In addition, his wife was diagnosed with MS, and he began to wonder if he could help her. Dr. Zamboni was an expert on ultrasound, so he applied this expertise to the veins of the head and neck. In particular, he focused on the internal jugular veins, vertebral veins, and those veins observable within the brain with ultrasound.

Dr. Zamboni went on to describe five factors that were additive in the potential diagnosis of significant venous drainage from the brain. At the time, he coined the term chronic cerebrospinal venous insufficiency (CCSVI). Then he published a paper in which he compared MS venous drainage from the brain with that of normal controls. He admitted this was not a prospective trial but only a pilot study. In the pilot study, he and his neurologist colleague documented the status of the MS patients before and after they underwent venous balloon angioplasty. Many of the patients, including his wife, clinically improved. Fairly frequently, approximately one third had symptoms relapse. If venous angioplasty was repeated, it was found that almost all of them had restenosed.

In reality, this is close to the restenosis rate seen in arterial and venous angioplasty—something we do daily in cardiology artery intervention and wrist arterio-venous shunts in patients with kidney failure. In the latter, this is in treating the venous narrowings secondary to the venous hypertension caused by the arterio-venous shunt. These patients require treatment of these venous narrowings, including the internal jugular vein valves, three to four times a year. Unfortunately, this regular treatment of venous problems in renal failure patients is virtually unknown to many physicians, including neurologists. It is these differences in knowledge base between different specialties within medicine that has created much of the pain and angst that has occurred since 2009 with respect to CCSVI.

When the CCSVI story was told in documentary fashion on a Canadian television network in November 2009, it was like an explosion among Canadian MS patients. Even though Dr. Zamboni admitted that more research was required, many patients throughout Canada acted on this new sliver of hope.

On a personal note, I initially had my internal jugular veins checked with my stroke neurologist friend. He had his top ultrasound technician check my veins for stenosis. This was done only in the supine (lying flat) position, as that was the routine for looking at the common and internal carotid arteries. Ultrasound of the carotid arteries is a critical examination when evaluating someone for stroke risk, because approximately 60 percent of strokes originate from this area. However, even though this was a very experienced carotid artery ultrasound technician, I believe it was her first evaluation of jugular veins. This is very important for anyone having the neck veins evaluated with ultrasound. First, the person doing ultrasound needs to be well trained in the specific area of assessing jugular veins. If this is not the case, it is quite easy for him or her to call a variation of anatomy a normal jugular vein.

Second, as well described by Dr. Zamboni, this jugular vein examination must occur in both supine and sitting positions.

Classically, the flow in the jugular veins is much better in the supine position. Meanwhile, when you sit up, the jugular veins should almost be collapsed, as the majority of flow should occur through the vertebral veins into the azygos vein. A later study of my jugular veins indicated that I was virtually the same in both positions, which is a distinct abnormality.

I do not fault the first technician, as she was extremely good at what she was trained to do. However, an ideal future possibility would be that patients examined for their carotid artery could also have an examination of their jugular veins. This would require minimal additional training and then would be performed by the group with the most expertise in ultrasound of the neck blood vessels. It would require including the sitting position. An important side note is that optimal neck ultrasound is very observer-dependent; hence, it requires someone with good training, time, and patience. Also, one cannot evaluate the azygos vein with ultrasound, because it lies between the heart and the front of the vertebral column.

Stroke prevention and treatment following a stroke often involves interventional radiology of the carotid artery. An angioplasty of the carotid artery is a high-risk procedure due to the risk of any displaced plaques or clots causing another stroke. I believe this is one reason neurologists are so anxious about interventional radiology treatment for CCSVI. This is not difficult to understand if one recognizes the major challenges that occur when we get a stroke or loss of blood supply to a region of the brain. Recovery from a stroke can vary dramatically. We know it is critical to prevent the next stroke.

In contrast to this, interventional radiologists recognize that angioplasty of veins is a relatively safe procedure, because it deals with a low-pressure system. In addition, plaque hardly ever occurs in the venous system, and if a blood clot should occur, it travels to the heart and is pumped to the lungs. In the lungs, small blood clots are filtered and dealt with routinely and create no major troubles. Once again neurologists have described blood clots to the lungs as a devastating and potentially lethal outcome of CCSVI angioplasty. However, the risk of serious blood clots to the lungs is almost completely due to large blood clots from the leg or pelvic veins. These are large enough to restrict or almost eliminate the heart function and so represent a large risk factor. The size of the blood clot generated from the jugular or azygos veins is relatively minimal and has little acute risk to stopping heart function. If one looks at the concerns of some neurologists, we realize their anxiety is somewhat misplaced. We must remember to compare apples to apples and oranges to oranges.

Following my evaluation with ultrasound of the neck in the supine position, I was assessed by a keen young MS neurologist. He described Dr. Zamboni's article as incomplete and poor-quality science. Unfortunately, he had not ventured into the research literature about similar discussions of restricted outflow of blood from the brain or excess iron deposition in the brain. In fact, I felt scolded by the exchange. I journeyed home with my tail between my legs! However, within a few months, I was asked to participate as a master of ceremonies at an information gathering of several hundred people suffering from MS and their families. Five people with MS who had the CCSVI procedure of ballooning by venous angioplasty were on the panel. Most of them had improved, some dramatically; this rekindled my interest in the concept. Subsequent to this, Sandra Birrell and Landon Schmidt began a society to enhance knowledge of this in the public domain. Later, this became the Canadian Neurovascular Health Society (www. CNHS.ca). I helped organize six of their annual conferences and spoke at eight of them.

Next, I travelled to a centre with expertise in looking at CCSVI in Buffalo, New York. On September 1, 2010, in Buffalo, I began my day with a 100-minute MRI. This was at least double the length of any previous six MRIs in Canada. Then I had the ultrasound of my neck that included the transcranial Doppler. This was performed in the Zamboni fashion, as the technician had been trained in Italy and was now training others, including Canadians. Hence, it was very thorough and was performed in the sitting and supine positions.

After the ultrasound, I had a two-hour session of neuropsychologic testing, as I was participating in an overall larger study. Needless to say, I was exhausted by then, as anyone who struggles with the fatigue of MS or other health challenges will understand. The next morning, I had a thorough interview, examination, and discussion with a superb MS neurologist, Dr. Weinstock Guttman. She went over the results of my ultrasound, MRI, MRV, and iron assessment of the brain. This included a pictogram of the iron map and iron data graph that demonstrated how multiple sclerosis patients have more iron than average. I had more than the expected brain iron, based on my age and my MS. That is not a good thing! Dr. Weinstock Guttman also reviewed my head and neck ultrasound with me. She described I had four of five of Dr. Zamboni's criteria.

Overall, it was the most complete evaluation I've had by any MS neurologist since my diagnosis in 1996 by Dr. Donald Paty at the University of British Columbia. Before leaving Buffalo that afternoon, I was fortunate to meet with Dr. Zivadinov and discuss his ideas about neuroimaging and many of the features of ultrasound diagnosis and CCSVI.

Denise and I had already committed to a three-week Rotary friendship exchange to Melbourne, Australia, and the state of Victoria in October. Therefore, I contacted two people in Australia, one with MS and the other a long-time family friend. I had hoped I might be able to set up an angioplasty there, but this did not happen. However, I met with Kerri Cassidy of CCSVI Australia. Through her suggestion, I was able to meet two of the key players in venous angioplasty research in Australia. These are Ken Thomson, MD, and Helen Kavnoudias, PhD, of the Alfred Hospital, Melbourne, Australia. These relationships have been inspirational continue to the present day.

Later in the fall of 2010, I was invited to speak at a seminar on CCSVI in Vancouver. Dr. Joseph Hewett, an interventional radiologist from California, was also going to speak. I did some further research on this group of interventional radiologists, Drs. Hewett and Arata, and felt confident in selecting them for my own procedure.

I was very impressed with Dr. Hewett's talk as he spoke about handling standard cases and problem cases, including misplaced or clotted stents and incomplete treatments.

Finally, he outlined three symptomology areas that respond especially well to angioplasty of CCSVI. These include fatigue, headaches (especially upon waking), and sleep disturbances. I had all three and realized that if even one improved, it would be worth the treatment. My procedure was booked for November 29, 2010.

On November 28, I had my consultation at 8:30 with Dr. Michael Arata. I liked him immediately. He explained things thoroughly and was patient with our questions. I learned more about his approach to angioplasty for CCSVI, which includes valvuloplasty (expansion of the jugular vein valves) as well as close assessment and similar balloon angioplasty of the azygos vein. Dr Arata mentioned stents and stated these were best avoided in the jugular veins. My family and close friends encouraged me to have the procedure but to avoid stents. My personal attitude was that I needed to trust the person doing the procedure and listen to their best advice. I believe this is a piece of angioplasty for CCSVI that has gradually changed over the last eight years. If one needs a stent, then it should be as large as possible and is better tolerated in the azygos vein or the left renal vein.

I was impressed and pleased with my preoperative, operative, and postoperative care at the facility. I was unable to watch the procedure and do not remember the angioplasty of my jugular veins, but I could feel the work inside the azygos vein. In summary, all three veins were treated. I noted an immediate reduction of pressure inside my head on the operating room table. This impressed me. In addition, I appreciated the intravenous sedation with fentanyl and midazolam, two of my old friends from anesthesiology! I also received intravenous fluids, supplemental oxygen, and monitoring by ECG and pulse oximeter. It was modern care, and I appreciated this.

My postoperative course was reasonably uneventful. Perhaps one of the most important observations was Denise noting that my face and forehead were dramatically pinker immediately. A headache occurred the following morning with a similar outcome by two in the afternoon. However, since then I have had virtually no headaches for eight to ten months. This is critical, as I was previously experiencing four to five headaches per week. In addition, my sleep improved almost immediately, and this has continued for several years. Within a few days, I noted that the hesitancy and urgency problem with my bladder had all but disappeared. I felt I had a bladder closer to what I had thirty years earlier.

Since my procedure, I have continued on my anti-inflammatory diet and supplement regimen. During my integrative medicine training with Dr. Andrew Weil, I learned the anti-inflammatory diet is critical. If one gets the nutrition correct, the body heals quicker and with less scarring. This is just as important for a new scar inside a vein as it is for one on the skin surface. An injury on the skin reacts with inflammation, including redness, swelling, heat, and pain. The more fully the inflammation is controlled, the more the scar and the scar contraction are reduced. Reducing inflammation was critically important to prevent the scar forming inside my veins from contracting down. I believe optimal nutrition can decrease the likelihood of needing a future angioplasty.

My personal regimen includes at least 3,000 mg per day of combined EPA plus DHA from molecularly distilled fish oil. I do not use cod liver oil or halibut liver oil, because this might provide excess vitamin A. In addition, I recommend 10,000 IU of vitamin D3 per day for a month prior to angioplasty and for at least three months thereafter. We know vitamin D is important in blood vessel health and is anti-inflammatory at or above 2,000 IU per day. In addition, it is safe to take 10,000 IU per day for six months. This is intuitively correct, as even modest sun exposure during the summer can produce at least 10,000 IU on our skin daily.

I used to take 40-60 g per day of quality micro-filtered whey protein isolate prepared at low temperature. I did this in two doses and usually included two tablespoons of ground brown flax. Ground flax is a valuable omega-3 source as well as a soluble and non-soluble fibre. I have been on this regimen for the last ten years and believe it has contributed to holding the ravages of MS at bay.

For anyone who has been relatively immobile, the extra vitamin D helps muscle strength and balance. In addition, whey protein is a valuable resource in rebuilding muscle strength and muscle recovery. Whey protein is high in bio-active cystine, which assists in wound healing. Quality whey protein isolates are recognized to raise intracellular glutathione (our master antioxidant) throughout the body and may assist in removing excess iron from the brain (Bounous 1988).

I continued to learn about chronic cerebrospinal venous insufficiency. I believe it is related to improper circulation, perfusion of the brain, and oxygen for the brain (Petrov et al. 2016). CCSVI may be a unifying factor in hydrocephalus, spina bifida, Chiari malformation, syringomyelia, and transient global ischemia. These factors may play a part in leukoaraiosis (LA), which is white matter lesions in the brains of the elderly with cognitive problems.

Another mystery to me is why nearly all my lower-back pain disappeared after my angioplasty. We know there is a major circulation connection with the azygos and hemiazygos veins that include the lumbar sacral plexus. Once again, it may all be about circulation.

Another important feature that bears mention is the excess iron in the brain of MS, Parkinson's, Alzheimer's, and stroke patients. Does this iron reduce in the brain after angioplasty? Alternatively, is it necessary to assist the removal through some chelation? I know that Dr. Mark Haacke is especially interested in this area and has developed a way to consistently measure and follow iron levels. I believe we may be on the verge of another set of treatment modalities for several cerebrospinal diseases.

In short, I believe CCSVI is the "real deal" and is a part of the critical puzzle for the signs and symptoms of MS. Historically, coronary artery bypass grafting and coronary angioplasty were developed for symptomatic relief of chest pain. Why not angioplasty CCSVI for relief of fatigue, headaches, neuropathic pain, sleep disturbance, muscle spasm, and balance problems in MS?

On November 29, 2017, I celebrated my seven-year anniversary of the above procedure. In the seven years since my first venous angioplasty, I have retained several benefits. I still have reduced cognitive impairment, less brain fog, although I am not as good as the first eight to ten months post procedure. My bladder symptoms improved but have again worsened. A urologist's assessment and cystoscopy at age sixty-four revealed this is primarily my MS. My rectal sphincter has continued to be more normal since the procedure. I've now completely lost my fear of pending rectal incontinence. Fatigue is still an issue, albeit somewhat better than before the venous angioplasty. Of note, my voice is still stronger but perhaps not as good as in 2011. My sleep quality improved dramatically for several months only. My headaches through the night and during the day dramatically reduced but have returned more often than I would like. In summary, I believe venous balloon angioplasty helped me. In addition, I have seen dramatic and sometimes lasting results in other MS people. However, I do not believe angioplasty is a panacea but rather a useful piece of the puzzle in understanding brain illnesses, including MS.

In my first CCSVI intervention, evaluating and treating left renal vein stenosis was not considered. In addition, my understanding of endothelial injury and healing had greatly advanced in those seven years. I felt several adjunctive (HBOT, GFT and PBMT as per later in this book) interventions post angioplasty would reduce my risk of recurrence after a second intervention. Finally, Dr. Sclafani is an expert at Intravascular Ultrasound (IVUS), which assists in venous assessment and treatment. IVUS was not included in my original CCSVI treatment in 2010, as it was in its relative infancy.

Denise and I flew to New York and I had my meticulous clinical assessment with Dr. Sclafani in November 2017. I underwent balloon angioplasty of both jugular veins and my azygos vein. Dr. Sclafani's IVUS assessment of my left renal vein revealed only a 25 percent stenosis, so a stent was not recommended. The following night, I experienced multiple benefits. Firstly, my bladder function was much improved with reduced urgency and frequency of urination. My energy and cognitive skills both improved several notches. Finally, my headache frequency and severity was reduced. My own efforts toward optimizing healing post-op included cancelling a speaking tour in Europe two weeks later. In addition, for a month, I did almost daily hyperbaric oxygen therapy, nightly oxygen therapy, and PBMT of my head and neck. In

March 2016 I had done GFT at Taymount UK. I believe this regimen, coupled with decreased stress and more rest, has helped my endothelium heal more optimally. I am glad I had the second procedure.

CCSVI and ISNVD, Italy 2011

Following my initial venous angioplasty treatment in November 2010, I decided to attend the first International Society of Neurovascular Disease (ISNVD) conference in Bologna, Italy, in March 2011. There I learned that vascular venous injury was even bigger than MS. Venous injury can be a part of MS, ALS, temporary global amnesia, traumatic brain injury (TBI), Parkinson's, and even Alzheimer's. In addition, we have models or examples of venous injury outside the brain. These include varicose veins and ulcers of the legs, May-Thurber and Nutcracker syndrome on the left leg and left kidney, respectively, female pelvic pain, and in men, hydrocele of the scrotum. Obviously, healthy venous drainage matters and is often treatable with balloon venoplasty and sometimes stents. It is worth noting that it is probably wisest not to use stents in the internal jugular veins. This is an issue of posture change resulting in minimal or no flow through the veins. The consequence of this is frequent clotting within those stents.

The brain and neck in humans adds some extra challenges to angioplasty of the venous system. First, some parts of vessels are surrounded by bone and, therefore, cannot be treated by catheter. Second, the internal jugular vein, ideally empty when we are upright, causes slow flow through an internal jugular vein stent with the risk of clotting and blockage. Third, the venous sinuses within the brain, which are formed by dura coverings, are not readily accessible or safely expandable in the brain by venous angioplasty.

The other major problem is that even if all venous flow problems are solved by surgery, we still have the problem of recurrence in approximately one third of people. Also, we still have some potential injury from venous reflux. This is compounded by venous atherosclerosis and venous hypertension injury. It is these two areas that we must dramatically address through diet and lifestyle. Coronary artery and carotid artery atherosclerosis is reversible with diet and lifestyle. Therefore, it follows that venous atherosclerosis should be as well. Hence, diet and lifestyle are a significant part of this book. I have also added other interventions, especially oxygen therapy, which should help us in the recovery and prevention of ongoing progression of our brain illnesses. I now consider oxygen therapy as an initial twenty to forty treatments and then an ongoing subsequent weekly treatment. This makes it an option for almost any brain illness that I am discussing within this book. If you're interested in reading further, *Oxygen and the Brain: The Journey of Our Lifetime* (James 2014) is an excellent place to start. An easier read may be available in late 2018 or 2019 as Professor James, Duncan Black and I are writing a book for the layperson on the new MS – Microvascular Syndrome.

Glymphatics: The Brain Lymph System

A final important detoxification method is the glymphatic system within the brain and spinal cord. Recent evidence from universities in the USA and Finland have confirmed that we have a lymphatic "drainage" or cleaning system within the brain and spinal cord (Xie 2013). This fluid link between the cerebrospinal fluid, the CSF system, and the lymphatic system is called the glymphatic system, which is a blend of the words "glial" and "lymphatic." Glial cells are also called astrocytes and are as numerous and important as neurons in brain support and function.

In descriptive terms, a flushing occurs with CSF along glial cells and in between brain cells. This flushing removes many of the by-products or "exhaust" of energy production by the brain cells' mitochondria. In addition, this "brainwashing" removes many toxins, such as heavy metals, artificial biologic toxins such as pesticides and herbicides, which, if not removed, further injure brain cells. We know this glymphatic brain wash, described earlier (Cook 2007), occurs best and almost completely during sleep. Therefore, be sure and read chapter 12 to learn how sleep can help optimize the glymphatic detoxification body function. Allow me to add that EMF (see Chapter 3) interferes with the glymphatic system as it interferes with optimal sleep.

10: The Microbiome: Linking Gut and Brain Health

Contributed by Dr. Teri Jaklin, ND

As a naturopathic doctor, the gastrointestinal system is central to the recovery and maintenance of human health. Often when I introduce this concept to patients, I get one of two responses—a blank stare or total agreement, punctuated with comments like "I have always had problems in my gut" or "I knew it! I just didn't know how to explain it!" The truth is, this understanding is not exclusive to naturopathic medicine. It is seen in many traditional medicine practices the world over. This almost intuitive historical understanding of the gut in health has been unraveling itself in the evidence base for decades. More recently, the explosion of scientific data, especially in the last decade, has put the human microbiome front and center in how we consider immunity, inflammation, changes in innate immunity (previously called autoimmunity), and ultimately the potential of the brain to heal and recover.

In 2008, the National Institutes of Health's Human Microbiome Project began to shine the scientific spotlight on how important the microbial environment of the gut is. The volume of research that followed makes it arguably the hottest topic in science and illuminates the significance of the micro-biome in human health. What may be most intriguing about the new science is how the brain affects the microbiome and how the microbiome, in turn, affects the brain in what has become known as the brain-gut (or gut-brain) axis.

You may be asking yourself, what exactly is the microbi-ome, and how does the gut affect the brain? At its core, the microbiome has a unique fingerprint, different layers of tissues with specific functions, that do not really change from day to day. It is populated by 100 trillion microbes, referred to as the microbiota, a dynamic part of the microbiome that can easily change within just twenty-four hours. Its structure and function can be influenced by what you eat and drink along with the state of your digestion, whether you were delivered via C-section at birth, your geographic location, emotional or physical stress, and medical practices, such as vaccination and antibiotic use. It is different depending on age, ethnicity, and possibly even gender, and can even be impacted based on your mood, what kind of a day you are having, or if you are jet lagged! If the microbiome is altered for more than five days, a proinflammatory environment is created in the gut. In fact, studies on EAE (experimental autoimmune encephalomyeli-tis), an experimental model of brain inflammation in mice, suggest these proinflammatory conditions in the gut result in the onset of "autoimmune diseases," among which is MS (Escribano 2014) in the traditional manner (see the New MS chapter 19).

Your microbiome contains an incredible number of genes responsible for everything from digestion and nutrient absorption to blood sugar balance, detoxification, and even the overall tone of the immune response. The microbiome pro-duces short-chain fatty acids, amino acids, neurotransmitters, and vitamins—building blocks for every essential function of the body. Its mucous membranes protect against pathogens, and the microbiome is central to the overall immune response, determining whether an immune response is tolerant or reactive, i.e., inflammatory in nature (Kranich 2011).

Centered in the gut, the microbial population of the microbiome reaches far and wide from the skin and sinuses through the urinary tract and even populates a woman's vagina. The intestines house several pounds of microbes, making it the most densely populated area of the microbiome. One gram of stool contains more microbes than there are stars in the sky! This is optimally the most diverse ecosystem on the planet, and it is exactly this diversity that is key. Bacteria, viruses, fungi, yeast, and parasitic elements, both good and bad, make up the veritable microbial soup. When there is an abundance of the different species, they work together to provide a powerful barrier between the toxins and foreign proteins within the intestines and the rest of your body and can play a significant role in disease prevention or recovery.

If that diversity is compromised, as it is by things like alcohol, food sensitivities, genetically modified foods, glyphosate, medications like acid blockers (protein pump inhibitors), NSAIDS, and antibiotics, sleep deprivation, thyroid dysfunction, or extreme temperatures, there are fewer health-promoting species and more pathogenic species. Thus, the gut is put in a state of dysbiosis, which alters the microbiome structure and plays a role in the inflammatory, functional hormone, and metabolic balance of the body. This dysbiosis can potentially enhance disease susceptibility. Dysbiosis causes different responses in different people. In one person, it may present as an itchy skin rash, while someone else may experience headaches, peripheral neuropathy, blood sugar imbalance, or inflammatory arthritis. Other symptoms common in dysbiosis can be fatigue, poor sleep, depression, brain fog (cognitive dysfunction), menstrual problems, motor function, and lack of strength. Do any of these sound familiar?

Structurally, dysbiosis causes the tight junctions between the cells of the gut barrier to break down and render the gut barrier permeable, i.e., "leaky gut." One of the biggest challenges of a leaky gut is that endotoxins, such as LPS (lipopolysaccharides) and food proteins can pass through into the blood, where they activate an immune response. This is a normal response, as food particles in the blood are foreign proteins to the body. This immune response causes a release of inflammatory chemicals called cytokines, which set up and perpetuate generalized inflammation, which can turn up anywhere in the body, from rheumatoid arthritis of joints, dermatitis or psoriasis of skin, or brain inflammation, presenting as depression anxiety or other neurodegenerative diseases.

The presence of LPS in the blood plasma provides a measurable value that correlates directly to the level of gut permeability. As such, it can also be considered, to some degree, a marker for inflammation. LPS has been measured and is visibly increased in mood disorders, ALS (Lou Gehrig's Disease) (Zhang 2009), and autism (Emanuele 2010), indicating the gut has become permeable and the resulting systemic inflammation is targeting the brain, increasing the permeability of the blood-brain-barrier (BBB), causing, you guessed it, leaky brain. Once the BBB is breached, the brain's immune cells are activated, causing one of the foundations of all brain injury, neuroinflammation. An additional link of the gut-brain/brain-gut communication occurs via the vagus nerve (Yu 2014), which senses changes in the microbiome and sends cytokines and other inflammatory chemicals to the brain. The conversation between the gut and the brain is incredibly important in the control of neuroinflammation, which has become a hallmark in neurodegenerative conditions (e.g., MS, Alzheimer's, and Parkinson's).

A 2015 study linked chronic intestinal inflammation to a reduction in hippocampal neurogenesis, the brain's ability

to create new neurons (Zonis 2015). The hippocan.
involved in learning, memory, and mood control. Rese
ers have shown that decreased hippocampal neurogenesis
ondary to neuroinflammation can lead to significant behavioural changes, cognitive impairment, and depression. This
neuroinflammation also damages mitochondrial DNA, affecting energy production in the electron transport chain that
controls energy production in brain cells. Together, neuroinflammation and mitochondrial dysfunction further damage
neurons through increased production of reactive oxygen
species and are thought to play a fundamental role in the
pathogenesis of neurological disorders, such as MS, Alzheimer's, Parkinson's, and stroke (Witte et al. 2010). Ultimately, we
rely on neurogenesis, healthy mitochondrial function, and the
production of BDNF (brain-derived neurotrophic factor) to
keep our brains healthy. This can now all be linked to having
a healthy gut.

In case you were wishing you had never taken those NSAIDs
or had not had such a thing for junk food, rest assured, that is
only part of it. The formation of the microbiome begins long
before neuroinflammation can actually damage the brain in
an in-utero exchange between mother and fetus. It is richly
inoculated as the baby passes through mom's vaginal microbiota on the way out. Breastfeeding passes more beneficial
microbes from the mother through the breast milk, and so
the creation of the precious, omnipotent microbiome evolves.
You can imagine then, how a C-section birth would impart
a dramatically different population of microbes. Rather than
picking up mom's microbial contribution, the microbiome is
instead seeded by the microbes on the skin of the attending
physician and nurses, the air in the delivery room, and any
other microbes the newborn may come in contact with. If a
baby is born by C-section, it has been shown to be more susceptible to allergies, asthma, celiac disease, type 1 diabetes,

and inflammatory bowel disease, all because the microbiome is seeded differently at birth (Funkhouser 2013).

So, if you were a C-section baby and/or not breast fed, and/or if your mom was given antibiotics during her pregnancy, chances are you have a very different and disadvantaged microbiome. To take it one step further, a recent study published in the journal *Microbiome* adds that early adverse life events (like trauma) can cause an altered microbiome and correlates those events with an abundance of certain microbial species and distinct changes in brain structure, suggesting a possible role for gut microbes and their metabolites in the development and shaping of the gut-brain axis early in life (Labus 2017). If you were unlucky enough to have been one of those kids with constant ear infections or chronic tonsillitis, requiring round after round of antibiotics, guess what? More bad news. That negatively affected your microbiome too! As you can see, the brain pathologies we develop may actually have their grounding at the beginning of our lives in situations we have had no control over. However, despair not. We can change tomorrow by changing what we eat, probiotics, prebiotics, and, if need be, fecal microbial transplant (FMT) now called GFT, Gut Flora Transplant.

At this point in history, western cultures have largely eliminated bacterial pathogens through hygiene, antibiotics, and rigorous sanitation practices. This is now playing itself out in the dysbiosis, leaky gut, neuroinflammation, and neurodegeneration of our population. I would venture to say that the biggest issue in most neurodegenerative conditions is failure in the gut-brain axis.

Individual studies implicating gut dysfunction with neuroinflammation and the pathogenesis of neurodegenerative conditions like Alzheimer's (Fox 2013; Daulatzai 2014), Parkinson's, ALS, traumatic brain injury, and MS are too numerous to mention. But I encourage you to take a look at the simple search engine instruction "dysbiosis and multiple sclerosis." This will yield a weekend's worth of reading.

Since the diversity of the microbial population is the most important feature of a healthy microbiome, a healthy immune response, and ultimately a healthy brain, we can begin to take corrective action under the premise "heal the gut, heal the brain."

While pharmaceuticals cannot improve the biodiversity of the microbiome and its eventual neuroinflammation and mitochondrial dysfunction, there is abundant evidence supporting modifiable lifestyle factors that can. What follows are five simple but powerful steps you can start to take today to begin to restore your microbiome.

1. Food changes the microbiome for better or worse. Diet rapidly alters the microbiome. Think about your diet as eating to seed. Include prebiotic foods like chicory root, dandelion greens, garlic, jicama, and Jerusalem artichoke. Include probiotic foods like sauerkraut, kimchi, kombucha, and kefir. Eat whole, unprocessed food and strive to consume fifty different foods each week. Avoid sugar. Not only does it promote pathogenic species in the gut, consumption of it has a direct correlation to increased incidents of dementia (Crane 2013).

2. Many studies show that exercise improves microbial diversity and immune function. Some studies even show that changes due to exercise are independent of changes made via diet. This is important, because that means changing both can have an additive effect. Studies show that cardiorespiratory fitness is a good predictor of gut microbial diversity in healthy humans, and the microbiome in high cardiorespiratory fitness individuals seems to favour decreased LPS pathways (Estaki 2016; Kang 2014; Cook 2015).

3. Avoid genetically modified foods (GMOs) and glyphosate. This herbicide is associated with GMO foods, is used as a desiccant to harvest wheat, potatoes, sweet potatoes, and other

foods, and is known to cause changes in the microbiome by acting as an antibiotic and a mitochondrial toxin, deactivating vitamin D3, and impairing liver detoxification (Samsel 2013).

4. Like every other system in the body, stress hormones change the microbiome (Panda 2014), and the anxious or negative thoughts we have during times of stress further impact it. Building stress resiliency is key. Tranquility promotes a healthier microbiome by calming the gut-brain axis. Find time each day for stillness, whether that be meditation, prayer, deep breathing, walking in nature, or any other gentle activity that will calm the brain to heal the gut.

5. Take a probiotic supplement. If you are uncertain how to begin, speak to your health care practitioner.

Increased diversity of the diet and more exercise independently alter the wellbeing of the gut microbiome and reveal independent associations with anxiety and cognition (Kang 2014). Most of the time, the job of the immune system is to *not* respond! I mean by this that if the microbiota is healthy and diverse then our immune system, which is 70-80 percent gut based, is also calm and healthy. Therefore the immune system will not need to respond to minor adverse events.

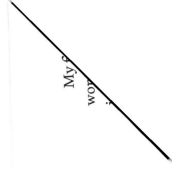

11: Thyroid, Iron, and Other Important Lab Investigations

I have included a chapter on hypothyroidism in this book about brain recovery for one important reason: cognitive dysfunction. The thyroid gland controls the metabolic function of mitochondria, or energy production, in the cell. When your thyroid hormone is lower than it should be, it feels like your energy "dimmer switch" is turned down. The consequence of this is cognitive dysfunction, memory loss, anxiety, and even depression. Optimal function of the thyroid is a key component in maintaining optimal brain health and function.

In my opinion, low-functioning thyroid is the most commonly undertreated medical issue today. How did we get here? I believe this occurred over the last forty years. During this time, our clinical evaluation of people's thyroid function has been superseded by lab values. Lab values, especially thyroid-stimulating hormone (TSH), have become near absolute in the eyes of most MDs. The consequence is that many sincere complaints by patients, especially women, have been shrugged off or even belittled. As a result, many of these same patients have had to struggle on their own. Sadly, many are put on antidepressants or tranquilizers, which may mask or even compound the problem.

...irst major example of this involves a fifty-five-year-old ...nan who was experiencing cognitive problems. D.J. is an ...ntelligent, well-educated individual with a master's degree. She did her research especially well and noted she had twenty-one of the many signs and symptoms of hypothyroidism. After her third child, twenty years previously, she was diagnosed with postpartum depression and started on an antidepressant. At age fifty-two, she had been investigated twice for a rapid heart rate with the resting pulse usually at 95–100 bpm (beats per minute). She had been seen twice by a cardiologist, who did the three-day Holter monitor (monitor that records your EKG continuously) and reassured her that everything was normal. She continued to see her family doctor, who was quite capable and empathetic. Finally, her physician agreed to a short trial on Synthroid, which is eltroxin (pure T4). D.J. actually felt worse on this medication. Hence, after nearly a year on Synthroid, she returned to her family doctor, stating that she felt no better and, in fact, in some ways felt worse. Her doctor suggested that she next try hormone-replacement therapy, and if that did not work, to see a psychiatrist.

D.J. disagreed and, fortunately, found an integrated physician in a nearby city. This physician recommended temperature monitoring. D.J.'s temperature measured at 35.0°C or about 96°F. The integrative physician suggested a compounded T3 replacement rather than the Synthroid. T3 is the active form of thyroid hormone. Synthroid mainly contains T4, which must be converted to T3 in the body. The benefits were dramatic. D.J.'s resting pulse within 48 hours consistently stayed at 70 bpm. This impressed D.J. She started to feel as if she was waking up from a long sleep. Her body temperature gradually increased to normal. Her brain function improved, and she felt she could problem solve and function much better than in the previous few years. She was able to return to work, which included a forty-five-minute commute on a busy highway. All her other symptoms also improved. D.J. firmly believed that she would not have been able to cope at work without thyroid replacement therapy. She tapered off her antidepressant and has never needed them again in fifteen years since. I wonder how many women are in a similar scenario?

Now that I have your attention, allow me to describe some key points about thyroid function. First, the thyroid gland is a butterfly-shaped tissue just below the hard notch under your chin. This is the thyroid cartilage of the windpipe or trachea. This gland takes up the iodine absorbed from the food and mixes it with a number of key proteins to make the compounds T1, T2, T3, and T4. T1 only has one iodine molecule and T4 has four iodine molecules. T4 is the storage form of thyroid hormone. It has minimal action directly on the body's receptors and cells. Instead, T4 must be converted by enzymes in the body into the active form of T3. This enzyme conversion process occurs primarily in the liver and is both zinc- and selenium-dependent. Therefore, if you are deficient in zinc or selenium or both, then you feel hypothyroid. The other third of the conversion of T4 into T3 actually happens in the gut within the microbiota.

The major control of the thyroid hormone production within the body is done by the pituitary gland. When this small gland, at the base of the brain, senses an inadequate amount of circulating T3, the pituitary gland secretes more TSH. TSH (thyroid-stimulating hormone). TSH travels through the bloodstream to the thyroid gland, triggering the production of more thyroid hormones (T1, T2, T3, and T4). All of this would work relatively well except for the "evil twin," reverse T3. Reverse T3 cannot be used by the body. T4 can be converted into T3 or reverse T3 or both. Both of these compounds are recognized by the pituitary gland, and this suppresses or minimizes the amount of TSH produced. Unfortunately, when your MD only measures TSH to assess your thyroid function, lab interpretation trumps clinical acumen. This means that if the TSH is within the lab's normal range, all the patient's clinical signs and symptoms tend to be disregarded. The signs and symptoms include a considerable list of psychiatric symptoms. Consequently, many of these patients end up on mental health treatment when, in reality, they are only hypothyroid.

An important point to make here is that only T3 activates the metabolism of virtually every cell of the body. Reverse T3 has none of these effects. That is why my mentor and colleague, Dr. Louis Cady, an integrative medicine psychiatrist, calls reverse T3 the evil twin. Dr. Cady has been my favourite teacher regarding optimal treatment of thyroid illness. He speaks regularly at the Integrated Medicine for Mental Health Conferences, hosted by Great Plains Laboratory in Lenexa, Kansas. Over production of reverse T3 from T4 occurs primarily when we are chronically stressed. Chronic stress causes our adrenal gland to produce more and more cortisol to cope. The result is adrenal fatigue and excess reverse T3 from T4. This adrenal fatigue must be kept in mind when treating a patient with thyroid replacement if he or she seems to be unresponsive to therapy. It is often useful to add an adaptogen, such as rhodiola, which helps the adrenals.

To summarize, in the presence of ongoing and chronic stress, the body produces more reverse T3 than the active T3. Reverse T3 and T3 both have an effect on the feedback to the pituitary gland. Consequently, the pituitary gland interprets that everything is okay when it is not. As a result, testing thyroid function by only measuring TSH, the physician ends up shortchanging the patient and possibly adding unnecessary medications.

The other concept I learned from Dr. Cady is that of optimal health. With regard to thyroid function, I aim to have people's free T3 and free T4 in the upper half of normal range if they already have symptoms of hypothyroidism. This often means

upper 1/3 of normal

treating a TSH of 2.0 or even 1.0. Meanwhile, the TSH laboratory guideline is to start treatment when the TSH is 4.5 to 5.5. This blind belief, that everybody is the same with respect to the normal range advocated by the laboratory, does not serve patients well.

Only recently has this disconnect been reviewed by endocrinologists. I am happy to report that some endocrinologists are now requesting more than the standard TSH test. They are treating patients to achieve lower TSH values. In addition, those well-trained in functional and integrative medicine are responding by treating hypothyroid symptoms with the measured TSH of 2.0. By measuring the free T3 and free T4 as well as reverse T3, many more patients can be treated for optimal health if they have the symptoms of hypothyroidism.

Considerable knowledge has been written about thyroid problems for the lay public. I particularly like the summary by Jill Carnahan, MD. She lists sixteen signs that you might be hypothyroid. They are as follows:
- Trouble conceiving a baby
- Have had one or more miscarriages
- Feel depressed most of the time
- Feel restless or anxious
- Puffiness and swelling around the eyes and face
- Moods change easily
- Difficulty concentrating or focusing
- Feelings of sadness
- Loss of interest in normal daily activities
- More forgetful lately
- Hair is falling out
- Cannot seem to remember things
- No sex drive
- Frequent infections that last longer than usual
- Dry, gritty eyes
- Eyes sensitive to light

- Difficulty swallowing or feeling a lump in the throat
- Hoarse or gravelly voice
- Tinnitus or ringing in the ears
- Light-headedness or dizziness
- Severe menstrual cramps and heavy flow

Dr. Carnahan lists other conditions that may be associated with thyroid dysfunction. These include acne, high cholesterol, irregular periods, fluid retention, difficulty swallowing, respiratory difficulties, iron deficiency, and frequent headaches. She also lists family history that might suggest you have a higher risk for hypothyroidism. This includes a history of hypothyroidism, celiac disease or gluten intolerance, goiter (enlarged lump on the thyroid), prematurely grey hair, type 1 diabetes mellitus, Crohn's disease or ulcerative colitis, MS, elevated cholesterol, and autoimmune diseases, such as rheumatoid arthritis, lupus, sarcoidosis, and Sjogren's syndrome.

Hypothyroidism is much more common than hyperthyroidism (Graves' disease). The main cause of both illnesses is felt to be autoimmune in origin. I believe this immune dysfunction is primarily based on leaky gut, with the foreign proteins entering the bloodstream and subsequent attack on them by the immune system. Because the foreign proteins resemble the thyroid tissue, the immune system also begins to attack the thyroid. This is referred to as molecular mimicry and triggers one of the two thyroid diseases mentioned above.

As noted, hyperthyroidism (Graves' disease) is much less common than hypothyroidism. However, Graves' disease is increasing in incidence and is especially common in women twenty to forty years of age. It often occurs after giving birth. Other autoimmune illnesses that are felt to predispose an individual to Graves' disease are Addison's, lupus, pernicious anemia, rheumatoid arthritis, type 1 diabetes mellitus, and vitiligo. The common physical signs associated with hyperthyroidism are protruding eyes, swelling or enlargement of the thyroid, goitre, and abnormal nerve sensations. These nerve sensations can include tingling, burning, and pins and needles in any or all of the four extremities. These patients often have an increased heart rate. One way to remember hyperthyroidism symptoms is the three a's. The first is arrhythmia, meaning a rapid and often uneven heart rate. The second is agitation, meaning a short fuse or easily irritated temper. The third "a" denotes anxiety. Further symptoms reported by Graves' patients include feeling nervous, jittery, difficulty sitting still, problems sleeping at night, or all of the above. In extreme cases, sufferers report weight loss.

Early treatment of Graves' disease was surgery, which was risky in the presence of high-circulating thyroid hormone. More recently, treatment includes either propylthiouracil or the use of radioactive thyroid. However, a careful history might suggest an easier solution in some cases. If the patient is using a large amount of aspartame, one of the most frequently used artificial sweeteners, stopping this may have a dramatic beneficial effect. A low-grade infection, such as mycoplasma, is another possibility and can aggravate Graves' disease. Finally, healing the gut is critical. Once the gut is healed, much of the ongoing trigger of autoimmune illness can be minimized.

Hashimoto's thyroiditis, another form of hypothyroidism, is much more common than Graves' disease and is estimated to affect as much as 2 percent of the population. This thyroiditis is named after Hakaru Hashimoto, a Japanese surgeon, who described it in the twentieth century. Hashimoto's thyroiditis symptoms can often begin with some hyperthyroid symptoms, such as increased heart rate, nervousness, and uncontrolled abundant energy. These initial symptoms are often due to inflammation and swelling of the thyroid gland, which squeezes excess thyroid hormone into the bloodstream. However, once these initial phase symptoms disappear, they are replaced by typical symptoms of hypothyroidism. These include fatigue, coldness, loss of hair, dry skin—especially on the lower legs—and can progress to sadness, depression, and cognitive dysfunction.

Hashimoto's thyroiditis (hypothyroidism) can affect people of all ages, but it is most common in women in their thirties and forties. It is associated with other autoimmune illnesses, such as adrenal insufficiency, chronic active hepatitis, diabetes mellitus type I, Graves', lupus, rheumatoid arthritis, and Sjogren's syndrome. Blood tests frequently reveal antithyroid antibodies in 90 percent of patients and anti-microsomal antibodies in about 80 percent of patients. At least 10 percent of all of these patients will demonstrate neither of these antibodies. Therefore, treat the patient, not the lab value.

The clinical diagnosis of low thyroid function include the symptoms list given previously as well as poor eyebrow growth—especially the outer third—periorbital edema, or swelling under the eyes, and a lower basal body temperature. This final sign is not always employed, but it is a useful adjunct and is of no cost, other than the purchase of a thermometer. This is probably easiest with a digital thermometer. Ideally, take your temperature before you get out of bed in the morning and record it five days in a row. In women having menstrual cycles, it is best to measure it on the second day of the cycle. Thyroid function is normal when temperatures are in the range of 36.6-36.8°C or 97.8-98.2°F when taken under the armpit. This will be closer to 37°C or 98.6°F when done orally. A body temperature half a degree or more below this may well suggest hypothyroidism if there is no other reasonable explanation.

Thyroid hormone resistance can also cause hypothyroidism. This should be considered when an individual needs considerably more thyroid hormone replacement than would be anticipated. An analogy to thyroid hormone resistance is insulin resistance, as in type 2 diabetes mellitus. In this type of diabetes, the pancreas is secreting enough insulin, but the cells are resistant to its effect.

In thyroid hormone resistance, it is common to have normal thyroid blood tests despite consistent signs and symptoms of hypothyroidism. Common association of thyroid hormone resistance is a diagnosis of fibromyalgia, chronic fatigue syndrome, or both. This entity is quite treatable, and my preference is desiccated thyroid. As stated previously, this may require seemingly large doses of desiccated thyroid, so instead of 30-75 mg per day, you may need 125-250 mg per day. These clients rarely show signs of thyrotoxicosis, which is excess thyroid hormone. Most of these clients respond to the thyroid hormone replacement along with nutritional supplementation of iodine, zinc, and selenium and exercise to tolerance. Some patients will benefit from increased B vitamins, particularly B12, and sometimes vitamins E, D, and A.

Thyroid hormone resistance can occur from multiple factors. These include 1) genetic anomalies of thyroid hormone receptors, 2) autoimmune, oxidative, or toxic damage of thyroid hormone receptors, and 3) competitive binding to thyroid hormone receptors by pollutants, such as food additives, pesticides, and perhaps even plastic components, as in estrogen hormone disruptors. Glyphosate is an additional thyroid toxin to be minimized. It chelates (binds) minerals, so one can be deficient in zinc and selenium, both important to thyroid health. Artificial sweeteners (e.g., aspartame, sucralose) should also be eliminated.

The second thyroid case study is a young woman (B.F.), whom I have followed for several years. B.F. is an intelligent woman in her early thirties with a PhD. However, she was diagnosed with thyroid cancer in her early twenties and was being followed by an endocrinologist following her cancer treatment. The treatment of her thyroid cancer was surgical removal, which virtually eliminates any further thyroid function. Her endocrinologist persisted in using Synthroid, chemically synthesized T-4 (eltroxin), but she felt she still had many symptoms consistent with hypothyroidism. When I reviewed her in an integrated medicine consult, I suggested she go on a small amount of iodine replacement and change from Synthroid to desiccated thyroid. In Canada, this thyroid is of porcine origin and is distributed to pharmacies by the pharmaceutical company ERFA. This animal product contains T1, T2, T3, and T4 (approximately twice as much T4 as T3). The presence of T3 supports the direct action of the T3 without any enzyme transformation. This change in thyroid hormone worked well for B.F. She has maintained this for five years and has had two successful pregnancies. During pregnancy, it is particularly important to closely monitor thyroid function as the needs change. It is critical for the health of the mother and the baby that these be optimized.

The above discussion reminds me of an MS client of mine from the southern United States. In reviewing her story, I learned she had received a diagnosis of hypothyroidism at the Mayo Clinic. She was started on Synthroid, and it worked well for nine or ten months. Then she noted that she was once again getting many of the signs and symptoms of hypothyroidism. She returned to the Mayo Clinic. In view of her story, they changed her to desiccated thyroid, the Armor brand. She improved dramatically and has stayed well on this regimen. In my practice, I tend to prescribe only desiccated thyroid for the treatment of thyroid illness. In fact, this is one of the few prescription medicines that I still prescribe. I also advise my patients that they may be asked a question by their pharmacist when they take in this prescription. The pharmacist frequently asks, "Doesn't Dr. Code know there is a new synthetic thyroid without the variability of the biologic animal thyroid?" I tell my patients ahead of time that, yes, I do know. We have had synthetic thyroid for more than thirty-five years.

Thus, practitioners need to recognize the many symptoms associated with hypothyroidism. It is also important for physicians to treat the symptoms, not the lab values. In this way, more people will be treated more optimally for thyroid dysfunction. The result will be reduced symptoms, improved quality of life, and better brain function. If you want to read more, I suggest a book by David Brownstein, MD, called *Overcoming Thyroid Disorders*, now in its third edition (2008).

Hemochromatosis

If you know about hemochromatosis already, skip to the end of the chapter. If not, read carefully, because more cases of hemochromatosis are diagnosed in a year than ALS, MS, and muscular dystrophy combined.

Hemochromatosis is a common, inherited condition that is rarely diagnosed. Three quarters of patients have no symptoms. Excessive iron accumulations are found in affected brain areas of people with Alzheimer's, Parkinson's, Huntington's, MS (Stankiewicz 2014), and even epilepsy. The question arises of whether the iron deposition in the brain or inflammation comes first, as discussed in MS patients (Zivadinov 2011).

Even in normal adults, people with higher brain accumulations of iron perform poorer on cognitive tests than do those with lower brain iron concentrations (Bartzokis 2011). This brilliant study by George Bartzokis et al. at UCLA confirmed that limiting lifetime exposure to iron can reduce iron accumulation in the brain. The study showed women after hysterectomy soon achieved iron concentrations equal to men. One protective effect of monthly periods in women is less iron accumulation. Of course, women also need careful evaluation to avoid anemia from low iron, especially during pregnancy.

Hemochromatosis is genetic, and more than one in 250 people carry this gene—especially Caucasians, often of Irish origin. Today, testing is done by most labs to determine your iron genetics, particularly if you have a close relative (parent, sibling, or child) with a hemochromatosis diagnosis or if you have excessive iron. Undiagnosed and untreated hemochromatosis increases the risk for diabetes, irregular heartbeat or heart attack, arthritis, osteoporosis, liver cirrhosis or cancer, gall bladder problems, depression, impotence, infertility, hypothyroidism, small testes or ovaries, and even some cancers. Chronic fatigue and joint pain are the most common complaints of people with hemochromatosis, but 75 percent have no symptoms! The classic joint pain of hemochromatosis is pain in the knuckles of the pointer and middle finger and the so-called "iron fist." Memory problems, brain fog, and heart flutters or irregular heartbeat are suggestions the body iron must be checked to rule out hemochromatosis.

Measurement of body iron is relatively inexpensive and available. I start with ferritin on everyone, because if it is low, it is important to remedy. If ferritin is elevated (greater than 300 ng/ml in men and greater than 200 ng/ml in women), I measure fasting serum iron and total iron binding capacity. If these are awry, then the blood test for your iron genetics is indicated. Happily, liver biopsies are no longer indicated. Simple reference charts available at www.irondisorders.org will help both patients and clinicians follow iron safely and long term.

Treatment of hemochromatosis is quite straightforward. First, reduce your iron intake. No men and no post-menopausal women should take iron-containing multivitamins unless they are iron deficient. Similarly, reducing your intake of red meat (beef, lamb, bison, emu, ostrich) will help. The iron in these meats is easily absorbed. This is why I recommend them to individuals with iron deficiency anemia. Finally, giving blood every few weeks lowers iron stores. Serum ferritin drops about 30 ng/ml with each unit (500 cc) of blood removed. You may need a prescription from your physician, or you can donate at a blood clinic if you pass their screening criteria and assessment.

Once iron levels reach normal, you may be able to donate every two to four months for life. If hemochromatosis is diagnosed early and treated before organs are damaged, a person can live a normal life expectancy. To follow up on diet, including meal and food planning suggestions and a list of iron content in foods, see www.irondisorders.org/diet.

Other Key Lab Investigations

I began this chapter with two commonly missed problems—low thyroid and excess iron, which can only be determined with laboratory assessment. I would be remiss if I did not include some other important assessments that specialized laboratories can now perform.

First, let me address genetic testing. This can be as simple as 23 and Me (www.23andme.com) or the often more useful MTHFR evaluation and interpretation. My personal preference for laboratory assessments is Great Plains Labs (GPL). They do a quality assessment but also include a personal discussion with the patient, clinician, or both. This is critical, as their expertise in explaining what the results may mean for each individual is extremely helpful.

The components included in GPL's genetic evaluation can explain your individual ability to use the detoxification pathways. This can be critical in explaining why you are unwell while those around you on the same diet, drugs, and environment appear healthy and stay healthy. Sometimes a single

SNP (single-nucleotide polymorphism) makes you into a "canary in the coal mine." In addition, this assessment might explain why you have a dramatic or even dangerous response to a medication. You can read a bit more of this chapter 15.

A third useful screening is hair metal analysis. This can highlight a needed intervention in either heavy metal toxicity or trace metal insufficiency. This is not a comprehensive, complete evaluation of heavy metal problems, but it is a relatively inexpensive starting point. If you want further detailed assistance, then I direct you to Dr. Christopher Shade at Quicksilver Scientific.

The fourth investigation I frequently find useful is IgG evaluation of food sensitivities. This is done on a blood spot on special paper from GPL. When this is done in conjunction with a careful and detailed functional medicine history, your clinician can glean a tremendous amount of information. Multiple food sensitivities are commonly associated with many conditions involving excess inflammation. These conditions range from hypothyroidism to depression, anxiety, MS, schizophrenia, and even dementia. Solutions are available if one heals the leaky gut that triggers this problem. In cases of severe gut problems, a Gut Flora Transplant,GFT,also called fecal microbial transplant (FMT) should be considered.

Testing for gluten sensitivity is a further possibility. The world experts for this test are Cyrex Labs. Many clinicians simply test for alpha gliadin. This is insufficient. Cyrex, in their Array #3, identify twelve different components of wheat that can promote inflammation and negatively stimulate the immune system. This test can be quite expensive. Consequently, I often suggest complete withdrawal of gluten for three months. However, if the client is resistant, and men often are, objective evidence from a lab test may improve compliance.

My favorite go-to test if I am struggling with a complex client is the organic acid test (OAT). The OAT, which evaluates urine, was pioneered at the Centre for Disease Control by Dr. William Shaw and further perfected by his lab, GPL. However, its benefits can be used widely. This test explains oxalic acid abnormalities, neurotransmitter deficiencies and excesses, and even nutrient deficiencies, such as B12, coenzyme Q10, and cysteine for glutathione synthesis. Especially valuable is the personal evaluation of the lab results by GPL staff.

Finally, some of the most recent additions to testing at GPL are their glyphosate and manmade toxin measurements. These can document and explain a heretofore unsolvable dilemma.

The above tests are rarely in the available toolbox of most clinicians. I will now list the lab tests I do routinely when I see a client. Almost all these are covered by health care plans in Canada. Within hematology, I do a profile of hemoglobin, white blood cells, red blood cells, hematocrit, and platelets. I include ferritin as my iron excess or deficiency screen. Blood sugar is key with fasting and hemoglobin A1C, which reflects an average blood sugar over a period of three months. If these are borderline, I measure fasting insulin. I also test total cholesterol, mostly to see if there is enough for optimal brain function.

For thyroid function, I request TSH, free T-3, free T-4, and reverse T-3. I do an electrolyte screen that includes creatinine glomerular filtration rate (GFR) for kidney evaluation. For liver evaluation, I include prealbumin, albumin, alkaline phosphatase, ALT, GGT, bilirubin, and total protein. I always check vitamin D (25-OH) and C-reactive protein, shown as a prognostic biomarker in ALS (Lunetta 2017), and diet can make a difference (Nieves 2016) as a marker of inflammation. I also check serum homocysteine for stroke and Alzheimer's prevention (Carlsson 2007) and vitamin B12 as useful screens for neurological problems, including risk of dementia. Further tests are possible if areas of abnormality are suggested. I do not always follow the "normal" guidelines of the local laboratory.

Rather, I coordinate the clinical picture with the lab result. We must remember to treat the client, not the lab result.

12: Sleep Issues, Snoring, and Sleep Apnea

"To sleep, perchance to dream." Shakespeare said it well. Have you ever had insufficient sleep so that you cannot think clearly? I have any number of times. Mine was often related to being on call and up at night, either as a family physician or as an anaesthesiologist. Similarly, if I sleep soundly for seven to eight hours, I am ready to take on the world. In this chapter, I discuss how you can improve your sleep and rest, why you need sleep, and sleep problems, including CPAP (continuous positive airway pressure) and sleep apnea. Combined, each of these can have a tremendous impact on your health. I also discuss oxygen supplementation and improved sleep. This is noted in a cerebral palsy and HBOT study (Long 2017).

If you want to weaken or "break" someone's resistance, sleep deprivation is a big step toward success. We also know that if you are awake for a twenty-four hour period, your mind function is equivalent to being impaired by .08 percent alcohol in your blood, the legal impairment level in many countries. Is it any wonder that teenagers like to party all night? They can achieve a giddy or drunk-like state without any drugs! Thus, lack of sleep does affect us. In fact, chronic sleep deprivation has significant consequences to our health. Research has established that sleep deficit rushes you toward chronic illness. Lack of sleep can weaken your immune system, accelerate cancer and type 2 diabetes mellitus, and seriously impair your cognition. This cognitive impairment includes reduced executive function, short-term memory loss, and reduced coping skills with mental and physical tasks. Lack of sleep increases your risk of dying from all causes.

Sleep is one of the great mysteries of life. However, we know more about it now, how it enhances well-being, and how to optimize our six to eight hours of quality sleep. To begin, I will talk about stages of sleep, which include the ones that are most critical for brain recovery. Sleep is classified on the basis of electroencephalogram (EEG) and electro-oculogram (EOG), the electrical activity captured from the muscles in movement of the eyes. This includes stages 1–3 as well as REM (rapid eye movement) and non-REM sleep.

Stage 1 sleep is dozing from which one can awaken easily. The EEG of this stage is low-amplitude waves with mixed frequency but mostly fast waves. Stage 2 sleep is similar to stage 1 but has episodes of sleep spindles, where the frequency is 12-14 Hz between large biphasic waves of characteristic appearance. One starts to see large-amplitude (delta) waves in stage 2 sleep. In stage 3, these delta waves are more dominant, and sleep spindles nearly disappear. In stage 4 sleep, which is often called deep sleep, the EEG is mainly high-voltage, more than 75 µvolts, and more than half is slow, delta frequency. Recently, stages 3 and 4 sleep have been combined into simply stage 3 sleep—one less for you to remember.

REM sleep is quite different. The EEG pattern is the same in stage 1, but the EOG shows frequent rapid eye movements. Other forms of activity during sleep occur here as well. Non-REM sleep does not show rapid eye movements but does have rolling eye movements, which are distinctly different.

Through the night, the stages of sleep vary among individuals. Sleep patterns can also vary night to night for the same individual. You may have noticed that if you are extremely tired, you seem to dream less. This is often the case. Sleep begins by entering stage 1 and often progresses through stages 2 and 3. REM or dreaming sleep is the brain activity actually increasing. Curiously, the body in general becomes more relaxed and our muscles more immobilized during this stage. Episodes of REM sleep alternate with non-REM sleep throughout the night, with more of these occurring toward morning. On average, there are four to five episodes of REM sleep per night, with the duration of these increasing toward morning. If we are extremely tired, we do not have as much REM sleep. On the next night of rest, however, the body seems to catch up, and there is considerably more REM sleep. It is often stage 3 sleep that dominates snoring and sleep apnea. The sleeper can pass from any stage into stage 1 or fully awake.

While we sleep, our metabolic rate decreases by about 10 percent below our base metabolic rate. You may have noticed you are hungrier and eat more if you have insufficient sleep. I noticed this in my long call nights while awake for twenty-four to thirty-six hours. A similar reduction of 10 percent in the metabolic rate occurs during anaesthesia. As we age, or if we are affected by drugs, such as anaesthetics or narcotics, transient episodes of low blood oxygen occur during sleep, even in healthy people. The depth of our breathing decreases with deepening levels or stages of non-REM sleep. Tidal volume, the amount of air we move in and out of our lungs in a single breath, is the most minimal in REM sleep, about 25 percent less than awake. Remember this concept when I talk about snoring and sleep apnea.

Why do we need sleep? Sleep benefits our health. Some of the theories of why we sleep include:

1. Being inactive keeps us out of harm's way and encourages energy conservation.

2. Restorative functions like muscle growth, tissue repair, protein synthesis, and growth hormone release mostly occur during sleep.

3. Sleep rejuvenates the brain's cognitive function. Perhaps sleeping on an idea is a reasonable thing to do.

4. Brainwash occurs. This concept suggests that during the deep stages of sleep, the brain contracts and squeezes itself like a sponge. This helps to remove the fluids, by-products of metabolism, and toxins by squeezing them into the cerebrospinal fluid on their way out of the body. This idea is further supported in recent years as scientists report that this system can help remove the toxic protein beta-amyloid from brain tissue. Other research has confirmed that brain levels of beta-amyloid fall during sleep. (Further details can be found in the journal *Brain* (July 2017). This brain wash occurs via the glial cell-controlled lymphatics, sometimes called glymphatics. Sleep enlarges these channels around the blood vessels so that pressure, which is much faster than just diffusion, can wash away these toxins. In short, sleep drives or enhances metabolite clearance from the adult brain (Xie 2013). This has implications in traumatic brain injury, Alzheimer's, MS, and stroke.

5. Sleep is important for brain plasticity. I find brain plasticity theory, neuroplasticity, quite compelling (Doidge 2007). There is significant brain activity during sleep. Although sleep appears to be a passive and restful time, it actually involves a highly active and well-scripted interplay of brain circuits, which results in sleep's EEG stages. Much of this reorganization of neurons seems to occur during REM sleep.

What interferes with falling asleep or reaching optimal sleep stages? Our physiology has been developed over several thousands of years. However, the last 200 years or so has given us a dramatic increase in the amount of light at night.

This change has been particularly profound since the development of screens on our television, computer, smart phone, or tablet devices. Most often, these are high in blue light, typical of the dawn, and is wakeful to us. This is why it is important to either not use these for one or two hours before sleep or at least have them reset into a mode of more yellow or orange lights and less blue. In addition, it is important to sleep in a dark room. Your room should be free of any significant light. Wearing a sleep mask does not work, because even if your hands or arms are exposed to the light, almost all melatonin production is stopped. Melatonin is a key sleep-optimizing anti-inflammatory hormone that rises through the night. Once you are exposed to light, the production of melatonin is stopped for the night.Melatonin is also important for sleep and brain function.

From reading the chapter about dirty electricity and electromagnetic smog, you will be aware of many of the devices that send intermittent electrical pulses through the airwaves. Our body does not know to ignore these. Consequently, optimal sleep patterns are interrupted and hampered. This seems to be a greater problem for anyone with an injured or poorly functioning brain. I am in this group and am extremely conscientious about turning off the Wi-Fi at night and not having a charging cell phone or other electrical device within two meters of my bed. At home, I only use phones with cords rather than hands-free devices, which are particularly damaging to sleep. In Sweden, I am told that they provide MS patients with a silver-fibre canopy surrounding their bed. This is certainly less expensive than moving a decent distance from a cell phone tower. One of my sons purchased one of these canopies, because he is right beside a cell tower. In his opinion, this improves his quality of restful sleep. For a photo, see page 30 at the end of Chapter 3.

Snoring

Snoring can happen at any stage but is predominant in our first, fifth, and sixth decades of life. Snoring in children is often allergy-triggered and occurs due to polyps in the nose and/or enlarged tonsils and adenoids. Snoring is more common in men than women and is aggravated by obesity in both sexes. Snoring can be present in all stages of sleep, but it predominates in deep non-REM sleep and is minimized in REM sleep. At least 25 percent of the population snores, and it is the dominant reason for couples having separate bedrooms. There is a strong association between snoring and many health problems. These include hypertension, heart and lung disease, arthritis, diabetes mellitus, and depression. All snoring is worsened with obesity, smoking, and alcohol intake. In obesity, all neck tissues and the tongue increase in fatty tissue. This increase in fatty tissue also occurs with aging. This increases the likelihood of obstruction of the upper airway, and snoring is the result, as snoring is the sound of partial obstruction. Remember, I was an anesthesiologist! The most serious impact of snoring is that it often progresses to sleep apnea.

Sleep Apnea

This is the next logical progression from snoring. Snoring happens first and many, but not all, snorers progress to sleep apnea.

There are three main types of sleep apnea: 1) obstructive sleep apnea (OSA), 2) central sleep apnea (CSA), and 3) a mixture of 1) and 2), which is a combination of obstructive and central sleep apnea. The well-documented health effects of untreated sleep apnea should have each of us who snore be investigated by a sleep lab or equivalent. People with sleep apnea have a higher risk of hypertension, heart attack, chronic heart failure, arrhythmia, and stroke. This makes OSA a major public health problem by affecting patients' health and quality of life, including brain changes on MRI (Kim 2013).

At least 4 percent of adult men and 2 percent of adult women in the general population are diagnosed with OSA. Of everyone with the characteristic symptoms of OSA but not daytime sleepiness, this incidence climbs to 24 percent and 10 percent respectively. This tells us that over one third of people are on the verge. In obese and elderly populations, these values rise to 60 percent.

The possibility of having OSA goes up to 60 percent after an acute heart attack. I already mentioned the increased cardiovascular risk factors related to OSA. Oxidative stress and inflammation are two major mechanisms to explain this. The trigger of both of these is intermittent hypoxia or lack of oxygen. If you stop breathing or stop moving air in and out, your oxygen drops precipitously. In addition, when you restart breathing, as the oxygen returns to the tissues, you relieve the hypoxia, and this is followed by a reperfusion injury. This is the increased health risk time, because the excess free radical production occurs as the tissues are reperfused. This is similar to muscle that has had blood flow cut off with a tourniquet, as is occasionally done during orthopedic surgery or after heart surgery when the heart has been stopped to permit surgery. These changes tend to affect the brain and heart the most, because these tissues need the most oxygen. Oxygen therapy is reviewed by Mehta (Mehta 2013).

Therefore, if you snore and wonder if you have sleep apnea, get it checked out as soon as possible. I routinely asked patients preoperatively if they snored. Even better, I asked their sleeping partner if they snored or had pauses in their breathing. All the drugs used in anesthesia aggravate these issues. The life you save by intervention may be your own. For example, I was in an audience of farming people in Washington state. I noted one of the farmers kept falling asleep. He was a big man, somewhat obese. I approached him at the break and asked if he had ever been evaluated for sleep apnea. He said he had not but wondered if he should. I highly recommended he see a pulmonary specialist. He phoned me a month later and thanked me for saving his life. He saw the specialist, was put on a CPAP, lost fifty pounds, and regained his quality of life. The weight gain of OSA is classic, because eating is the only thing left in life that makes a person feel better.

CPAP helps the airway remain open, so the frequency of obstruction and secondary hypoxia is reduced. The morning headache disappears, and alertness returns. Suddenly, the person is a better employee and less likely to nod off while driving. All these are good results.

The other central sleep apnea and mixed sleep apnea groups are slightly more complicated to treat. Yes, CPAP is still useful. However, if there is a heart attack, heart failure, or stroke history, they might also benefit from 2-3 litres per minute of oxygen added to a T-piece of their CPAP machine (Pokorski 2000; Gottlieb 2009). This will further protect them and usually reduces the central sleep apnea episodes (Friedman 2001). This latter suggestion is less known, but I recommend it, because it will harm no one and will help protect the brain and heart function and improve quality of life (Lavie 2015).

Improved Sleep

We all know that rest is good for the body, but researchers have also found evidence that sleep is good for learning and

memory. When you nod off at night, your bra
day's events. During this replay, brain regions
store memories talk to each other. Scientis
replay and regional "talking" is how the brain 1
ories from temporary storage to long-term sto1
need quality sleep if we are going to have a quality memory.
Furthermore, sleep can also help integrate new information,
leading to creative insights, hence the concept of "sleep on it"
to assist decision making.

To optimize your sleep, I recommend a visit to Dr. Mercola's website, http://articles.mercola.com/sites/articles/archive/2010/10/02/secrets-to-a-good-night-sleep.aspx. I have provided a summary below.

1. Sleep in complete darkness.
2. Keep the temperature of the bedroom less than 20°C (70°F).
3. Remove EMF fields (see the chapter on EMF).
4. Move alarm clocks from beside your bed to two meters or more away. Make the time difficult to see, as clock watching does not help you.
5. Consider a gentle dawn or light-increasing alarm clock.
6. Use your bed for sleeping, not for work or television.
7. If your partner or pet impairs your sleep, consider separate rooms.
8. Aim for bed about 10:00 p.m., no later than 11:00 p.m.
9. Keep a consistent bedtime.
10. Establish a bedtime routine.
11. Avoid fluids for two hours before bed.
12. Go to the toilet just before bed.
13. Avoid bedtime snacks, especially grains and sugars.
14. Take a hot bath, shower, or sauna before bed.
15. Try wearing socks to bed, as it may reduce night waking.
16. Wear an eye mask, if necessary.

. Quit your work one to two hours before bed.

18. No TV or blue light from the computer or smartphone screen before bed.

19. Listen to relaxing music.

20. Read a calming book or journal before bed to prevent your mind from racing.

21. Minimize drugs, avoid caffeine after midday, and avoid alcohol, as it costs you sleep during the night.

22. Exercise regularly.

23. If necessary, learn about EFT (Emotional Freedom Technique).

24. Increase your melatonin by exposure to bright sunshine or a full-spectrum fluorescent bulb in winter.

Section Four
Pharmacology

13: Anesthesia and Post-operative Cognitive Dysfunction

A general anesthetic affects brain function. I am sure that sounds like an outlandish or scary thought, but what if it were true? In my days as an academic anesthesiologist teaching residents in training and doing research on general anesthesia, I thought this was false. At that time, about 1990, I often encountered MS patients who were concerned about their pending surgery and anesthetic. I told them that they had nothing to worry about. I would answer differently today, more than twenty-five years later. At the same time, in the early 1990s, many of my anesthesia colleagues were anxious about using regional spinal, epidural, or nerve-block techniques in people who already had a neurological illness. When I reviewed the literature about MS and anesthesia or surgical impact at that time, the articles reinforced my statement. In summary, the belief was that there was no problem unless the patient developed a fever. The fever would exacerbate the symptoms of the existing neurological illness, which, in many cases, was MS. It is now well known that an injured brain or spinal cord does poorly in the presence of fever. Hence, MS patients are advised to avoid taking hot baths or spending time in a hot tub. In addition, most MS patients know that excess heat worsens their symptoms. Fever or excess heat in our surroundings may not cause an attack, but it can certainly aggravate symptoms. In those earlier days, my MS anesthetic patients listened to me, nodded appropriately, but were still concerned. Now I believe they were right, and I was wrong.

If you fast-forward some eight to twelve years later, I had my own general anesthetics for different fractures. This followed the diagnosis of my own MS in 1996. In 1998, I had a complex fracture of my right lower leg (tibia and fibula). This fracture occurred in a back alley off Davie Street in Vancouver, so I was taken to St. Paul's Hospital. No, I was not buying or selling drugs, as might be suggested by my location, I was trying out a recumbent bicycle! After thirty hours of waiting in the queue, my anesthetic flattened me. However, I was on many drugs, probably had a compound fracture (later developed osteomyelitis), and needed a bladder catheter to relieve urinary retention. In summary, I learned little about anesthetics and MS responses because of all the other issues involved.

Fast-forward to 2004, when I fractured my hand. This happened at home when I was kicked by an emu. I had to go to a nearby city to have my surgery (open reduction and internal fixation of a fractured metacarpal). The anesthesiologist I was assigned was young, keen, and well trained. He asked me my preference between regional nerve block and a general anesthetic. I chose the latter for two reasons. First, I still believed the standard diatribe about MS and anesthetics. Second, I knew that having an awake physician/patient in the room, especially an anesthesiologist, makes everyone anxious and uptight. No one performs optimally in this operating room milieu, so I chose a general anesthetic. I received just under an hour of general anesthesia using the most modern drugs of the time. Imagine my surprise when my brain felt like absolute crap for eight days thereafter! My thinking was sluggish, and my cognitive skills were further blunted, i.e., even worse than usual.

The science of brain function after surgery and anesthesia had advanced since the 1990s. However, my knowledge of it had not. When doing a literature search for this book, I found a superb review and discussion of this topic. It is written by Ann D. Liebert et al. of Australia and is from the *Journal of Experimental Neuroscience* (2016). The official term for this symptom complex is "postoperative cognitive dysfunction" (POCD). It is a neurodegenerative condition acquired after surgery and anesthesia and is similar to Alzheimer's disease in terms of symptoms and risk factors, such as age and education level (Fodale 2010).

POCD manifests often as a subtle deterioration in cognition, including a loss of the ability to perform everyday tasks. Does not that strike fear into you? It certainly does in me. Living independently and knowing who I am is part of what drives me to stay well.

POCD may affect several different functional components. These include memory, speed of information processing, orientation, concentration, psychomotor ability, fine motor skills, and attention span. This condition is suggested if suddenly you are unable to do crossword puzzles or Sudoku. It is diagnosed by a variety of neuropsychological testing. These are essentially the ones used to also diagnose MS cognitive problems and dementias, including Alzheimer's. It is suggested to wait at least a week after surgery, so immediate postoperative issues and most pain drugs are gone, because they can affect the outcome.

Major factors that influence POCD include age (greater than sixty years, although some use sixty-five or seventy years), preoperative cognitive condition, and education. Additional factors include length and complexity of surgery (cardiac surgery is riskier) and a history of alcohol abuse, previous stroke, diabetes mellitus, hypertension, athero-sclerosis, and postoperative complications, especially lung problems or postoperative infections. Women are more at risk than men, just as in Alzheimer's disease. Recent prospective studies have placed a risk in all people between 1.35 and 1.99 times normal, which is roughly double the risk of people without an anaesthetic.

Although age is a factor in POCD, the concern extends to young people as well. Since the risk of dementia increases with age, we must minimize the risk of dementia in several ways. First, we need to regain optimal health by controlling our personal risk factors. Second, we need to avoid unnecessary surgery or anesthesia. This latter problem can be minimized by having a regional component to your anesthetic. This improves your POCD risk, reduces postoperative pain, and speeds your recovery. In addition, it is now known that the "worry" of not doing a regional in the presence of a neurological illness, such as MS, is not a significant risk once the benefits are appreciated. In short, I believe the benefits outweigh the risks. Third, because the risk of dementia increases as we age in virtually all Western societies, we must work to minimize it. Otherwise, our health care system will implode. I hope you will choose some of the interventions mentioned in this book, such as oxygen therapy or PBMT (photobiomodulation therapy) preoperatively to reduce your risk of POCD.

The incidence or frequency of POCD is listed at 10-40 percent of people for one week after surgery and up to 15 percent after three months, if non-cardiac surgery. A major international study found that in patients over age 60, 26 percent had POCD at one week post operatively and 10 percent had POCD at three months. I believe this is too large a number to ignore. Recovery from POCD, though it will be slower, is similar to the recovery that occurs within hours after cortical spreading depression. This cortical spreading depression, a widespread depolarization of neurons, is the phenomenon that accompanies and follows migraines with or without aura and cluster headache. I am very familiar with this phenomenon, having experienced it a large number of times.

What causes POCD? This is almost certainly multifactorial, as is dementia. Contributing factors include inflammation, pain, and secondary illnesses. Particular risks are changes in cerebral blood flow, such as stroke or migraine, cardiopulmonary bypass, lack of oxygen in the blood, and microemboli (see chapter 20). Sleep disturbance after surgery is worsened by narcotic pain relief, which is also a significant risk factor.

POCD has similarities with other forms of dementia, including Alzheimer's. For this reason, the two areas frequently "collide" when an individual who already has some cognitive challenges needs surgery and anesthesia. The MS patients that I spoke of, including myself, are already in this category, as at least 70 percent of MS patients already have cognitive impairment.

The exact mechanism of anesthesia is still unclear. I should know this, having spent two full years in a neuropharmacology lab researching this in the 1980s. Relatively minimal progress in this field has occurred since. Many of the same receptors that general anesthetics block are known to affect memory. These include NMDA (N-methyl-D-aspartame) receptors, with ketamine and nitrous oxide, or enhancing GABA-A receptors with agents like isoflurane, desflurane, and possibly Propofol.

An expert group attending the British Journal of Anaesthesia seminar in Salzburg in 2012 reviewed POCD. They concluded that general anesthesia can reduce cognition in the elderly and the very young. The depth of anesthesia may have an impact, with deeper anesthesia causing more risk. Finally, elevation of inflammatory markers is a significant risk factor in POCD. Once again, an anti-inflammatory diet and lifestyle may be one of our best defenses. A further possibility is additional oxygen for up to twenty-four hours immediately postoperatively. Patients already receive oxygen with a mask in the recovery room, the post anesthesia care unit (PACU). If this was maintained for several hours, then the brain might recover better. Surgical wounds are known to heal better with additional oxygen postoperatively (Greif 2000).

14: Drugs: To Do or Not to Do

As a medical student, I was very naïve. I thought that once a physician determined a diagnosis, the correct drug would solve the problem and make the person well. This was quite a few years ago, as I was born in 1953, and the post-World War II era's thinking was "better living through better chemistry." Now I realize that this was a complete fallacy. Almost all drugs have a major downside or risk scenario, and often we need one or even two drugs to handle the side effects of the first drug. This has led to the fact, in North America, that people in their seventies or older, are on an average of ten to twelve drugs. This is definitely not healthy, because it creates potential drug interactions that may have huge costs to our health and well-being. Some drugs in particular bother me, and I will outline them here.

Before starting on a new prescription drug, I hope everyone asks, "Is this the best thing for me long term?" We must be very aware of the downsides or risk/benefit ratio of any medication that we take. Many drugs have significant downsides if they are used repeatedly or on an ongoing basis. I will give you several examples of these drugs. I will also describe a few drugs that you should probably never use. Again, I will discuss the risk/benefit ratio, which has been my practice ever since my training in anesthesiology and pharmacology.

When possible, I will give you references that you can read if you want to look into this further.

Even pharmacists, with their extensive drug knowledge, respect anesthesiologists for their drug wisdom. While I was in an academic position at the university, I held a joint appointment in pharmacology. I was one of the professors teaching courses to medical students and pharmacy students. The above experience, coupled with my prior four years in family practice and my twenty years since, which included my integrative medicine training at the University of Arizona and chronic pain treatment of patients, makes me very comfortable in making suggestions about medications.

NSAIDs and Aspirin

People with pain, especially headaches, usually begin here. These drugs, available to everyone over the counter (OTC), include ibuprofen (Advil and Motrin) and naproxen (Aleve). Many other NSAIDs are available by prescription only. These drugs work by reducing the number of prostaglandins in the body. Prostaglandins have the following functions: 1) promote inflammation toward healing, 2) support blood clotting, especially platelet stickiness or adhesion, 3) protect the stomach lining from stomach acid, 4) maintain the gut lining, reducing permeability and leaky gut syndrome, and 5) maintain healthy ovulation in women.

Whenever we take an NSAID, all the above prostaglandin effects are potentially jeopardized. Every year, a considerable number of people die secondary to gastrointestinal bleeds, triggered by NSAIDs. We also know that leaky gut syndrome, aggravated by NSAIDS, is a severe trigger of inflammation within the body. This affects not only the joints with arthritis but also the brain with potential changes in mood, memory loss, and even Parkinson's. One simple alternative to these drugs is turmeric. I suggest 1-2 g of turmeric extract, called curcumin, every 1-3 hours, as needed. The second alternative to NSAIDs is cannabis, another herb which may be optimal if it contains approximately equal amounts of THC and CBD.

Acetaminophen (Paracetamol)

According to the title of a 2013 article by Dr. Shaw, there is "Evidence that Increased Use [of acetaminophen] in Genetically Vulnerable Children Appears to be a Major Cause of the Epidemics of Autism, Attention Deficit with Hyperactivity, and Asthma" (Shaw 2013). In these people, the consequence of taking acetaminophen reduces the body's ability to detoxify many toxic chemicals in our environment, which increases oxidative stress, and then we need more antioxidants to counteract this. Acetaminophen also acts on the prostaglandins, somewhat similar to NSAIDs, and on the endocannabinoid system. (More on this can be found in chapter 16). New information confirms that when acetaminophen is combined with NSAIDs, the incidence of gastrointestinal bleeds increases accordingly. In addition, acetaminophen causes dose-related kidney injury. Finally, a considerable number of people die each year from acetaminophen overdose, secondary to liver failure. Acetaminophen is probably not the best choice for osteoarthritis knee pain or lower-back pain. One concern is its lack of benefit, but it also triggers a number of increased adverse cardiovascular events, similar to NSAIDs. It was reported in the *Lancet* in 2014 that up to 4 g of acetaminophen per day was no better in resolving back pain than a placebo. A similar lack of benefit was shown in osteoarthritis knee pain.

In summary, while it may be reasonable to reach for these occasionally, it is unwise to do it daily or even several times a week. Other alternatives should be sought. The discussion of these can be found in chapter 19.

Statins

To many of my medical colleagues, my view on statins will sound sacrilegious. In fact, I have a confession to make. In 1974, after learning that I had the highest cholesterol level in my medical school class, I studied this area intensively. In the last forty years, I have never taken a statin drug, even though my family doctor has suggested it to me numerous times. Happily, I have now been fully vindicated, as I believe statins do much more harm than good. Despite this, they have become the standard of care in cardiovascular disease and diabetes.

I suggest that we have been hoodwinked by the unfair use of statistics. In fact, if 100 people take regular statin drugs, they will only have one less heart attack than the same 100 people taking a placebo. This has been sold to us as a 50 percent reduction in heart attacks by using the term "relative risk." In reality, there is no such thing. This is well described in a 2015 paper from the journal *Expert Review of Clinical Pharmacology*. The name of the paper speaks for itself: "How statistical deception created the appearance that statins are safe and effective in primary and secondary prevention of cardiovascular disease" (Diamond 2015). In this article, they describe that drug promoters transform the 1 percent reduction using the term "relative risk" to suggest that there is a 30–50 percent reduction in myocardial infarction (heart attack). They also mention some 300 adverse side effects related to taking these drugs. These include muscle and nerve damage, reduced brain function, and an increased risk for diabetes mellitus, heart disease, and depression.

In addition, new evidence suggests that a low cholesterol level is linked to memory loss and depression and worsens symptoms of autism spectrum disorder. Low cholesterol is even associated with an increased amount of violence to oneself and others. Almost all body hormones have their base in the cholesterol molecule. Hence, we need it in our diet. The simplest way to increase our cholesterol intake is to eat an egg yolk, which is equivalent to 250 mg in pill form. Please, give up eating egg-white omelettes. An egg is as close to a perfect food that we have. I routinely eat three eggs for breakfast, and I recommend to my ninety-two-year-old mother that she have two eggs daily. (Women typically only need two eggs.)

Protein Pump Inhibitors

Nexium, Prilosec, Prevacid, and Protonix are drugs that reduce acid production in the stomach. They are designed to treat heartburn and upper-abdominal indigestion, which is also called gastroesophageal reflux disease (GERD). Their design and label suggest use for a maximum of twelve weeks. However, it seems that everybody forgets to read this. This twelve-week window is for your own safety and well-being. Prolonged use of the drug dramatically reduces your B12. In fact, the higher the dose of the protein pump inhibitor, the greater the B12 deficiency. B12 is critically important for optimal nerve and brain function, white blood cell production, and performance. It is also a factor in atherosclerosis. Taking protein pump inhibitors (PPIs) eliminates 99 percent of the stomach acid. However, we need acid for optimal digestion and absorption of food. Taking PPIs eliminates mineral absorption, including iron, selenium, zinc, magnesium, and calcium. A side effect of long-term use of PPIs is worsening osteoporosis. In addition, PPIs dramatically alter the gut flora, your microbiome, for the worse. This occurs even within one week of taking these drugs.

A multitude of solutions exist to help replace PPIs. One secret is to eliminate gluten in your diet. Regular use of digestive enzymes is another option. These are particularly helpful for breaking down fats, which often reduce the closing of the valve at the bottom of the esophagus. Years ago, I learned I could still eat chocolate without heartburn if I took one of these enzymes. Now I rarely need extra enzymes, because I use a lot of probiotics and follow a gluten-free diet. Some people have tremendous success by taking either apple cider vinegar or aloe vera juice regularly.

It is unlikely that you will be able to stop taking protein pump inhibitors suddenly or "cold turkey". Unfortunately, these drugs only come in one size and are quite difficult to taper or reduce gradually. Another alternative is to switch to ranitidine, 150 mg gradually or one day per week. After seven weeks, you will be on ranitidine only. Then you can start to taper these every second day until you're able to get down to a much lower amount. During this time, you should use your alternative treatment methods. This may seem tedious, but is well worth it for long-term health benefits.

Steroids

You may know these better as prednisone, Decadron, or methylprednisolone. The brothers William James and Charles Horace Mayo, both doctors, founded the renowned Mayo Clinic and they received the Nobel prize in the early 1950s for their discovery and use of prednisone.Of course, humans produce a corticosteroid, called cortisol. In fact, Addison's disease is caused by almost a complete lack of cortisol, which is life threatening. Our cortisol is made inside our adrenal glands, and an increased amount is made during times of stress. However, the same glands can quit making cortisol when the body is regularly given corticosteroids as medication. This is why it is critical to taper off these medications gradually and your clinician will help you do this once you are feeling better.

Corticosteroids are best used for a few days of acute treatment. They are almost never helpful in a long-term chronic illness. Steroids are particularly useful in acute, life-threatening, upper-airway swelling or asthma attack. Occasionally, corticosteroids are useful in an acute brain swelling. However, corticosteroids have been shown to be of zero long-term benefit in arthritis, MS, or brain trauma. Yes, zero benefit in the long term! Even though they are still used in three-day bursts in MS or even monthly, supposedly to prevent attacks. I know several MS patients who have lost their hip joint as a secondary side effect to the steroids they were given. My stance on MS attacks and corticosteroids is unchanged from my earlier book. I suggest that if you wake up and are blind from an MS attack, have no help from a spouse, family, or friends, and have two small children under your care, then use corticosteroids in this acute phase. Otherwise, I suggest you avoid them.

More than twenty years ago, when I was in active anesthesia practice, I did epidural injections for back pain using the long-acting corticosteroid methylprednisolone. Knowing what I know now about other modalities, I would not do these epidural injections. They may help initially, but they will not last. Relief will be shorter and shorter in duration, and you still run the risk of losing your hip joint and worsening your osteoporosis risk.

Immune Modulators

Because this book is about the brain and nervous system problems, I will confine this commentary to the drugs that have been used in MS-relapsing remitting patients for over twenty years. These include the interferons 1a (Avonex and Rebif), 1b (Betaseron), and glatimer acetate (Copaxone). These drugs cost $20,000–$40,000 per year.

Three comprehensive reviews, including one by Dr. Ebers at Oxford, UK, have confirmed that these drugs do not delay the onset of disability in people with MS (see www.mshope.com). Hence, they have no real upside but have considerable side effects, including fatigue, depression, and increased risk of cancer. This poor risk/benefit ratio seems obvious; however, these drugs are still prescribed today for young MS patients. I believe this is a travesty perpetuated by lack of knowledge and aggressive marketing. In 2017, Matt Embry produced a superb documentary film called *Living Proof*, which is a no-holds-barred exposure of MS drugs. You can find more information at his website, www.mshope.com. Please, watch the film. One of the stars is Dr. Ebers, mentioned above, now retired.

The final drug I would like to mention is natalizumab (Tysabri). This drug was first released in 2005 for some patients with MS and then withdrawn within a year, as a number of people developed PML (progressive multifocal leukoencephalopathy). This is a disease of the white matter of the brain, which can cause vision loss, weakness, and even death. Thirty to 50 percent of people will die within months of diagnosis of PML, and the rest may face serious permanent disability. As of September 7, 2016, 683 patients with MS have been diagnosed with PML after receiving Tysabri. The drug was reintroduced in 2006 with strict prescribing guidelines, which stated that patients could only be on it for two years. Then they must have recurrent testing to see if they are developing antibodies to the Jacob-Creutzfeldt virus. This drug has not cured MS in anyone. I suggest the poor risk/benefit ratio is obvious and would not take it, as we have a considerable number of other avenues to walk down, albeit without drugs.

Opioids/Narcotics

The original opioids were from the opium poppy. These include morphine, heroin, and codeine. Codeine is changed into morphine within the body, and this accounts for some people's extra sensitivity to this agent. Some fifty years ago, the first narcotics were synthesized, the first one being meperidine/pethidine (Demerol) in the UK. Later, in the 1970s, fentanyl was synthesized, and it was particularly popular within anesthesiology. When I trained in anesthesiology in Calgary in the 1980s, I was nicknamed one of the "fentanyl twins," because I found that if I used a considerable amount of it during anesthetics, I could almost always wake up the patient pain free.

Later, a number of derivatives of fentanyl were developed, including one called carfentanil, which is incredibly potent. A tiny amount on the end of a dart is enough to anesthetize a polar bear or an elephant. It has become the gold standard as far as a mu-opioid agonist by pharmacologists and works at such a low concentration as Avogadro's number. Avogadro's number is 6.02 times the twenty-third power, so a very large dilution. In 1811, Avogadro first proposed that the volume of a gas is proportional to the number of atoms or molecules, regardless of the nature of the gas. The potency of carfentanil enabled me to understand how homeopathy could be much more effective than a regular allopathic physician had suggested. Opioids are terribly addictive and quite lethal, because they cause a depressed respiration in the brainstem, resulting in death. One of the biggest crises within regular medicine today is addiction from prescription drugs, particularly opioids. This has been magnified recently, because carfentanil has been synthesized illegally and is available on the black market. This is causing a huge number of deaths over and above what were already occurring. It is difficult to control drug action when it is this potent. It is estimated that a few grams or ounces could anesthetize four million people.

What can we learn from this, and how might we counteract this huge problem? One method is enhanced education about the use and non-use of opioids in the treatment of acute pain, especially chronic pain. Opioids do not work well in chronic pain, but many physicians are not aware of alternatives. For many years, I have advocated to physicians and dentists to use a combination of NSAIDs and acetaminophen in place of two codeine/acetaminophen tablets. The equivalent dose would be Ibuprofen 400 mg and acetaminophen 1,000 mg. This would work in most short-term acute pain situations. Another straightforward solution is the use of cannabis extracts. (I talk about this in detail in chapter 17. I have already mentioned turmeric with the extract of curcumin when talking about NSAIDs.) Finally, I encourage physicians to learn more about other modalities, such as photobiomodulation therapy (PBMT), discussed at the end of chapter 19 and in its own chapter as well.

Low-dose Naltrexone (LDN)

Before leaving opioids, I want to mention an opioid antagonist, low-dose naltrexone (LDN). It can have useful attributes in chronic illnesses, such as AIDS, cancer, MS, and fibromyalgia (Younger 2014) and inflammatory bowel disease. Patients with these chronic illnesses have low circulating endogenous opiates, met-enkephalin, and beta-endorphin. LDN triggers the body to produce more of these. Naltrexone typically comes in a 50 mg tablet. Low-dose naltrexone is prepared by a compounding pharmacy in capsule or liquid form, creating from 0.5 mg to 4.5 mg naltrexone. LDN is taken at bedtime. In chronic illness, the circulating endogenous opioids are usually depressed to around 20–25 percent of normal. By giving this small dose of antagonist (LDN), the body creates more of the endogenous opioids. This typically enhances one's feeling of well-being, modulates the immune system, and usually improves quality of life. I have used LDN in a large number of people with chronic illness, with virtually no downside. In addition, complications are rare, and I reassure patients that this small dose will not affect the regular use of opioids. I realize many physicians are not aware of this, and they fear it will block any opioids they prescribe. This is not the case. In fact, some of the new oral opioids combine either of the two antagonists, naloxone or naltrexone, with a strong opioid to minimize the side effect of constipation when these are given together orally.

Anesthetic Drugs

Before ending this section on drugs, I want include a discussion about anesthesiology and its general anesthetics, including isoflurane, desflurane, and the earlier prototypes, halothane and ether. These agents are not as fully reversible as we had hoped. Their effects can linger for months and may even be permanent in some. Please read chapter 13 for a better understanding of this.

In summary, I hope my discussion helps you work at your diet and lifestyle changes, so you need fewer drugs. Your brain and the rest of your body will certainly appreciate this in the long term.

15: Benzodiazepines, Antidepressants, Sleep Medications, and Point of Return Withdrawal Wisdom

As stated previously, I took prescribed antidepressants for almost twenty years. My first prescription was for imipramine, the original tricyclic antidepressant, which I began at age twenty-eight. At that time, Denise and I had two young sons and were living in a small town in Saskatchewan. I was one of three busy family medicine practitioners. My practice included emergency room work, administration, family practice, and a heavy obstetrics load. Also, I was the sole practitioner for anaesthesia.

I was diagnosed with depression by a young psychiatrist in Saskatoon. The initial prescription plan was to take an antidepressant for six to twelve months and then taper off. I did this and was drug free after twelve months. My well-being was reasonable until our daughter was born. Denise developed a postpartum depression a few months later. Some months after that, my depression returned. I am told this is not uncommon when the initial challenges of the caregiver, in this case me, are resolved. Once again, a psychiatrist started me on imipramine. By that time we were living in Calgary, and I was part of the anaesthesiology residency training program. Denise and I were both working full-time with three young children, ages one, four, and six.

The Calgary psychiatrist felt I might be a bipolar depressive and suggested adding lithium to the imipramine. The feeling at that time was that a patient with a two-year cycle of bipolar depression would have less of a recurrence problem with lithium. After three years on both medicines, several changes occurred. First, my imipramine was increased twice and was at 250 mg at bedtime. This is a relatively large dose. Several years later when I had genetic testing done for my metabolism, I found that I was a rapid metabolizer of this group of drugs. This individual variation of drug metabolism is now much better understood, and many labs can test for this. This can be an incredible assist for safety in many drugs and should be considered as an option whenever someone has an unusual response to any drug. I use Great Plains Labs for this, but there are many choices, and the team at Point of Return can suggest other lab choices. Second, I developed a considerable tremor in my right side, which was especially evident when I was holding a long needle with one hand. This did not instill confidence in the operating room! When I talked this over with my psychiatrist, he stopped the lithium. Fortunately, he recognized that the potential benefit of the lithium was outweighed by its cost or side effects. I was able to stop the lithium "cold turkey" and did not suffer any significant withdrawal problems. Not everyone is so fortunate. Now, many years later, I take a much smaller dose of lithium, 10 mg per day versus 600 mg per day, with no tremor.

I was still on imipramine when my world was turned upside down with a diagnosis of MS in August 1996. I had to leave the practice of anaesthesiology to permit some recovery. After several months, I made enough progress to make another attempt at working in the operating room. However, that trial ended after three weeks as my symptoms of MS worsened.

Some years later, I began taking a quality whey protein and successfully reduced my fatigue. Because of the benefits I experienced from this whey product, I began giving a number of talks on this topic around North America. In 2005, I was asked to meet two young women in California who used a similar whey protein in their business. One of these women, Alessandra Rain, had written a book, *Deeds of Trust* (2005), about her own challenging journey withdrawing from a large number of psychiatric medications. She joined efforts with another young woman, Andrea Crocker, to form Point of Return, a non-profit organization dedicated to helping others in a gradual and safe tapering method from antidepressants, tranquilizers, and sleep medications. They connect online or by phone, counselling individuals on how they can gradually taper off these drugs one at a time. The use of supplements and ongoing personal support are important elements to success. Every client remains under the care of his or her own health care practitioner. Their model is to use some key supplements to help restore body health through detoxification.

Before starting people on their withdrawal program, they use a number of supplements and protocols to optimize the individual's metabolism. Clients begin by taking an individualized amount of the Point of Return quality bioactive whey protein, Support. This is not a standard whey protein but one that contains an increased amount of the amino acid cysteine and is well absorbed into the body. Cysteine is the rate-limiting step of the three amino acids required for the cells to build glutathione. Glutathione is present in the highest amounts in the liver, kidneys, and lungs. In fact, glutathione is present in every human cell. It helps the cells break down or remove any potentially damaging toxin. This includes most drugs and all the psychiatric drugs that I have mentioned, including antidepressants, tranquilizers, and most sleep medications. Prior to withdrawal, individuals are advised to take a high-quality fish oil supplement with large amounts of DHA and EPA. This is important for several reasons. First, these oils help stabilize the cell membranes, especially in the brain, as these are primarily omega-3 based. Second, omega-3 oils are anti-inflammatory. This is fitting, seeing as depression and anxiety are occasionally called the "brain on fire" (inflamed brain). Third, the omega-3 oils on their own frequently help reduce depression and anxiety.

Initially, Alessandra and Andrea wrote a manual, and then a book, in which I contributed a portion. This book is called *Point of Return* (Rain 2006). It includes a description of many foods and supplements that might interfere with the withdrawal process. In addition, they describe the benefits of their whey protein product, encapsulated fish oils, melatonin in a cherry extract, and a protein from casein that helps people relax. This book and the Point of Return protocol can be found at their website, www.pointofreturn.com. When I first met Alessandra and Andrea, they had already helped hundreds of patients. Now, several years later, they've helped over 20,000 people on their journey. Alessandra and Andrea have assisted people in their withdrawal from opiates and antipsychotics on a case-by-case basis. Point of Return provides frequent contact by telephone or email to assist clients down an often lonely and bumpy road.

Alessandra and Andrea were interested in hearing my personal journey with antidepressant medication. They asked me to work with them partly because of my own health journey and also because of my interest in an integrative medicine approach. I felt there was a good synergy within this, as many people with a chronic health journey end up on psychiatric medication, which, on occasion, becomes part of the problem. By this time, I wondered if I had been truly depressed or if it was some of the early severe fatigue and cognitive problems were early MS or even hypothyroidism.

Any brain illness can show some of these same symptoms of fatigue and cognitive problems. In fact, most people with MS end up on antidepressants and sleep medication. An additional medication used in MS is clonazepam to reduce muscle contractions and spasms. Unfortunately, few people knew that clonazepam, marketed as a muscle relaxant, is a close cousin to Valium. The generic name for Valium is diazepam. This group of drugs, benzodiazepines, is especially addicting and one of the hardest from which to withdraw. It is now established by the work of Professor C. Heather Ashton, DM, FRCP, from Newcastle upon Tyne in England that it is best to taper this drug by 5 percent per week and occasionally by 2.5 percent per week. Sleep medication is in this same group as benzodiazepines with similar challenges of addiction. It is interesting to note that sleep medications do not provide truly restful sleep. Individuals who take them often feel that they have slept better, but in reality, the drug is helping them to forget the times that they woke up!

Antidepressant medications can often be tapered at 10 percent per week. However, most of these medications are available in one or two dosages. How does one taper 10 percent per week? The safest and best answer is with the assistance of a compounding pharmacist. However, patients must convince their doctor about the need for this decision. It is not always an easy task. If the individual is able to find a trained integrative medicine or functional medicine physician, they are more likely to obtain help for a gradual tapering off of their medication. Hopefully, this same clinician can help resolve the problem that triggered the prescription. Medications can interact and can affect taper rates, so an even slower taper may be required. An example of this is the fact that Ambien increases lorazepam, so standard taper rates might be too fast, as the individual can be essentially feeling withdrawals from two drugs even though they are only tapering one at the time.

For this reason, it is helpful to have an experienced guide in this process. Not much of this wisdom exists among physicians or even pharmacists, so Point of Return is often a helpful starting place.

My own experience with the antidepressant imipramine has taught me the advantages of a slow taper. If I ever forgot my medication, I would spend a terribly restless night with graphic dreams and unpleasant feelings. These side effects could be minimized at a taper of 10 percent per week. The same holds true for most antidepressants, although some drugs are more challenging to withdraw from than others. However, the experience and ongoing support by Alessandra and Andrea helps most people through these difficult times.

Since the start of Point of Return, we have seen the ongoing development of integrative and functional medicine throughout North America and the world. Both groups are entry points for physicians for the newest specialty in the USA, integrative medicine. Please refer to chapter 26 to learn why fewer people may need these antidepressants, tranquilizers, and sleep medications. I believe it is much better to peel away the layers of the onion and solve the underlying problem than to add a drug "Band-Aid" to mask the symptoms.

Over time, Alessandra and Andrea have increasingly suggested that their clients have genetic testing if they have particular problems in their withdrawal process. The science has moved forward tremendously in the last fifteen years. We can now determine the ability of an individual's body to break down drugs and, hence, their individual tolerance. This allows for more appropriate individualized dosing of medication. An example of this is a generally healthy woman, aged fifty-five years old, who just lost a loved one and was having major problems sleeping during the grieving process. She was prescribed a small number of sleeping tablets. She took one and developed a psychotic episode. This episode was severe enough that she was admitted to a psychiatric hospital. This psychotic episode was the first and only one in her entire life, suggesting it was drug-induced. You may think this is a rare event related to prescription drugs, but it is not.

Genetic studies of the metabolism of a new medication are done on humans exposed to the drug. This helps the drug company determine how the drug is handled and metabolized. It is also how the knowledge of the response of the drug, as well as its side effect profile, are determined. All this knowledge is required before acceptance by the FDA, Health Canada, or equivalent governing bodies. Because of many years of testing, we know that approximately 7 percent of people will not be able to metabolize these drugs in the normal fashion. Consequently, these people have a profound, usually negative, response after a single dose or a few doses of the medication. This creates huge problems for that individual. Often their health care practitioner does not believe the adverse reaction has occurred. Unfortunately, this fact is rarely known by either family medicine practitioners or many other medical specialists, including psychiatrists.

Several different paths have led us to the large number of these medications being prescribed. These include hypothyroidism, grief, personal trauma, body inflammation, and even variations in sex hormones. Low testosterone is often a precipitating feature in men. Similarly, estrogen and progesterone irregularities in women are a frequent source of mood problems. This can be aggravated as simply as starting on oral contraceptives or the insertion of a hormone-containing IUD (intra-uterine device).

Hormone-replacement therapy became the next panacea for perimenopausal women in the 1980s. Pharmaceutical companies started to use pregnant mares' urine (PMU) as a source of estrogen and progesterone. They packaged this into pills and gave it to millions of women. Unfortunately, this does not simulate the natural hormones. Consequently, women on hormone-replacement therapy sustained much higher risks of heart disease and cardiovascular disease, including stroke. Also, many women became obese. Finally, many developed secondary mood and sleep challenges.

Now we realize that female sex hormones, in excess, have long-term negative impacts. This can include anxiety and depression. So began another part of the story of "better living through better chemistry" from the 1950s. Initially, we solved the anxiety problems with barbiturates, such as Tuinal. Then in the 1960s, pharmaceutical companies released drugs called Librium and Valium. These last two drugs were from the benzodiazepines family. All these drugs were initially presented and promoted as being safe and non-addictive. Soon we realized that nothing was further from the truth. Some readers will remember the book *Valley of the Dolls,* which graphically told about the perils of these drugs.

The first antidepressants, MAOIs (monoamine oxidase inhibitors), and tricyclic antidepressants had some unpleasant and even dangerous side effects. Psychiatrists used them with considerable discretion. However, the floodgates opened once Prozac, the early prototype for SSRIs (serotonin selective reuptake inhibitors) arrived on the scene. Many will recognize serotonin as the "feel good" hormone. Another group of drugs are SNRIs (serotonin norepinephrine reuptake inhibitors, or if in Canada or the UK, serotonin noradrenaline reuptake inhibitors). They help elevate serotonin and noradrenaline. They are not just used as an antidepressant or antianxiety drug. Other indications are: OCD (obsessive-compulsive disorder), ADHD, chronic neuropathic pain, fibromyalgia, and relief of menopausal symptoms. Some of these drugs are even recommended for gastrointestinal problems, such as irritable bowel syndrome. These latter two drug groups were welcomed and promoted with reckless abandon. In the last two decades, millions of people in North America have been started on these medications.

Today, nearly 30 percent of all people are on an antidepressant at some point in their life. Nearly a third of women in the perimenopausal time in their life, between forty and fifty-five years of age, are on an antidepressant. Even our young people are not left out, with 5-10 percent of them on one of these agents.

Now that I have described how we got into this mess with tranquilizers, barbiturates, benzodiazepines, and antidepressants (SSRIs and SNRIs) you will understand the importance and value of the Point of Return organization. We know that if you are on such ongoing medications, the brain cells adapt. In fact, the cells add a large number of receptors in an effort to maintain their normal function. The new norm is a brain continually bathed in the medication. Therefore, if you withdraw suddenly from this status quo, your brain goes through some very unpleasant side effects. These can vary from headaches to anxiety, depression, gastrointestinal problems, and even shooting electrical pains (brain zaps) and sleeplessness. Slow and careful tapering off of these medications minimizes the problems of withdrawal. It may still be a significant challenge, but it is certainly much more tolerable. Such gradual reduction, along with the assistance of informed people, means withdrawal can be done at home. Almost all the Point of Return clients (more than 20,000), have been able to do this at home with the help of their health care practitioner. A similar protocol can be followed for withdrawing from sleep medications.

16: Cannabis

You may wonder why I talk about cannabis when I talk about brain recovery. One compelling reason is that virtually no new medications are being produced or even researched to assist in brain recovery. The major pharmaceutical companies have determined that this is a non-fruitful road to travel after decades of trying. Hence, I suggest it is time to look at old established choices, particularly cannabis. My goal is to help you understand how cannabis is used by the body, including the brain. Research in the last few decades has shown us the body's own "inside the body" or endocannabinoid system (ECS). Also, this system is one of our major neuroprotective components when we sustain a stroke or a traumatic brain injury. In this chapter, you will learn many items that, even though they are well researched, are not uppermost in the minds of many Canadians, Americans, or even Europeans. You will also learn how this important herb might be a powerful addition to your personal wellness toolbox.

Cannabis as Medicine: A Rich History

The history of cannabis for medical use is long and has occurred in almost every civilized culture to date. In Siberia, cannabis seeds have been found inside burial mounds dating back to 3,000 BC. Because the plant originated in Asia, it is not surprising that the Chinese were the first to use cannabis as medicine. In 2,037 BC, Shen Neng, often described as the father of Chinese medicine, wrote about some 100 different ailments that cannabis helped. He is also believed to have been the first to write about ginseng, ephedra, and tea. Shen Neng described cannabis as possessing both yin and yang. This is consistent with its ability to be stimulating and calming. According to ancient Chinese medicine, cannabis was described as being analgesic (pain relief) and helpful in childbirth as an anaesthetic, and providing relief from migraines, indigestion, and insomnia.

Cannabis was used widely on the Indian subcontinent. Ayurvedic medicine (a system of healing originating in ancient India) mentions cannabis in its original materia medica between 1,100 to 1,700 BC. The materia medica described the cannabis resin as being like a narcotic but without causing nausea, constipation, or headache, as opium does. The Egyptians' materia medica, Ebers Papyrus, written in approximately 1,550 BC, also included cannabis. Cannabis pollen was also found on the mummy of Ramses II. Much later, Spanish explorers were credited with taking cannabis to Chile in 1545. In fact, the British mandated the growing of hemp in most colonies, because it was required for sails and rigging and, therefore, critical to their navy.

Cannabis was also introduced in North America. George Washington grew hemp on Mount Vernon. Thomas Jefferson grew hemp as well. Always the economist, Jefferson stated that hemp was of the first necessity to the wealth and protection of the country. Once again, he was addressing the ropes and sails of warships. Nothing has ever replaced this powerful plant fibre, which comes from the cannabis plant. The early *Cannabis sativa* grew up to fourteen feet high and was composed of strong, long, and powerful fibres.

In 1804, Napoleon and his soldiers were credited with bringing cannabis back to France from Egypt. Then, in 1839, William Brooke O' Shaughnessy, an Irish physician working on the telegraph across India, reintroduced cannabis to Britain. Sir Russell Reynolds wrote glowingly about cannabis in *The Lancet* in 1894. He described cannabis as the treatment of choice for Queen Victoria for her dysmenorrhea (menstrual cramping). At approximately the same time, Sir William Osler (1849–1919), one of the four physicians who founded Johns Hopkins in Baltimore, wrote in his famous book, the *Principles and Practice of Medicine*, that cannabis was the best treatment for migraine headaches. Osler is deemed by many to be the father of medicine in North America, and, as a Canadian, I am proud to tell you that he was from Canada.

This era was certainly the peak of cannabis use within medicine in the United States. It became a popular component within patent medicines, which were huge in the United States between 1825 and 1915. In the 1920s alone, physicians wrote 3 million prescriptions per year that contained cannabis. In 1927, J.P. Remington's *The Science and Practice of Pharmacy* described cannabis as an analgesic and calmative.

Everything started to change after the Flexner report, funded by the Carnegie family, which suggested that herbal medicine was not as modern or standardized as pharmaceuticals. This report boosted the rise of allopathic medicine and the decline of herbalists, homeopaths, and patent medicines. This, along with the wish to tax hemp, coupled with prohibition issues, paved the way for the Marijuana Tax Act of 1937. This legislation was masterminded by Harry Anslinger, who was the director of the Federal Bureau of Narcotics from its creation in 1931 until 1962. He testified in Congress that marijuana was the most violence-causing drug in the history of humankind. This was an entire fabrication, "fake news," but very successful politically. The American Medical Association opposed the marijuana tax, because there was no objective evidence for its harmful effects. Despite this, the act was passed.

The Marijuana Tax Act made it cumbersome but not illegal to use cannabis in medicine. However, its impact was tremendous. In 1943, cannabis was removed from the US pharmacopeia, and this reinforced the notion that cannabis was not a useful therapy. In 1944, Mayor LaGuardia of New York commissioned an investigation into the reality of the potential risks and benefits of cannabis. This report stated that cannabis was not associated with any increased risk of criminal activity, addiction, or insanity, as had been claimed. Although there was no real basis for Anslinger's statements, he was able to minimize the contribution of cannabis to medicine and research for nearly seventy-five years! Consequently, until recently, most of the research has been done outside the United States and Canada.

It wasn't until 1949 that research into cannabis began again with the publishing of a paper by H.H. Ramsay, MD, and Jean Davis, MD. They wrote about the value of using cannabis for intractable seizures, helping five of the seven in the study.

In 1964, Rafael Mechoulam, PhD, at Hebrew University in Israel, characterized the structure of delta nine THC. This dedicated and brilliant scientist went on to discover the first cannabinoid receptor on the surface of human cells in 1988 and named it CB1. This discovery resulted in an explosion of information. Mechoulam and other scientists have helped transform cannabis's 6,000-year history of medical use into a modern understanding to how it acts on the human body.

In 1970, marijuana was classified as a Schedule 1 drug in the USA. Other Schedule 1 drugs include heroin, LSD, mescaline, and most recently, gamma-hydroxybutyrate. Schedule 1 drugs are distinguished as having no accepted medical use. In addition, they are substances with a high potential for abuse. The 1970 Act further stymied the investigation and research of cannabis as a medical therapy in the United States and Canada. Fortunately, other countries continued to research cannabis and this led to significant breakthroughs.

Different countries have demonstrated a variety of responses to the cannabis plant. Uruguay has legalized marijuana, and Portugal has decriminalized it. Israel, Canada, and the Netherlands have all developed medical marijuana programs. These have been extremely successful. In Canada, I have been one of the small number of physicians, about 16 percent, willing to use medical marijuana in my treatment of chronic pain, neuropathic pain, muscular spasms, and in many brain injuries, including MS. Each of these treatments has been validated as recently as June 2015 in the *Journal of the American Medical Association* (Whiting et al. 2015). It stated there was sufficient medical evidence for this type of practice. Another article in this same journal, June 2015, outlined that one-half of the fifty states in the United States had either a medical marijuana program or a recreational use permit. Today, twenty-nine out of fifty states have medical marijuana programs. California, Washington, Colorado, and Oregon permit recreational purchase as well. This is probably where Canada will be in late 2018 as the current Government has committed to legalizing marijuana for recreational use.

The "Inside the Body" Endocannabinoid System

Humans and almost all animals, including some invertebrates, have two cannabis receptors within the body. This interaction of cannabinoids within the body and its receptors is known as the endocannabinoid system (eCB). In this section, you will learn the difference between endocannabinoids, phyto-cannabinoids, and synthetic cannabinoids, taking you on a journey that will help you understand why cannabis can help treat some of our most difficult conditions. These include chronic pain, particularly neuropathic pain, migraines, epileptic seizures, major depression, bipolar illness, and MS—including MS-related pain, spasticity, and headaches. I will help you understand how cannabis can help reset or optimize neuroplasticity or how the brain is able to change itself.

Modern acceptance of the role of cannabis within medicine changed dramatically in 1988 with the discovery of the CB1 receptor in mammals. This has since been confirmed to occur in humans and almost all animals, including a number of invertebrates. Soon after, in 1993, a second cannabinoid receptor, CB2, was discovered. The discovery of these two internal cannabinoid receptors put cannabis on a foundation similar to the importance of the three opioid receptors: mu, kappa, and delta.

Just as the body has internal opioids or endorphins, namely beta-endorphin and met-enkephalin, we now know of two inside-the-body cannabinoids, i.e., endocannabinoids. The first of these was found in 1992 and was called anandamide (AEA), after the Sanskrit word for "bliss." We now know that exercise elevates AEA. This may be the best explanation for the "runner's high." This AEA molecule plays a role in basic functions, such as memory, balance, movement, immune health, and neuroprotection.

A few years later, the second endocannabinoid, 2-arachidonoylglycerol (2-AG), was discovered. AEA works primarily on CB1 receptors, and 2-AG works primarily on CB2 receptors. Research on this entire system and on the cannabis plant with its components and even the synthetic cannabinoids has taken us from 6 scientific citations in 1993 to more than 6,000 in 2014.

CB1 receptors are found primarily in the central nervous system (brain and spinal cord), the reproductive system, and in connective tissue. In the brain, the largest concentrations are in the basal ganglia, cerebellum, hippocampus, and cerebral cortex. The major focus of the body for this receptor is in the central nervous system and peripheral nerves. There is almost a complete absence of any cannabinoid receptors in the brainstem. This area is responsible for breathing and heart control. The absence of cannabinoid receptors means there is almost no lethal dose from these agents. This makes them much safer than many drugs, such as opioids, benzodiazepines, and barbiturates. The CB1 receptors interact with the brain through a G protein-coupling mechanism. CB1 receptors account for short-term memory, cognition, mood and emotion, motor function, and nociception (unpleasant sensations).

CB2 receptors are generally much more widely distributed throughout the body. When it was first identified in 1993, it was initially found in the gut of dogs. The highest concentration of CB2 receptors is located on B lymphocytes and natural killer cells, suggesting a significant role in immunity. CB2 is very important in immune modulation, inhibiting inflammation, reducing visceral pain, and in controlling gut motility, especially in the inflamed gut.

Both endocannabinoids, AEA and 2-AG, often work in synergy throughout the body to control many functions. These functions include neuroprotection, autonomic regulation (blood pressure and pulse control), antinociception (reversing unpleasant sensations), and even retrograde synaptic transmission (a feedback loop on neuron-to-neuron transmission). The endocannabinoids also work in synergy with the opioid system and improve bone replacement, combatting osteoporosis. The endocannabinoids have a similar benefit in preventing cartilage destruction, reducing connective tissue inflammation, and even dampening the inflammatory component of atherosclerosis (hardening of blood vessels). The synergy with the opioid system is dramatic, as ingestion of cannabis will enhance the action of opioids by four to ten times!

Pharmacology of Plant-based Cannabinoids

A significant resource for this section is the excellent review by Ethan B. Russo and Jahan Marcu in *Advances in Pharmacology* (Russo 2017). In addition, I want to credit much of the following information to the excellent presentation at The Medical Cannabis Institute (TMCI) by Laura M. Borgelt, Doctor of Pharmacology. She initially spoke about the current drugs available in the United States, namely Marinol, the derivative of delta nine THC, which is a Schedule 3 drug. Next, she talked about Sativex, which is a drug composed of 50 percent THC and 50 percent CBD. Each spray releases 2.7 mg of THC and 2.5 mg of CBD. It is documented to be helpful in MS spasms and neuropathic pain. Sativex is available by pharmacy prescription in over twenty countries, including Canada. I suggest this is a reasonable starting point for people living in those sixteen countries to determine whether cannabis might help them.

Dr. Borgelt goes on to discuss the cannabis plant, which has more than sixty active compounds. Each compound has a partial effect on the others and this is probably why there are fewer problems with psychoactive side effects when a component of the whole cannabis plant is used. Dr. Mechoulam, Dr. Ethan Russo, and others like to emphasize the "entourage effect." This describes the interactive synergy between the multiple compounds within the whole cannabis plant. This includes THC, CBD, other cannabinoids, terpenes, and others. I liken this to the benefits of eating whole foods rather than just part of the whole food, as in processed foods. This is the secret to optimal health, including cannabis, which can be used as an excellent green vegetable.

THC

THC is the most well-studied cannabinoid, with more than 100 published articles. THC is produced in the cannabis plant via an allele codominant with CBD (cannabidiol). THC acts on both the CB1 and CB2 receptors, which explains its activities in modulating pain, spasticity, sedation, appetite, and mood. In addition, it is a bronchodilator and widens airways, as in asthma. Furthermore, THC is a neuroprotective antioxidant (more powerful than vitamins C and E), is anti-itching in jaundice (yellow skin from liver disease), and has twenty times the anti-inflammatory power of Aspirin and twice that of hydrocortisone.

The key psychoactive and appetite stimulation target for THC is the CB1 receptor. AEA is the body's cannabinoid, which acts primarily at this receptor, which is mostly in the brain and the nerves. The CB1 receptor is also found in the eye, gut, nervous system, immune system (bone marrow, thymus, spleen, and tonsils), and many other organs. THC's action at the CB2 receptor is associated with pain relief and anti-inflammatory activities. The CB2 receptor is also prevalent in the immune system but especially in B lymphocytes, monocytes, natural killer cells, mast cells, and large white blood cells, including the brain's white blood cells, the microglial. The number of CB2 receptors increases significantly during inflammation or injury. See the possibility of cannabinoids to help traumatic brain injury, stroke, MS, Alzheimer's, and Parkinson's in their respective chapters.

Now I would like to discuss the relatively non-psychotropic, that is,much less psychoactive, cannabinoids. To assist in this, I will include the pie chart that I frequently share with patients. It is from a 2009 *Trends in Pharmacology* article (Izzo 2009).

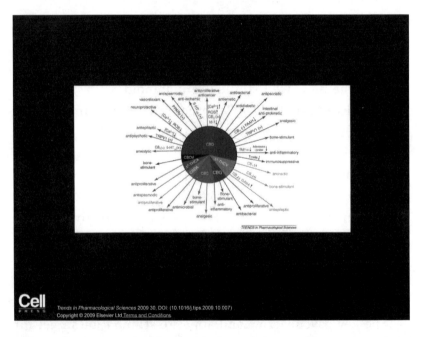

Trends in Pharmacological Sciences 2009 30, DOI: (10.1016/j.tips.2009.10.007)
Copyright © 2009 Elsevier Ltd Terms and Conditions

Pharmacological actions of non-psychotropic cannabinoids (with the indication of the preoposed mechanisims of action) Abbreviations: D9-THC, D9-tetrahydrocannabinol; D8-THC, D8-tetrahydrocannabinol; cannabinol; CBD, cannabidiol; D9-THCV, D9-tetrahydrocannabivarin; CBC, cannabichromene; CBG, cannabigerol; D9-THCA, D9-tetrahydrocannabinolic acid; CBDA, cannabidiolic acid; TRPVI, transient receptor potential vanilloid type I; PPARg, peroxisome proliferator-activated receptor g; ROS, reactive oxygen species; 5-HTIA, 5-hydroxtryptamine receptor subtype IA; FAAH, fatty acid amide hydrolasse. (+), direct or indirect activation; ↑, increase; ↓, decrease.

Cannabidiol (CBD)

Cannabidiol (CBD) is one of the two relatively non-intoxicating phytocannabinoids, along with its acid precursor, cannabidiolic acid (CBDA). CBD has little activity at the CB1 and CB2 receptors. Instead, it works on other receptors to produce a wide range of activities, including anti-convulsive, anti-inflammatory, antioxidant, and antipsychotic effects. Included in this is a neuroprotective effect of CBD, which supports its role in the treatment of a number of neurological disorders, including epilepsy, Parkinson's, amyotrophic lateral sclerosis, Huntington's disease, Alzheimer's, and MS. CBD possesses the unique ability to counteract the intoxicating and adverse or unpleasant effects of cannabis, such as anxiety, tachycardia, hunger, and sedation. Recently, CBD demonstrated its strong anti-inflammatory and immunosuppressive properties in a study on organ transplants in a phase 2 trial (Yeshurun et al. 2015). If CBD was started at 300 mg per day a week before the procedure, there was an associated reduced mortality and complications. There is no evidence to support the lab studies suggesting that CBD converts to THC under acidic conditions within humans.

Restated, CBD has little binding affinity for either the CB1 or the CB2 receptors. Instead, it suppresses the enzyme FAAH, which breaks down AEA (anandamide), the body's CB1-activating endocannabinoid. This relatively increases the action on the CB1 receptor. In addition, CBD opposes the action of THC at the CB1 receptor and thereby helps reduce THC's psychoactive effect. Finally, CBD stimulates the release of 2-AG, which acts primarily on the CB2 receptor. In this way, CBD is like a direct stimulator of CB2 receptors. This is why CBD can provide pain relief and anti-inflammatory activities in addition to immunomodulatory effects. Therefore, when used in combination with some THC, CBD can be quite helpful in traumatic brain injury, stroke, MS, Alzheimer's, Huntington's, and Parkinson's. CBD is also active in the receptors TRPV1 and 5-HT-1A. These additional receptor actions help explain the wide set of actions of CBD, including its anti-anxiety, antidepressant, and antipsychotic effects.

Cannabigerol (CBG)

Cannabigerol (CBG) was purified from cannabis the same year as THC, 1964. However, CBG does not have psychoactive effects. CBG stimulates a range of receptors important for pain, inflammation, and antidepressant effects. Its antagonism toward the receptor TRPM8 may make it useful for prostate cancer, hyperactive bladder (detrusor overactivity), and bladder pain. Its ability to relieve pain, reduce red skin rashes, and block lipoxygenase may even surpass that of THC. CBG has also been shown to have modest antifungal effects. In addition to being a strong ADA uptake inhibitor, it is a powerful agent against MRSA (methicillin-resistant staphylococcus aureus). Finally, CBG acts as a potent adrenoreceptor agonist, which further supports its analgesic capability.

Cannabichromene (CBC)

While cannabichromene (CBC) may only represent 0.3 percent of standard cannabis in some varieties, it may be significantly higher. These CBC-rich cannabis strains were created by selective inheritance of a recessive gene. This particular extract is not included under the list of scheduled drugs by the DEA. CBC can cause potent anti-inflammatory effects through non-CB receptor mechanisms. It can be a significant factor in the "entourage effect" in some particular strains of cannabis.

Cannabinol (CBN)

Cannabinol (CBN) is a time-related oxidation by-product of THC. It is most commonly found after prolonged storage, especially at higher temperatures. CBN was the first cannabinoid to be identified and isolated from cannabis, as early as 1899. CBN maintains about a quarter of the potency of THC. CBN can be sedative, anticonvulsant, and has significant properties related to anti-inflammatory, antibiotic, and anti-MRSA activity. CBN has potential as a component in topical applications, possibly to minimize scarring by inhibiting keratinocyte proliferation. CBN also stimulates the recruitment of dormant mesenchymal stem cells in marrow, promoting bone formation.

Tetrahydrocannabivarin (THCV)

Tetrahydrocannabivarin (THCV) is frequently found in low concentrations that can be up to 16 percent by prior weight. THCV can have positive and negative effects at the CB1 receptor. THCV produces weight loss and can decrease body fat and serum leptin concentrations with increased energy expenditure in obese mice. THCV is a fractional component of many southern Africa cannabis types. THCV can suppress the appetite and the intoxicating effects of THC.

Tetrahydrocannabinolic Acid (THCA)

Tetrahydrocannabivarin acid (THCA) is not psychoactive and does not activate CB1 cannabinoid receptors in the brain. THCA does not turn into THC within the human body. To turn THCA into psychoactive THC, it must first be heated. This can be done by vaporizing raw flowers, baking edibles, or heating cannabis in a process known as decarboxylation. THCA is present in the raw plant, and this is what many people are talking about when they talk about juicing cannabis. One important point is that almost all fat-soluble components remain within the pulp and are not transferred into the watery green fluid. Therefore, you should also use the pulp over the course of the day in smoothies, salads, or another mode of intake.

THCA is a potent antiepileptic agent, working at 0.1–1.0 mg per kilogram of body weight per day. Preclinical research suggests that THCA may be anti-inflammatory and may reduce nausea. Fortunately, THCA may be able to work in small doses. THCA is 10–100 times more potent for treating nausea than is THC. A dose can be as small as 0.1–1.0 mg/kg of body weight per day of THCA. THCA is relatively available, because the marijuana plant leaves or early buds can provide this. A higher dose of THCA, when combined with some THC, can occasionally be effective for treatment of resistant seizures, pain, and arthritis. In addition, THCA only impacts the 5-HT1a receptors and not the CB1 receptors, where THC acts.

Clinical studies are at an early stage, but a number of individual case reports are quite hopeful. Daily consumption of 10-20 mg of THCA was effective in reducing pain in some patients with arthritis and irritable bowel syndrome. Perhaps this is due to the fact the THCA inhibits MAGL (the enzyme that breaks down 2-AG), which results in higher levels of the endocannabinoid 2-AG acting on the CB2 receptor. Both

THCA and CBDA block COX 1 and 2 enzymes, accounting for their anti-inflammatory effects. In an Alzheimer's patient, THCA improved cognitive symptoms, and in one teenager, a low dose of THCA prevented severe refractory migraines. THCA is typically administered along with the other components of cannabis in a tincture by an under-the-tongue dropper or spray.

The value of small doses is particularly enticing and suggest a practical approach of using the raw plant as a food. If one uses the dosage suggested above, then for a child weighing 25 kg, this amounts to 2–23 mg of THCA per day. In contrast are the studies with Epidiolex, the antiepileptic drug soon to be released in the United States, which is 99.5 percent pure CBD. Epidiolex sublingual spray starts at a dose of 5 mg/kg per day and may increase up to 25 mg/kg per day. Note that the THCA dose is one tenth to one hundredth of this pure CBD dose. One seven-year-old patient weighing 20 kg has been seizure free for over two and a half years since being on a dosage regimen of 50 mg per day of CBD and 10 mg per day of THCA. This is a fraction of the above dose.

Cannabidivarin (CBDV)

Cannabidivarin, an analog or cousin of CBD, engages the endocannabinoid system by inhibiting the breakdown of AEA and 2-AG, two endogenous cannabinoids. This happens at minimal concentrations and is enhanced by the CBDV's ability to inhibit the cellular uptake of AEA. Both effects enhance the endocannabinoid system. There is strong evidence that CBDV has significant anticonvulsant properties, even rivaling those of CBD. It seems to be particularly useful in partial onset or focal seizures. It may also be useful in the treatment of nausea and vomiting.

Cannabidiolic Acid (CBDA)

Cannabidiolic acid (CBDA) is a natural precursor of CBD in its acidic form and is found in the leaves and bud in the raw form. This compound can inhibit endocannabinoid degradation enzymes. In addition, CBDA can inhibit Cox 1 and Cox 2 compounds. This action has a significant anti-inflammatory effect. CBDA is particularly active at the 5-HT1A receptor. In fact, CBDA is a much more effective 5-HT agonist then CBD, helping it be active against nausea and vomiting, anxiety, depression, and pain. This may make it particularly valuable for the production of serotonin and dopamine. Significant antiemetic effects have also been demonstrated in lab animals. Clinical benefits are still undergoing research, as this is available in raw cannabis and is only recently being investigated.

Cannabigerol Monomethyl Ether

Cannabigerol monomethyl ether is a component commonly encountered in cannabis. However, it has not yet been researched for its pharmacological activity. Because it is present with relative frequency, it should be a research priority.

The above is a brief summary of the non-psychoactive components that I have listed since the THC discussion. The presence of many, or all, of these components explain the importance of the entourage effect. It is my impression that in almost all cases we should concentrate the whole cannabis plant for optimal benefits and minimal side effects. Next, I will discuss the terpenes, which are other key components in the entourage effect.

Cannabinoid Chemistry and Biology Review, Including Terpenes

Cannabinoids are a group of compounds produced uniquely by Cannabis sativa and Cannabis indica. Contrary to popular opinion, there is virtually no difference between these two species. In the last few years, there has been so much intermingling and interbreeding of these two that no one, including one of the experts, Dr. Ethan Russo, can tell the difference visually. The only real recognition is when they are tested in the lab for their constituent amounts of THC, CBD, or other components, including terpenoids.

The acceptance of cannabis as a potential medical compound changed dramatically with the discovery of the CB1 receptor in 1988. This receptor was initially found in the brain, with the largest concentrations being in the basal ganglia, cerebellum, hippocampus, and cerebral cortex. This receptor has since been found throughout the body, but it is particularly focused in the central nervous system and in peripheral nerves. Neuropathic pain (nerve pain) should come to mind with this fact. CB1 receptors began with vertebrates. These receptors are known to regulate calcium channels, and this regulates other systems within the body. In combination, CB1 and CB2 receptors make up the endocannabinoid system and are overall regulators of almost all biochemical flow within humans. In short, the CB1 receptor is the psychoactive receptor.

In 1993, a second cannabinoid receptor, CB2, was identified, initially in the gut of dogs. Today it is known that the highest concentrations of CB2 receptors are located on B lymphocytes and natural killer cells, which are key components of our immune system. This suggests a possible role for cannabis in immunity. You may recall that almost the entire immune system, 70 percent, is found in the gut lining. This brings the significant brain-gut connection to the fore. This is particularly evident for the cannabinoid receptors. In short, the CB2 receptor is immunomodulatory and the primary pain-relief receptor.

The next question you may ask is, are all these receptors simply there for the need of the cannabis plant? No, they are not. As previously mentioned, in 1992, the first cannabinoid produced inside the body, anandamide, was discovered. Since then, 2-AG (2-arachidonoylglycerol) has also been confirmed as part of the body's cannabinoid system. These cannabinoid receptors act through a G protein-coupling mechanism (as displayed in Figure 8.2 on page 252 of the *Integrative Oncology* book by Donald Abrams and Andrew Weil (Abrams 2014)).

One of the two major components within the cannabis plant is CBD or cannabidiol. It is not very intoxicating and is only somewhat psychoactive. Its psychoactive effects are both antianxiety and antipsychotic. A study in France showed that it was as effective as a potent antipsychotic drug but with almost no side effects. I suggest physicians consider a trial of CBD before beginning the regular antipsychotic drugs, because the side effects are much more tolerable. CBD is known to boost the painkilling benefit as well as the anti-inflammatory component of THC. CBD is also known to be neuroprotective and act as an antioxidant better than vitamin C or E. In general, CBD is a modulator of the endocannabinoid system. It has a direct antiseizure component. In fact, in late 2017 in the United States, it was released as a prescription product by GW Pharmaceuticals as an antiseizure medication. It is also known that CBD stimulates bone fracture healing and is probably useful in osteoporosis treatment. We know that CBD prevents prion accumulation (think mad cow disease) and reduces neuronal toxicity.

Finally, it is important to clear up a couple of misconceptions about CBD. First, it does not tend to induce sleep but is somewhat stimulating. It is probable that the strain that people think is simply high CBD helping sleep has actually got a fair amount of B-myrcene, a terpene described below.The terpene is the component helping sleep, not the CBD Second, it is now confirmed that CBD does not turn into THC within the human body.

Terpenes

Terpenes are small molecules that are made within the cannabis plant. They tend to be water-soluble, and if you squeeze the juice out of leaves and buds, you get a dark, green, watery substance. The main active ingredients within this juice are terpenes. The fat- or lipid-soluble components, namely THC and cannabinoids, are in the pulp left behind. The terpenes are particularly interesting, because they provide many of the subtle components of the cannabis plant that are not readily explained by the presence or absence of THC and cannabinoids. In general, the terpenes tend to be antibiotic, anti-inflammatory, and synergize particularly well with THC. Most quality cannabis labs can now evaluate how much and which terpenes are in a particular strain of cannabis. This will become increasingly important as we strive for the unique properties of particular terpenes.

Alpha-pinene and Beta-pinene

Alpha-pinene is a bicyclic monoterpene and is the most widely distributed terpenoid in nature. It is found in low concentrations in most modern cannabis strains but is prevalent in the "Blue Dream" strain of Southern California. Although it is scarce in most modern strains of cannabis, it permits clear thinking despite the short-term memory troubles present from THC. It is known to be an acetylcholinesterase inhibitor. This means it can maintain the acetylcholine present between neurons for a longer period. This is probably why it enhances clear thinking. One way to remember this is the concept of "forest bathing." This refers to sitting or walking in a pine forest, which helps clear the mind. This may help it serve in the treatment of dementia. Similarly, alpha-pinene has also been suggested as a modulator of THC overdose events. Its pharmacological effects are legion: anti-inflammatory via PGE-1, widening of the airways (bronchodilator) in humans at low concentrations, an antibiotic as effective as vancomycin against MRSA, and it also treats cryptococcus and Candida albicans.

B-Myrcene

The second terpene is B-myrcene, which induces sleep. Its nickname is the "couch lock" terpene, and it is largely responsible for the idea that cannabis can make some people disinterested in their surroundings and life. B-myrcene is quite common in modern strains of cannabis in North America and Europe. Its effect is reversed by naloxone, which also reverses opiates (i.e., narcotics). Once again, we see the interaction between the endogenous opioid system and the endocannabinoid system. Myrcene is also one of the sedative agents of hops (Humulus lupulus). In lab research, B-myrcene has notable effects against peptic ulcers by increasing mucus production and enhancing antioxidants in the tissues, which helps with healing. Similar benefits are suggested within the brain, so this terpene can add tremendous synergy neuroprotective benefits when combined with the effects of THC and CBD. B-myrcene's multiple effects may make it an excellent addition to THC and CBD in the treatment of traumatic brain injury or even stroke.

D-limonene

Perhaps it is best to think of lemon and citrus fragrances, because this terpene, D-limonene, is equated with cleanliness and bright thoughts. D-limonene has powerful antidepressant effects and is also a powerful immune stimulant. D-limonene also has an impressive support historically as an antidote to excessive psychoactive adverse events produced by THC. This terpene also has significant antibiotic effects against Staphylococcus aureus, Pseudomonas aeruginosa, and Propionibacterium acnes (the bacteria of acne). Concentrations of 400 μg/ml inhibit biofilm formation from the dental pathogen Streptococcus pyogenes and mutans. Limonene increases mitochondrial formation and has any number of positive effects on fat cells, suggesting it may have a role in obesity treatment.

D-linalool

The effect of D-Linalool is similar to lavender essential oil. This means it has an antianxiety application and is an excellent local anaesthetic. This allows you to put it on burns directly with considerable pain relief. In addition, it has anticonvulsant and anti-glutaminergic effects. This is important in brain injury from trauma or stroke, because huge amounts of glutamine are released at once, which is very toxic. This terpene can moderate or calm that injury considerably. Finally, linalool acts as a sedative, antidepressant, and anxiolytic, and has immune-potentiating effects.

Beta-ocimene

Beta-ocimene is commonly found in nature. Its properties include anticonvulsant activity, antifungal activity, antitumour activity, and pest resistance. It is also a volatile pheromone important for the social regulation of honeybee colonies. Commercially, we are seeing the development of "cannabis honey." This is also being used by law enforcement agencies to detect illicit drugs by "trained honeybees," which were proposed to replace sniffer dogs at some borders in 2015.

Gamma-terpinene

This terpene is common to eucalyptus and cumin but a minor component in cannabis. Other terpenes present to a minor degree within cannabis include alpha-terpinene, alpha-terpineol, camphene, terpinolene (may help against atherosclerosis), alpha-phellandrene, gamma-cadinene, delta 3-carene, cymene, fenchol, and 1,8-cineole (eucalyptol). They only become significant in the use of cannabis when a strain of cannabis is bred for higher amounts within the new strains.

Sesquinterpenoids

One key subset of terpenes is called sesquinterpenoids. The most important within this group is B-caryophyllene, which is the most common terpenoid in cannabis extracts and it is also quite common in foods. It is an excellent anti-inflammatory and also provides gastro-protective effects. It works on CB-2 receptors with strong potency. A recent publication confirms its therapeutic potential to protect against fatty liver disease from alcohol (Tam et al. 2011). It does this with its anti-inflammatory effects and by reducing the number of metabolic disturbances. It is especially useful to fight addiction. For example, it dramatically reduces cocaine requirements.

Caryophyllene Oxide

Caryophyllene oxide is also found in lemon balm and eucalyptus. It is nontoxic and non-sensitizing. It is the component responsible for cannabis detection by drug-sniffing dogs. This compound works well as a broad-spectrum antifungal in plant defence and as an insecticide.

Humulene (alpha-caryophyllene)

This substance provides some defence to plants in their products, and this compound inhibits fruit fly mating.

Beta-elemene

It is reported in some cannabis strains and is common to myrrh. I emphasize it here due to its versatility as a potential anti-cancer agent. This makes it worthy of selective breeding in cannabis plants to increase the amount in a particular strain and then to combine it with chemotherapeutic phyto-cannabinoids for a synergistic effect.

Other sesquinterpenoids include guaiol, eudesmol isomers, nerolidol, gurjunene, gamma-cadinene, and beta-farnesene.

Triterpinoids—from Cannabis Roots

Early research is just now starting to talk about the use of cannabis roots. One of the first mentions of the medical use of cannabis root was by the Roman historian, Pliny the Elder. He wrote that "a decoction of the root in water relaxes contraction of the joints and cures gout and similar maladies" (Ryz 2017). Researchers are now discovering a number of potential benefits from terpenoids. The main one so far seems to be an anti-inflammatory benefit. Cannabis roots have relatively little THC or CBD or even most of the terpenes. Of interest to gout patients are the compounds within roots, which can be quite successful at treatment of gouty arthritis.

In Summary

The overall potential physiologic responses of the cannabis plant are improved sleep, antiseizure effects, neuroprotective effects, reduced intraocular (inside the eye) pressure, helping PTSD, dilating the airways, relaxing muscles, reducing muscle spasms, reducing inflammation (especially in IBS and arthritis), and finally, reduced pain, especially neuropathic pain. In addition, the combination of substances within the cannabis plant can dramatically help osteoporosis, incontinence, dystonia, sleep apnea, hypertension, gliomas (a type of brain tumour), itchy skin, diabetes mellitus, Hepatitis C, and even methicillin-resistant staph infection (MRSA).

The adverse effects of the cannabis plant derivatives are relatively uncommon. However, they do include the possibility of increased heart rate, occasional palpitations, and sometimes a brief raising of blood pressure. The respiratory effects are primarily those of cough and sputum production increase, particularly when it is smoked. The main central nervous system effects are tiredness, a change in memory, a change in coordination and focus, and sometimes visual disturbances, which are almost always transitory. Most of these occur with pure THC when used alone. So, remember the entourage effect.

Cannabis formulations can come in six different varieties: raw, vaporized, oral, buccal (under the tongue), topical (skin), and rectal delivery. Each of these has their own relative benefits and problems. I will outline some of the most significant ones. But first, I would like to give you two definitions here that are important when talking about a drug or herb entering the body. The first of these is pharmacokinetics, which is what the body does to the drug. This includes the absorption, distribution, metabolism, and excretion. The second definition is of pharmacodynamics, which is what the drug does to the body. One example of pharmacokinetics is when cannabis is vaporized through the lungs. This delivery method is almost like an intravenous injection. However, only 10 or 20 percent is absorbed and metabolized in the liver, lungs, and brain. The elimination from the body is 65 percent into the feces and 20 percent in the urine, with the other components lost in the breathing side stream effect or combustion. If 1 gram of cannabis is used, and it is a 10 percent THC plant, then 16.3 mg is delivered into the bloodstream.

The second example is the oral use of dried cannabis, where three to five times as much is needed as in vaporization. In evaluation through over 165 studies, a minimum or low dose was 7 mg, a medium dose was 7-18 mg, and a high dose was greater than 18 mg of THC. It was also found that 30-120 minutes are needed for effect. Tolerance may develop. Also, this is the primary area of drug interactions, because a larger amount travels to the liver after absorption in the gut and influences the metabolism of some other drugs, although not dramatically so, unless this is an extremely high CBD preparation.

When taking cannabis orally, drug interactions should be considered. Happily, these are almost never dramatic. First, cannabis and tricyclic antidepressants may result in an increased heart rate and delirium, much like taking twice as much of the drug. Tricylic drugs are rarely used anymore and are probably best avoided in combination with high-CBD preparations. The second group of drugs are SSRIs, as patients may become somewhat manic, but the key thing here is to reduce the drug slightly. Another drug that should be used cautiously is sildenafil (Viagra or Cialis), because this may create a stress on the heart, even heart attack, and possibly bleeding within the lungs. Another important drug interaction to consider is that of coumadin or warfarin where the INR (a measure of clotting) may be increased so that the dose of the drug needs to be reduced. This is usually only an issue in the presence of the high-CBD preparations, which are used primarily in seizure control and anxiety. Finally, the group of CNS depressants, including alcohol, benzodiazepines, barbiturates, opioids, and antihistamines, may interact with cannabis. The effect of these drugs may be increased somewhat but certainly not dangerously so. The particular effect on opioids is improvement of pain relief with a suggestion that a small amount of cannabis can increase the morphine effect by four to ten times. This is more of a synergy phenomenon than a drug interaction.

In summary, as a group of clinical pearls, I suggest the following. If anti-retrovirals are to be used, you may need to decrease the cannabis dose. Second, you may need to reduce the dose of opioids, benzodiazepines (e.g., Valium, Ativan, and Klonopin), SSRIs antidepressants, and antiseizure medication. However, this is a small problem, as there has never been a case reported of overdose secondary to adding cannabis. Finally, as stated previously, it is probably best to avoid using them in the presence of tricyclic antidepressants. One other established feature is that there are no problems with drug interactions when raw cannabis or topical cannabis is used.

When prescribing dry cannabis, which has been the typical pattern in Canada until recently, the following dosages should be considered:

1. For smoking or vaporization, the dosage should be 1–12 grams per day. The terpenes actually vaporize at a lower temperature than the THC, but the entourage effect will still be present. This is a considerable advantage in that it reduces psychoactive side effects.

2. For oral ingestion, the dosage may be up to three (perhaps even five times) as much per day as smoking cannabis. As an example, 20 mg of THC taken orally is equivalent to smoking 7.5 mg. The maximum blood concentrations with oral ingestion may take up to six hours,

and the time for half the drug to leave the body could be as much as twenty to thirty hours. Oral ingestion also increases the effect of the liver metabolite 11-OH-THC. This increases the psychoactive effect and, due to the delay of liver breakdown of THC, accounts for the "second hit" many people notice. Concentrates can be created in coconut oil, which can be solidified and then cut with a knife into tiny grains, so the dose can start small and gradually be increased. The Rick Simpson protocol talks about one gram per day of a mixture that is 90 percent cannabis, which is equal to 900 mg per day (Simpson 2018). Almost everyone will have to gradually attain this dosage for the highly touted Rick Simpson's claims for recovery. If you are cannabis naïve, as I am, you will need to start gradually.

3. Under-the-tongue, buccal, or sublingual delivery has an onset at less than thirty minutes and lasts for approximately four to six hours.I use (for my MS) and prescribe Sativex spray. It provides measured dosing, is easy to repeat, and has a relatively long shelf life. This quick onset permits repeat dosing in twenty minutes, much like vapourization.Sativex is licensed for physician prescription in at least twenty-four countries including Canada,the UK and all of Europe including Norway. It is safe,available and a good starting point for physicians new to cannabis. I ask my physician colleagues "What are you waiting for?"

4. Topical delivery can be good for treatment of local symptoms, such as muscle spasms, inflammation, such as arthritis, or even neuropathic pain. It is also used for skin disorders and some peripheral pain problems. It minimizes the central effect and stimulates local cannabinoid receptors. The dose estimate is between .5–10 g per dose with the application one to four times daily.

New research on cannabis roots supports the several-thousand-year-old practice of the decoction, by putting the roots in water for one to two hours. The roots have no CBD or THC but contain a number of triterpenoids (friedelin and epifriedelanol), alkaloids (cannabisativine and anhydrocannbisativine), carvon, dihydrocarvone, trans-cinnamide, and various sterols, including sitosterol, campesterol, and stigmasterol. Since the latter part of the seventeenth century, herbalists have recommended cannabinoids to treat fever, inflammation, gout, arthritis, skin burns, and hard tumours. More details can be found in an excellent article by Natasha R. Ryz et al. in *Cannabis and Cannabinoid Research* (2017).

5. Raw cannabis delivery, often called juicing, is a relative problem due to stalactites, which are tiny leaf hairs that can irritate the mouth, throat, and stomach. In addition, sometimes the sticky resin on the bud sticks to the mouth. This cannabis preparation is probably medicinal due to the cannabinoid acids, CBDA and THCA. These are the non-psychoactive precursors in the plants. A juice regimen would use fresh cannabis four to five times a day and include the young tender leaves as well as the fan leaves and buds.

Dr. William Courtney (www.cannabisinternational.org) suggests twenty-five large fan leaves per day in juice, salsa, or pesto/salad. If using fresh bud, then he suggests one per day. In one report, 30 large leaves of a flowering cannabis plant, Omrita, yielded 11.5 mg of THCA and CBDA. Leaf mixtures of concentrates of cannabinoid acids yields range from 0.3 percent to 4 percent by weight. We also know the leaves have 10 percent of the cannabinoids of the buds. Success has been shown in treating chronic illness, particularly inflammatory bowel problems, using raw cannabis. Experience suggests it lasts some six to eight hours. It seems a good idea to be using food as medicine, as suggested by Hippocrates, "Let food be thy medicine and thy medicine be food." However, one needs a reasonably large fresh plant supply. Research has also shown that frozen leaves and bud can be used. I am hopeful that this may eventually permit people to grow larger amounts in the summer under their medical permit and then store excess in the freezer for the winter. As mentioned earlier, don't just squeeze out the watery green fluid, drink it, and then throw away the pulp. Why? The pulp has almost all the THC and CBD components, as they are fat soluble. Add the pulp to smoothies to be used over the day.

Tolerance or Reduced Effect of Cannabis

Tolerance is a recognized entity for a considerable number of drugs and herbs. Many people have experienced this effect with tea or coffee. Cannabis is no exception. It occurs due to the continued stimulation of receptors, which leads to a relative desensitization and down regulation of these same receptors. It certainly develops faster with higher potency cannabinoids. Also, CBD-rich strains have different tolerance-producing effects than do THC-rich strains, because each targets different primary receptors. In high-dose therapy, tolerance can require up to a tenfold increase in cannabis use. This is particularly common when it is being trialed as an anti-cancer agent, when the dose may go from 10–30 mg per day to hundreds of milligrams per day. One concept that may reduce tolerance is the so-called herbal holiday. This allows stopping the herb for a time to see if it is still needed. Several examples of this include:

- Stopping for one to three weeks every three to four months

- Stopping five to seven days every month
- Stopping one day every week
- If it does not seem advisable to stop the med entirely, then it might be advisable to use different strains of cannabis. The different strains often have different terpenes, altering the entourage effect, not just different amounts of THC and CBD.

Finally, a couple of cannabinoid dosing tips.

1. When a relatively non-psychoactive outcome is desired, better to use a high-CBD cannabis or cannabinoid acids or topical in addition. Yes, CBD has some psychoactive properties such as anti-anxiety although regular language often states it has no psychoactive action. I believe they are simply saying CBD has no trip inducing side effects .

2. If an antipsychotic (e.g., schizophrenia-resistant or intolerant of regular medication) and/or antianxiety outcome is desired, then it's probably best to use a high-CBD strain. When issues of sleep are of consideration, the best place to begin seems to be with a 1:1 ratio of THC to CBD.

Mental Health and Cannabis

Mental health challenges and cannabis were well outlined to me in a presentation at TCMI by Dr. Christopher G. Fitchener, MD, a psychiatrist. In his discussion of the "cannabis causing psychosis" controversy, he outlined a number of important points. To begin with, it is almost always a high dose of THC alone that triggers psychosis. It is more prevalent when the THC is used on its own in the absence of the modifying components of CBDs and terpenoids. Short-term observation of people experiencing this psychosis, occasionally for a few days, will help differentiate it from true psychosis. Follow-up has revealed that this is not triggering true schizophrenia but rather a temporary delirium. Recreational use of "shatter", a highly concentrated resin, an amount the size of a single grain of rice is usually the trigger.

In his discussion of PTSD, Dr. Fitchener talked about the reference of Dr. Tod Mikuriya, who cited that 80 PTSD patients in New Mexico had a reduction of overall symptoms by 75 percent. It seems the most useful in PTSD are the hybrid strains, where CBD and THC are present, so the entire cannabis entourage can provide benefit.

When Dr. Fitchener spoke of schizophrenia, he used an example in Europe where a high-CBD strain was as effective as one of the most potent antipsychotic drugs but without the tough side effects. In health challenges of mania and anxiety, he suggested primarily a high-CBD strain. Finally, in the diagnoses of ADD or ADHD, it is worth considering and trying a similar combination.

Before leaving this discussion, it is worthwhile to talk about cannabis use disorders. We have already talked about the occasional episode of psychosis precipitated by pure THC or a high-THC strain. The other important issue to mention is the severe recurrent vomiting syndrome, which occurs occasionally after prolonged and heavy use of cannabis. Acute treatment is recurrent hot showers. This disorder always responds to elimination of the cannabis itself.

Finally, I want to talk about an area that was discussed in the TCMI presentation I listened to from Mary Lynn Mathre, RN, MSN. She talked about cannabis as a harm-reduction agent and about using it as a substitute drug for the withdrawal of alcohol (Lau 2015), opioids (Lucas 2012), nicotine, cocaine (Socías 2017), and methamphetamine.

A corollary to the above is a study whereby it was shown that cannabis assisted in the methadone induction of narcotic-addicted patients (Scavone 2013). Also, there is a report of better naltrexone retention when used in heroin-addicted patients if cannabis is used (Raby 2009).

In summary, cannabis is a special medicine with a wide margin of safety. Cannabis has a rapid onset that enables people to self-titrate. It calms nausea and vomiting and improves appetite, has anti-inflammatory effects, reduces pain, and reduces or helps eliminate other conventional medicine.

I like to quote one of the pioneers in the use of medicinal cannabis, Dr. Tod Mikuriya: "we should be thinking of cannabis as a medicine first, that happens to have some psychoactive properties, as many medicines do, rather than as an intoxicant that happens to have a few therapeutic properties on the side."[10] I want to emphasize the important role of cannabinoids in modulating neuroplasticity. This includes control on neurogenesis, depolarization-induced suppression of excitation, and even neuroprotection. Studies have shown in animal models that AEA and 2-AG are produced in major amounts when the brain is injured by hypoxia, stroke, or mechanical trauma (Shohami 2011) These compounds can help reduce the problem of glutamate toxicity and so can reduce seizure activity and limit infarct (e.g., a stroke) or injury size by up to half. I know of no other body mechanism dedicated to these important problems.

I write this book from a Canadian perspective, where we have had medical marijuana available for patients under the auspices of Health Canada since 2001. I have completed many medical documents to enable people to apply to Health Canada for the use of cannabis in their personal health journey. These people struggle with a variety of conditions (e.g., chronic pain,

---

[10]   Dr. Tod Mikuriya, California psychiatrist, now deceased.

epilepsy, hepatitis C, HIV, MS, Parkinson's, Alzheimer's, PTSD, and cancer). These patients have taught me a great deal. These lessons, coupled with some of the literature over the last forty years, permit me to outline how you might use cannabis in your journey.

I will outline my personal medical practice in a consultative role, because medical marijuana has become very useful in this regard. I primarily see chronic pain patients, people with MS, and people with longstanding chronic illness. The predominant diagnosis is chronic pain. You will see more details about this in chapter 18. In particular, I am proud of the young people who have ended their addiction to opioids using medical marijuana. I believe this is one of the critical pieces in working toward the narcotic overdose and death crisis found throughout Canada and the United States. You may recall my saying that there is a 24.8 percent reduction in narcotic overdose deaths in US states that have a medical marijuana program. Most of these people start by using vapourized marijuana or smoking marijuana and then switch to ingestion of smoothies, oil, or other oral preparations, such as brownies or even gummy bears.

In addition to my chronic pain consultations, I've seen quite a few people with inflammatory bowel disease, ulcerative colitis and Crohn's disease, and inflammatory bowel syndrome (IBS). Many of these people have been able to get off toxic drugs, such as prednisone and methotrexate, with the use of cannabis. In addition, many MS patients get off several drugs, because medical marijuana has often helped them with their neuropathic pain, spasticity, and migraine headaches. The treatment of epilepsy, including in children, has been greatly enhanced with high-CBD preparations. Even dermatologic or skin problems have been greatly assisted with topical mixtures made from medical marijuana. On occasion, I have seen skin cancers resolve with these topical preparations. However, this is the only significant cancer that I might suggest is worth a try. That is, in the presence of basal cell carcinoma or squamous cell carcinoma of the skin. Otherwise, cannabis is primarily a useful adjunct in the treatment of cancer to allow the use of powerful medications or radiation by helping people cope with the side effects. A second exception might be the brain cancer glioma. Finally, I've seen many young men and women with ADHD, PTSD, or both eliminate other medications that have not worked for them. I now accept that regular medications do not help everyone. Therefore, I am willing to add medical cannabis to their choices and, if they are successful, have them follow up with their health care practitioner in the tapering of other medications, when indicated.

I would also like to acknowledge one of my key mentors in integrative medicine, Dr. Andrew Weil. He and his colleague, Donald Abrams, MD, edited a book together called *Integrative Oncology* (Abrams 2014). It includes a superb chapter on cannabis and its role as an adjunct in cancer treatment programs. In addition, I have gleaned a lot of knowledge from Dr. Ethan Russo, a neurologist, who is well versed in the clinical applications of cannabis. Finally, I would like to acknowledge the incredible contribution by Dr. R. Mechoulam in his discovery and publication of the cannabinoid receptor within mammals and humans. Dr. Mechoulam gave the final presentation of my online course from TMCI. This online course was incredibly thorough about the medical indications and use of cannabis and its components.

Marijuana Museum

Recently, on a trip to Barcelona, Spain, I toured the Marijuana Museum, which is one of two such museums, the first one being in Amsterdam, Netherlands. The museum depicts graphic and pictorial representations of the many ways cannabis has been accepted and used. These museums and the June 2015 edition of *National Geographic* magazine have also been helpful resources for me. National Geographic's cover page showed the cannabis leaf with the title "Weed—The New Science of Marijuana." The article described cannabis as a tonic to dull pain, aid sleep, and stimulate the appetite. The literature contains evidence that anorexia patients have a deficiency in one of the circulating endocannabinoids, a type of cannabis compound produced in the body (Jager 2014). If this deficiency is corrected with oral cannabis derivatives, these patients start to eat. Such articles will help to demystify cannabis to the medical profession and the public. Other articles have provided evidence that marijuana may help the body, especially the brain. Components of cannabis may protect the brain against trauma, modulate the immune system, and aid in memory extinction (forgetting) after catastrophic events. This latter factor suggests its use in treating PTSD.

Epilepsy

One of the more topical and controversial medical indications is epilepsy. You may have read the story of "Charlotte's Web" (not the children's novel of the same name) (Maa 2014). This story describes a young girl in the United States who had hundreds of seizures per day despite many heavy anti-epileptic drugs. She responded extremely well to a strain of cannabis high in CBD but with almost zero THC. This combination has been quite successful in many but not all children with seizure disorders. Several qualified pediatric neurologists have referred children to me for consideration of a prescription of medical marijuana. It has been very rewarding to see the gratitude of the parents and sometimes the children themselves to achieve near control of their seizures without the heavily sedating anti-epileptic drugs. When you look closely at seizure control, you see that nearly a third of people are unable to control their seizures despite multiple anti-seizure pharmaceuticals. Small wonder many of these folks want to try high-CBD strains of cannabis for better seizure control.

Marijuana Research

Happily, the use of medical marijuana continues to be investigated in a number of centers in the United States. Once marijuana is legalized for public use in Canada, it will open the door for more clinical investigation. Currently, investigation of cannabis in Canada is limited due to the difficulties of cannabis being regarded as a Schedule 1 drug, similar to opiates like heroin and hallucinogens such as LSD.

I have seen many young people, primarily men, who become addicted to narcotics after a motor vehicle accident or similar major injury. In an effort to control their pain, they develop a new problem of narcotic addiction. Some even turn to street drugs as a necessary follow up. Recent research in the United States has revealed that the states that permit the use of medical marijuana for pain have a 24.8 percent reduction in opiate overdose death. This must be a strong message to the rest of us. The sooner we adopt a way to provide marijuana for the control of post-traumatic pain, the better off our patients will be. As an anaesthesiologist and specialist in pain medicine, I have long advocated for the use of several synergistic medications (NSAIDs, acetaminophen, clonidine) or other physical means, such as TENS or acupuncture, to control pain. We have long known that opiates are poor for bone pain, neuropathic pain, and chronic pain. In addition, opiates suppress our immune system and, therefore, limit our healing capabilities. For a more complete discussion of acute pain and chronic pain, please refer to chapter 18.

History Revisited

By 1992, Mechoulam, in Israel, had discovered and described one of the endocannabinoids (ECB) in humans as being anandamide. He took this word from Sanskrit. It means supreme joy or bliss. We know that exercise elevates anandamide. This molecule plays a role in basic functions such as memory, balance, movement, immune health, and neuroprotection. However, Mechoulam also points out that we should not go down the path of finding individual molecules in a plant and use only those. He describes the synergy of different compounds in plants as the previously mentioned "entourage effect." We, in medicine and in the pharmaceutical industry, have forgotten this important principle. An important example is the compound isolated from the valerian plant to make Valium, a highly addictive medication. Usually, we go down this road to obtain a patent and to profit, forgetting our original intent of helping the patient.

When I discuss the possibility of prescribing medical marijuana with clients, I try to educate them as well. One diagram I use is thee is a pie chart shown previously, which shows the many possible responses to cannabis and its components. This chart is from a 2009 journal article in *Trends in Pharmacology*, produced jointly by universities in Italy and Israel (Izzo et al. 2009). The article reveals many of the most useful benefits provided by THCA, CBDA, CBD and other its derivatives. Not on this chart Much smaller is the list of benefits from THC. This is particularly important, because THC has almost all the "trip" side effects of the cannabis plant. Strains or preparations with no THC or almost no THC have many less trip-like side effects. This is especially important in the young or cannabis-naïve individuals.

Marijuana in Young People

It is important that I mention the controversial concept of using medical marijuana in young people aged twenty-three years or less. First, the study most frequently quoted has been re-analyzed, and there is considerable concern in how the data was collected and interpreted. Now that I have looked at the data more fully, I feel medical marijuana should be used with the same risk-benefit ratio of any drug. Hence, I'm willing to use medical marijuana with this consideration. We know that long-term use of drugs like Ritalin and alcohol have major brain problems. I suggest that these and many other drugs, including anaesthetics and antiseizure medications, need to undergo the same risk-benefit consideration. Suffice it to say I would rather use medical marijuana than Ritalin, antidepressants, antipsychotics, or powerful anti-seizure medications in young people. In addition, as parents, we need to look for many non-drug solutions in solving our own and our children's problems. This would even include the excessive use of alcohol as something to be avoided.

In 1999, the Institute of Medicine in the United States issued a report called "Marijuana and Medicine: Assessing the Science Base." This report concluded the following concerning the biology of cannabis and cannabinoids (Joy 1999).

Cannabinoids likely have a natural role in pain modulation, in control of movement, and in memory.

1. The actual role of cannabinoids in immune systems is likely multifaceted and remains unclear.
2. The brain may develop tolerance to cannabinoids.
3. Animal research has demonstrated the potential for dependence on cannabinoids. This potential is observed under a narrower range of conditions compared to benzodiazepines, opiates, cocaine, or nicotine.
4. Withdrawal symptoms, which are observed in animals, appear mild compared to those from opiates or benzodiazepines.

Pharmacology of Cannabis

If you are wondering about a definition for pharmacology, it would simply be how a compound enters the body and the response it creates in the body. How it enters the body is called pharmacokinetics. The response it creates is called pharmacodynamics. If cannabis is ingested orally, 6–20 percent of it reaches the bloodstream. The peak concentration is reached in the bloodstream in one to six hours. This concentration is maintained for quite some time, as it takes between twenty and thirty hours for half of it to be gone. This is called a terminal half-life.

Similarly, if only delta-9 THC is taken, a large proportion is metabolized in the liver to 11-hydroxy-THC. This compound is even more psychoactive than THC alone. However, the metabolism of delta-9 THC into 11-hydroxy THC is buffered considerably by the presence of either CBDs or several of the terpenes or both. I hope you are realizing the benefits of using whole-plant extracts rather than a concentration of THC alone. In contrast, if THC is inhaled, it peaks in the bloodstream in two to ten minutes. It also leaves in as little as thirty minutes.

Pharmacodynamics, the study of the action of the compound or drug in the body, can be understood by looking at the endocannabinoids anandamide and 2-AG. Anandamide works primarily in the brain areas by nociceptive processing. In other words, it helps modulate or calm unpleasant sensations, including pain. Meanwhile, the 2-AG works primarily outside the central nervous system on the CB-2 receptors. At least part of its ability to decrease pain is by initiating an anti-inflammatory effect by reducing both cyclooxygenase and lipoxygenase, two compounds which are highly inflammatory. In addition, 2-AG acts as a stabilizing effect on most cells, which could be a component of its bronchodilation and erythema- (redness) reducing effects.

Safety and Side Effect Profile

One important fact regarding the safety of cannabis is that cannabinoid receptors are not located in the brainstem, controlling respiration. Therefore, lethal overdoses due to respiratory depression do not occur. This makes cannabis much safer to use than opiates or benzodiazepines. Use of the whole plant is unlikely to cause a lethal overdose; however, great caution should be exercised when using cannabis concentrates like "shatter," which is almost pure THC.

Dosage Ranges

Individuals vary in their response to substances ingested. However, one does need a starting point when recommending an agent that is new to people. In my ten years of experience, I have learned to start with small amounts of cannabis and gradually increase. In cannabis-naïve individuals, I suggest a 1:1 ratio of THC to CBD. Many MDs could begin with Sativex, because it is close to this ratio and is available in sixteen countries worldwide by prescription. Each "pump" of this delivers 2.7 mg of THC and 2.5 mg of CBD. If this is not enough for the muscle spasms or other challenge, you can repeat in twenty to thirty minutes. Bedtime is often a good time to start using cannabis, because any grogginess will be gone by morning. In addition, most of us adapt quickly over one to two weeks to tolerate this herb.

My recommendation to clinicians is to begin with the 1:1 ratio, perhaps in the dose range of Sativex given above for MS, sleep issues, migraines, and pain. If insufficient for pain, then increase the THC component to a 4:1 ratio. Finally, if you are using cannabis for anxiety or epilepsy/seizure control, use pure CBD or a 1:20 THC to CBD ratio. With most new clients, I begin with the oils prepared by Health Canada-licensed producers, as these are measured and consistent mixtures.

Here are some examples from the literature and in my prescribing experience that show individual responses to different types of cannabis compounds.

> Example 1: A person with acute pain, such as post-dental surgery, will respond well to an oil with 2.0 or 2.5 mg of THC combined with 8 mg of CBDs. When this was given every four to six hours, as needed, the oil completely replaced narcotics and non-steroidal anti-inflammatory drugs.

Example 2: In a study with cancer patients, the dosages of pure THC for the best analgesia and anti-nausea response use was 15 mg and 20 mg. However, the 20-mg doses produced considerable sedation and a feeling of depersonalization.

Example 3: Another study suggests that 10 mg of THC was equal to 60 mg of codeine and that 20 mg of THC is equivalent to about 120 mg codeine. This latter dose of codeine would also make people feel unwell.

Example 4: A study tested whole-plant extract versus THC extract versus a placebo. It found that the combination of THC and CBD helped twice as many test subjects to reduce their pain by 30 percent.

Example 5: A neuropathy treatment study found that patients smoking cannabis reduced their pain by 34 percent versus placebos by 17 percent.

Drug Interactions

Drug interactions are particularly important in cancer treatment, because large amounts of opioids are often used. The addition of cannabis to medical treatment in cancer was reported by Abrams et al. (2011). In this study, patients were stabilized for pain on either sustained-release morphine or sustained-release oxycodone. Vaporized cannabis was then added to the patients' medical therapy, with no adverse side effects. The study did not look at pain; however, it noted that patients tended to have better pain control when using vaporized cannabis.

CNS effects (effects on the central nervous system) can be described in four different groups, which include stimulatory and depressive effects. These dominate if THC is used alone. These are:

1. Affective (euphoria and easy laughter)
2. Sensory (temporal and spatial perception alterations and disorientation)
3. Somatic (drowsiness, dizziness, and motor coordination)
4. Cognitive (confusion, memory lapses, and difficulty concentrating)

Other side effects for receptors throughout the body include rapid heart rate and low blood pressure, conjunctival injection (redness of eye blood vessels), bronchodilation, and relaxation and reduced gastrointestinal motility. Tolerance of unwanted side effects seems to develop rapidly. Almost all these are avoided with the entourage effect of the entire plant. Most benefit from a component of CBD along with terpenes.

The Addictive Potential of Cannabis

When discussing the risk of addiction with cannabis, I would refer you to the following agents. The relative risk of addiction for these are as follows: tobacco: 32 percent, heroin: 23 percent, cocaine: 17 percent, alcohol: 15 percent, and cannabis: 9 percent. These results are from the National Comorbidity Survey of 1994 in the United States (Degenhardt 2007).

Prescribed medications and substances of abuse, including heroin, nicotine, other opioids, and benzodiazepines, can be addictive. People often talk about the risk of marijuana as a gateway drug. In 1999, the United States Institute of Medicine addressed this, and reported, in summary, that there is no conclusive evidence that the use of marijuana is causally linked to the subsequent abuse of other illicit drugs. This supports the fact that marijuana does not necessarily lead to other drug abuse.

Symptoms and signs of withdrawal from cannabis include irritability, insomnia, hot flashes, restlessness, and occasionally nausea and cramping. These usually disappear in a few days. Marijuana compounds are stored in the fat, and this means it lingers in the body for a long time, with a half-life of one to three days.

Clinical Endocannabinoid Deficiency (CED)

This will be a new topic for many, as it was for me. However, it is of critical importance if you are to understand how significant the use of clinical cannabis might be. Earlier in this chapter, I described the receptors and cannabinoids produced in the body. These are constantly present and create an ongoing underlying tone. This tone is a function of the body's production of cannabinoids (i.e., endocannabinoids), their breakdown, and their relative concentration in the brain and throughout the body. If this tone is reduced, it follows that there would be a lower pain threshold. Also, there would be derangements of digestion, mood, and sleep. Perhaps the greatest evidence for clinical endocannabinoid deficiency (CED) is in migraines, fibromyalgia, and irritable bowel syndrome (Russo 2016).

The strongest evidence of CED and migraines is found in cerebral spinal fluid assays done in fifteen people with chronic migraines versus twenty controls (Sarchielli et al. 2006). In this study, a significantly reduced amount of anandamide was seen in the migraine population. It is believed that migraines may be due to a failure of the inhibitory role of AEA on the trigeminal-vascular system activation. The trigeminal nerve is the fifth cranial nerve, and it has three sensory branches to the face. It likely activates the blood vessels around the face and the outside of the brain as a trigger of migraines. Migraines affect 14 percent of Americans and are more common in women, with a 3:1 female to male ratio. ("Probable migraines" raise the rate to 28 percent of the population.) This is almost identical to the ratio for MS in women to men in North America. Migraine headaches certainly have a genetic predisposition for occurring in women, and the throbbing pain is frequently associated with nausea, photophobia (light sensitivity), phonophobia (sound sensitivity), and has hormonal and environmental triggers.

If one looks at the overlap between migraines, fibromyalgia, and IBS, one notices an interesting pattern. In a study that looked at 201 patients with fibromyalgia, 97 percent of them had a major headache history. In another study looking at chronic daily headaches, 36.5 percent had fibromyalgia, and 31.6 percent had IBS. Similarly, 32 percent of fibromyalgia patients also have a pattern fit for IBS (Russo 2016).

It is now suggested that each of the three diagnoses have a central or CNS-shared activation. This central activation also seems to be present in many chronic pain syndromes. Hence, because IBS is hypothesized as a visceral hyperalgesia (acute gut pain), this fits with the ECS as a primary target and CED as a rational explanation.

Other CED possibilities include cystic fibrosis, neonatal failure to thrive, causalgia, brachial plexus pain (arm and shoulder nerve pain), phantom limb pain, glaucoma, dysmenorrhea, PTSD, and bipolar disorder. Glaucoma is interesting, as the mechanism may be under tonic (balanced) ECS control. Glaucoma represents a vascular retinopathy (blood vessel injury at the back of the eye). In addition, cannabinoids lower intraocular pressure (pressure in the eye). Glaucoma diagnosis is predicated on raised intraocular pressure. In summary, many of the medical problems for which we have no explanation in regular medicine may be at least partially explained by a relative endocannabinoid deficiency. In the risk/benefit ratio analysis, it makes sense to try the cannabis mixture in this population. The downside is extremely small, and it may be very helpful for individuals in recovering their quality of life.

Additional conditions that suggest the use of CBD include motion sickness, epilepsy, MS (especially those with secondary-progressive MS), Huntington's disease, and possibly even Parkinson's disease. In a study of 46 survivors of the World Trade Center disaster diagnosed with PTSD, most were found to have reduced serum 2-AG compared to controls. Serum 2-AG is the second endocannabinoid discovered inside our body, whereas anandamide is the first one. In another study, major depression was described as being a disorder of CNS plasticity rather than a failure of body neurotransmitters, such as serotonin, norepinephrine, and dopamine. This reduced CNS plasticity is consistent with an inflammatory component, or possibly a degenerative disease, linked directly to CBD.

A discussion paper by E. Russo on the topic of CED sites the possible benefits of three interventions to raise the tone of the body's cannabinoid system (Sparling 2003). The first is a low-impact aerobics regimen, i.e. exercise. The second is dietary manipulations with probiotics and prebiotics to improve the microbiome diversity and optimize our microbiome. The third recommendation is a trial of whole-plant cannabis or mixtures thereof.

I hope the above discussion helps empower you to take control of your diet and lifestyle approaches. You should understand by now that *Solving the Brain Puzzle* involves a series of successful base hits. There are few, if any, silver bullets, or home run possibilities.

17: Addiction

I seriously debated whether or not to include addiction in this book. I finally realized it was time to step up to the plate and include it as a health challenge along with Alzheimer's, Parkinson's, MS, and TBI (traumatic brain injury). For many years, the World Health Organization (WHO) recognized addiction as a separate, distinct diagnosis and illness. In this chapter, I include my personal and clinical experiences and some of the newer treatment models. (e.g., Ibogaine, ayahuasca, and medical cannabis). Many people turn to substance abuse when frustrated with pain or gradual demise from illness. Finding solace in a bottle of alcohol or oxycodone is not a good solution.

Personal Story

I grew up on a midwestern prairie farm growing plants and domestic animals. My parents had changed location, moving 800 kilometres, to leave monoculture farming. Part of my father's vision for this move was that his six children would have many farm chores to do, so going to the mall or drinking with other bored teens would be less of an issue. I believe he was right, as none of us have a problem with addiction. My father's dictum was, "If you started having a drink of alcohol in the morning, you were well on the road to addiction." Binge drinking is also alcoholism, so Dad's dictum is not quite broad enough. Yes, alcohol is a drug, though many of us may not think of it as such.

Once I was in an established family practice in rural Saskatchewan, I was asked to be the rural physician on the Saskatchewan Alcoholism Commission. This meant a four-hour drive for monthly meetings with Dr. S. Cohen, a psychiatrist, who chaired the commission board. I served on the twelve-member board for four years. Half our meetings took place around the province in addiction treatment centers. I learned a great deal from these team players, half of whom had been addicted themselves. I learned that most alcoholics were bright, often covering up personal wounds or dealing with depression and anxiety with addictive substances.

I especially like Gabor Mate's book on addiction, *In the Realm of Hungry Ghosts* (Mate 2013). I also attended one of his three-day retreats in Mexico. He practiced medicine in Vancouver's lower east side, one of the highest concentrations of addicted people in Canada. Mate's premise is that emotional trauma, real or perceived, is often at the root of the pain. Perception can even begin with a small child's interpretation of reality. An example is abandonment, where the parent is away several hours, but the young child cannot relate and feels abandoned. The child begins to replay these "tapes" or repetitive thoughts. Often these occur before "memory," so we cannot even remember them without assistance. Expert counselling, breath work, mindfulness training, meditation, and even ayahuasca, a hallucinogen, can help people recover and resolve these deeply hidden pains.

During medical school, I spent a summer working on the surface in a copper mine near Whitehorse, Yukon. I stayed with my mentor and cousin, Don Branigan, MD. He helped introduce me to addiction and recovery by throwing me "in the deep end." He dropped me off at one of his long-term patients, G.Z., a serious alcoholic. G.Z. drank forty ounces (more than a litre) of vodka per day and was about to lose his family. After three hours of talking, G.Z. consented to hospital admission for detox. Dr. Branigan assisted his recovery with frequent acupuncture. This was in 1973, so Dr. Branigan was an early adopter of integrative medicine principles.

The above experience made me more aware of addiction issues in the rest of my medical training, and that persists with learning significantly more about addiction than might be ordinary for most physicians. I am not an expert, and I defer to medical specialists, psychologists, and addiction counsellors even today.

My personal journey and brush with alcoholism was in general practice in a small town with two and then three colleagues. Two of our spouses insisted that we must not talk shop when together outside of work. To me, this was needed to let off steam and discuss worries of work. Instead, I turned to alcohol. At the end of the work day, I would have a double scotch. Then, during evenings of curling, cards, or social events, I drank more alcohol. I took stock of myself after joining the alcoholism commission. At an average of four to five drinks per day, I was well on the road to full-blown addiction. I was lucky to learn this in a non-threatening educational manner and wise enough to change. I tapered off considerably. I also realized why so many small-town doctors, especially solo practitioners, became alcoholics.

A few years later, I was training in anesthesia and working in academic anesthesiology. I learned at Society of Education in Anesthesiology meetings that opiate addiction was rampant, with 10-12 percent of residents training in anesthesiology developing an opiate addiction. The reasons thought to contribute to this include:

1. Easiest access to opioids of physicians in medicine
2. Long stressful hours on call and difficult work schedule
3. Becoming drug experts and feeling in control of drug use
4. Pre-selecting a specialty based on the administration of medications

My most memorable case is a resident colleague who became addicted to fentanyl, unknown to the people around him. At that time, a 2-ml ampoule of fentanyl had blue writing. Unfortunately, another pharmaceutical company made the same-sized ampoule with the same colour of writing but containing pancuronium—a long-acting muscle relaxant, which paralyzes a person. This resident shot up one night in a small on-call room. A resident in the next on-call room heard a big thud as the drugged resident hit the floor, having accidentally taken pancuronium instead of fentanyl. Fortunately, the second resident rescued him immediately. The addicted resident woke up in intensive care and was suddenly "outed." He had a rough go with stumbling back into addiction several times but finally stayed clean of opioids. This salvaged his family and his career. I am proud to have been one of the three physicians who monitored and supported him through his final recovery. This transpired more than thirty years ago, but opiate addiction has become rampant today in general society, not just among anesthesiology residents.

Opioid Overdose Death Crisis

Currently, nearly 60,000 narcotic overdose deaths occur each year in the United States. To put that in perspective, that is more Americans than were killed in the entire Vietnam War. How did we get here? It is not a pretty story, but part of it was orchestrated by big pharma. Each time a new opiate was developed, it was suggested that the new drug was not as addictive as morphine. By the time we had fentanyl, sufentanil, and carfentanil, we realized these were more addictive than morphine and even heroin. Today, addicts prefer fentanyl injection to heroin. In addition, drug companies came up with new oral narcotics, such as oxycodone and Percodan, to replace codeine. In the 1980s, a shrewd pharmaceutical marketing team decided they could promote opioids for chronic pain, especially after trauma or surgery or both. Today, it is felt the most common road to addiction is based on excess post-operative prescriptions or chronic pain prescriptions. Part of this is based on physicians' belief that "one size fits all" and "let me prescribe a few extra, so they don't have to bother me again." Next, people quickly learn narcotics help them fall asleep, reduce nagging aches and pains, and even promote relaxation. Now these people are on the steep and slippery slope to narcotic addiction. Who brought them to the edge of the abyss? We physicians, cheered on by the pharmaceutical companies and financial gain. Yes, a significant number of physicians accept payment for prescribing opioids. Sadly, this sells more drugs and needs to be addressed.

When all the smoke is cleared away, physicians have inadequate training in pain management, especially chronic pain. In addition, staggering amounts of money have been made by multiple pharmaceutical companies. Finally, chemists have been highly paid to work for organized crime and now illicit fentanyl and carfentanil abound. Deaths will continue to skyrocket, because carfentanil is one million or more times as potent as fentanyl and is readily available on the street.

Alcohol and Benzodiazepines

In this chapter, so far, I have focused on opioids, because it is the topic on almost everyone's mind. I do not make light of other drugs, such as cocaine and alcohol. Alcohol is still the number one killer and cause of social ills in the world today. One in twenty people worldwide are addicted to alcohol. Other prescription drugs, besides narcotics, that are of great concern are the benzodiazepines: diazepam (Valium), Librium, clonazepam (Klonopin), and even antidepressants. Please see chapter 16 for discussion of this group.

The Science of Addiction

Great strides in understanding addiction have been achieved in recent years. A fine summary of this can be found in the September 2017 issue of *National Geographic* (Smith 2017). Smith's article "The Addicted Brain," begins with an excellent quote, "Addiction hijacks the brain's neural pathways. Scientists are challenging the view that it's a moral failing and researching treatments that could offer an exit from the cycle of desire, bingeing and withdrawal that traps tens of millions of people."

Scientists now better understand how addiction disrupts nerve pathways. Addiction causes hundreds of changes in brain anatomy, chemistry, and cell-to-cell signalling, including synapses, the gaps between neurons. It is these gaps where neurotransmitters, particularly dopamine, transport the messages between brain cells. Addiction uses the brain's amazing plasticity to give "extreme value" to cocaine, heroin, or gin. This is at the expense of health, work, family or life itself. A. Bonci, a neurologist at the National Institute on Drug Abuse states, "In a sense, addiction is a pathological form of learning" (Smith 2017). I suggest addiction has the brain developing different or aberrant neural pathways much as neuropathic pain and PTSD do. This principle should help us remember addiction is a disease, not a moral failing. This alone reduces most people's shame about their addiction and helps their acceptance, which is necessary on any journey to recovery.

Solutions for Addiction

Prevention is still important, because most of us are unaware when we are on the slippery slope. Three drinks per day can trigger liver cirrhosis in men. Only two drinks per day can trigger cirrhosis in women. Prescription-supplied opioids and benzodiazepines are still the major cause of these addictions. Once addiction is established, the solution must be individualized and tailored to what is available and affordable. These are valuable people, and recovery benefits everyone concerned.

The treatment of addiction follows the treatment patterns of other health challenges. For example, I learned in the 1980s that the more alcohol costs, the less alcohol people drink. Similarly, for every tax dollar taken in from government-sanctioned alcohol sales, it costs society two to three dollars to deal with the health and social costs created by alcohol. We must remember this when considering solutions to addiction.

Many people will have success with a twelve-step program, such as Alcoholics Anonymous. Much of this success is from the individual support and mentoring. Others will benefit greatly from mindfulness training. Transcranial Magnetic Stimulation (TMS) has shown success in Italy (Smith 2017). Some people will benefit from new uses of older medications, such as naltrexone and buprenorphine (Suboxone). These medications suppress the awful craving and withdrawal. Interestingly, these can help some addictions other than narcotics. Today, some people are advocating psychedelic herbs, such as Ibogaine, for opioid addiction. Other herbs, such as ayahuasca and peyote in the optimal setting of an experienced shaman, can often help with personal psychic and emotional pain, which may address the underlying trigger for addiction. Mate, MD, addresses the inner healing required in his book, *In the Realm of the Hungry Ghosts* (Mate 2013).

I have no magic solutions for addiction treatment. I believe we must tailor this to each individual. For example, if a person has physical, emotional, or psychic pain, we need to address it. One example that has worked many times with my patients is the use of medical cannabis for pain reduction. Subsequently, many of these patients have eliminated all their opioids and nearly eliminated their alcohol intake as well. I have been very impressed with this, hence my emphasis on medical cannabis in this book.

Section Five
Diagnoses

18: Chronic Pain

Many might ask why I would include a chapter on chronic pain in a book called *Solving the Brain Puzzle*. First, my previous book was called *Winning the Pain Game* (Code 2007). In that book, I presented an anti-inflammatory diet and lifestyle approach to reducing chronic pain. Since then, a considerable amount of research has been done, and my knowledge of solutions for chronic pain has increased. This chapter will give a summary of how this can improve one's quality of life. One major reason for including this chapter is that virtually all chronic pain is perceived in the brain. When we have an unpleasant sensation in the periphery, called nociception, it does not become pain until it occurs in the brain. This pain perception in the brain follows a complex series of events within the spinal cord and the brain pathways that, if they persist beyond the time of the injury or trauma, are called chronic pain.

Chronic pain is a huge detriment to our sense of happiness and well-being, placing incredible stress on us. Any constant, significant, ongoing stress is a detriment to optimal brain function. Depression, anxiety, and other mood disorders are common in chronic pain patients. My goal in this chapter is twofold. First, by reducing your chronic pain, I aim to reduce the stress on your brain and support your use of these same modalities to help reduce your chronic pain and thus improve and enhance your brain function.

Second, I feel compelled to write this chapter because my first major love in medicine was anesthesiology. Anesthesiologists almost always run the chronic pain centers in North America. In addition, anesthesiologists run acute pain treatment centers, mostly postoperatively, in hospitals. Treating pain is one of the most satisfying components of medicine when done successfully. There is no more obvious way of relieving human suffering. This alone drew me to the concept of relieving pain. Similarly, we know the treatment of chronic pain is often difficult and poorly handled by modern medicine. One consequence of medically treating the pain is the possibility of giving the patient a major addiction to narcotics. This problem may be equal to, or even surpass, the chronic pain problem. In my search for pain-relief possibilities and for pain-prevention techniques, I have learned a great deal. I want to share my knowledge with you, so you can help yourself or others around you in the journey to wellness without chronic pain.

On a more personal level, I have had my own challenges with chronic pain. Pain is an all-consuming entity when you are in the middle of it. For me, this includes severe migraine headaches, fractures of my leg, including osteomyelitis (infected bone), and neuropathic pain from my MS. Hence, I have much empathy for pain patients. In addition, as an anesthesiologist, it is inappropriate to be drug seeking, especially for opioids. I have had sustained migraine headaches since age twenty-six (I'm now sixty-five). I still get headaches occasionally. I have searched endlessly for pain relief and for pain-prevention techniques. I have learned it is better to stay out of problems, such as pain, than try to solve the problem once I am in great pain! Some of the earlier concepts were in my first book, as noted above, but there are enough new options that it bears presenting them here. As noted earlier, I can almost completely prevent my neuropathic pain from MS by avoiding gluten. Similarly, by altering what I put in my mouth, I've been able to reduce my headache incidence and severity to a considerable degree. Stress reduction is also important. However, I realize that zero stress is an impossibility while living in our world, so we must find modalities to control it.

Persistence of acute pain sends repeated messages to the brain and often triggers "windup." This is when the brain remembers the pain and perceives it even when the tissue message injury is no longer present. An excellent example of this is phantom limb pain. If a person has a local anesthetic block of all sensation from that limb before it is removed, phantom limb pain is almost nonexistent. For the same reason, I always encourage people anticipating surgery to request or agree to a combination of a regional anesthetic rather than a simple general anesthetic. It seems that if pain is prevented and not permitted to peak in persistent messages to the brain, chronic pain is minimized.

In my days on faculty on a tenure track at the University of Saskatchewan, I, along with others, conducted a number of studies on how to reduce pain after surgery by combining naproxen (NSAID) before surgery with regular surgical anesthetics, including opioids (Code 1994). These studies were published in the *Canadian Journal of Anesthaesia*. In fact, I was asked to write an editorial on other ways to minimize or control pain in an anesthesia journal. I titled it "Balanced Anesthesia, Why not Balanced Analgesia?" (Code 1993). Further to this, in 1996, I was asked to present on the topic of "non-opioid choices for pain" at the eleventh World Congress of Anesthesiology, which was held in Sydney, Australia, that same year (Code 1996). It was the first time that I had presented in front of thousands of people and remains imprinted on my brain as a consequence.

Prior to this presentation, I had sourced all non-opioid choices to the extreme. By combining two or more medications, herbs, or other pain-relieving substances, I was able to use a smaller amount of each drug, herb, or modality, so they were synergistic with one another. Recalling the concept of risk/benefit ratio, you can combine two, three, or four choices of small amounts with fewer problems than a single choice in large amounts. The best modern example of problems with a single solution is that of oxycontin addiction, which has become a widespread plague throughout North America. Contrary to this opiate or narcotic minimization is low-dose naltrexone as a novel anti-inflammatory treatment for chronic pain (Younger 2014).

For migraine headaches, my simple early formula to avoid opioids was using 1,000 mg of acetaminophen (paracetamol) combined with 400 mg of ibuprofen. This is thought to be equivalent to 60 mg of codeine (opioid) in combination with 650 mg of acetaminophen (ASA), which, in Canada, would be called Tylenol 3s or 292s, respectively. The last two products even include caffeine, which can be useful to treat headaches at times. My combination of acetaminophen and ibuprofen is popular with dentists and orthopedic surgeons, because they can send people home without a narcotic prescription. It also minimizes the slippery slope of opioid addiction. However, it does potentially injure the liver and kidneys. Therefore, I limit my intake of these medications and keep an eye on my liver and kidney function. Finally, NSAIDs, such as ibuprofen, also cause leaky gut and injure the microbiome.

In *Winning the Pain Game*, I spoke of a number of nutrient solutions for chronic pain. Many of these are anti-inflammatory in nature, and the list includes B vitamins, omega-3 fish oils, vitamin D, emu oil, and even boron and magnesium. Most of these are mentioned elsewhere in this book, so I will present only a brief summary in this chapter.

Three of the key B vitamins are vitamin B12, B6, and folate. Each of these are important, especially for peripheral neuropathy and nerve-related pain. If the B vitamin blood levels and the homocysteine concentration cannot be measured, then perhaps it is best to take a B-100 vitamin complex twice a day for three months. In most cases, this will solve the nutrient deficiencies of these particular B vitamins. Omega-3 fish oils are best from smaller fish and ideally will be cleaned of any heavy metals and dioxins. The recommended dose for any arthritis symptoms is 3,000 mg a day of EPA and DHA in combination. A major study from Australia showed that this reduced the overall pain by one half in chronic arthritis patients.

Vitamin D is recognized as an anti-inflammatory in its own right. It becomes anti-inflammatory on as little as 2,000 IU per day. I routinely recommend at least 4,000 IU of vitamin D, which is equal to 0.1 mg. If people have malabsorption problems, celiac disease, inflammatory bowel disease, or inflammatory bowel syndrome, I suggest more. Optimally, you should have your vitamin D measured several times a year. I suggest you keep it in the 125–200 millimoles (mmol)/L in Canada, Europe, and most of the world. In the United States, this is equal to 50–80 in their system of measurement. I have seen a considerable number of my clients with dramatic reduction in their constant muscle and joint pain within three or four days of taking this supplement.

I recommend emu oil in dosages of 1,500–2,000 mg per day to my chronic arthritis patients who have no success with the aforementioned suggestions. It is a recognized anti-inflammatory but works on a different pathway than omega-3 oil. I have written a book on emu oil as well as chapters on it in each of my previous books. We raised emus for over twenty years, and I've given talks on it on several continents. This includes two talks in Australia, with the first at the World Congress of

Anesthesiology (Code 1996). My second presentation in Australia was at the World Poultry Congress in Brisbane in 2008.

Finally, I want to mention two minerals, magnesium and boron. Magnesium is tremendous in reducing nerve irritability and muscle spasms. Boron is a much less known, but is an important trace mineral recognized as essential in human nutrition in 1990. I learned about it recently from a friend and client, A.T. He learned of it from a retired PhD nutritionist. A.T. began taking 20 mg boron per day and noticed within a month that almost all of his painful psoriatic arthritis pain was gone. I've had several clients with similar benefits. This is a supplement best avoided if you have reduced kidney function. If you notice no benefit on taking boron within a month, then I suggest you discontinue it, as it occasionally has some serious side effects.

Oxygen delivery is another consideration in the treatment of chronic pain. You will note in my discussion of hyperbaric oxygen therapy (HBOT) that I've had more than 350 such treatments in the last three years. Oxygen therapy reduces my migraines as well as my lower-back pain. In others, I have seen reduced back, hip, and knee pain. I now believe that a component of pain relief, even from chronic pain, is providing more oxygen to the tissues. The best way to do this is to provide 1.5–2 atm (atmospheres), which will treat the brain and the peripheral tissues at the same time. We certainly know that HBOT reduces inflammation and enhances healing. Is it also possible that some of this pain is ischemic in nature? Ischemia is the lack of blood flow and secondary hypoxia. I now suggest to clients that they consider a trial of HBOT. This is best done simultaneously with photobiomodulation therapy (PBMT). (I discuss this further later in this chapter.)

One of my recent synergies for pain relief is the combination of opioids and the THC (tetrahydrocannabinol) and CBD of cannabis. Even minimal amounts of cannabis increases the effect of morphine or codeine by a factor of four to ten. In addition, a study published in 2014 in the *Journal of the American Medical Association* showed that, in the USA, the incidence of deaths from opioid analgesic overdose dropped by 24.8 percent in states that have legalized medical marijuana (Bachhuber 2014). Suffice it to say that opioids alone are a poor solution for chronic pain and create the risk of addiction and even the risk of overdose or death.

In this discussion of synergy, multiple components within some plants, such as cannabis, in combination, are quite good at reducing pain. Within cannabis this includes THC, CBDs (cannabinoids), and even terpenes, such as myrcene and B-caryophyllene. By being present in combination (the entourage effect), they become synergistic and improve pain relief. They also reduce the unpleasant side effects of a single agent, such as THC. THC alone can be much more psychoactive, trippy, and downright unpleasant, especially in cannabis-naïve individuals. I learned of the value of cannabis in conjunction with narcotics recently with my own migraine headaches. In view of my MS, I have a medical license to purchase marijuana. The marijuana alone helps reduce a headache, but when I add 15 mg of codeine, the headaches are virtually gone. This is at least one quarter of the amount of codeine that I would need to take the edge off a headache if used on its own.

Finally, I would like to discuss what photobiomodulation therapy can do for neck pain. My neck pain had no effective treatment whatsoever until PBMT arrived on the scene. Yes, I have neck pain and follow my own suggestions. However, Denise, has had major neck pain for more than twenty years. She has tried many different solutions including acupuncture and massage therapy, physiotherapy, and chiropractic therapy. These have helped a little, but none have made a significant difference. In recent months, Denise began eight treatments of PBMT over a period of three weeks. A few days later, she flared dramatically. However, after two to three days of aggravation of her pain, she improved greatly. Sometimes, we have to go through the pain of healing on the way to being healed. Now she is able to garden and carry on with the activities of daily living without the constant neck pain.

PBMT (Photobiomodulation Therapy)

By James Carroll

Photobiomodulation Therapy (PBMT) is a light therapy that improves tissue repair and relieves pain. It has been shown in randomized clinical trials to be effective on a wide range of acute injuries and chronic degenerative diseases. Whilst it is not known to most practicing medical doctors, it is well known to medical schools who have published over 500 randomized controlled clinical trials in peer-reviewed medical journals. A further 4,000 laboratory studies have been published by scientists reporting on the mechanism of action and dose response. This treatment is now appearing in some medical guidelines, though insurance companies have yet to include it as a reimbursable treatment.

The strong evidence for PBMT is on musculoskeletal pain (tendon injuries),[11] osteoarthritis,[12] back pain,[13] neck pain,[14] and oral mucositis,[15] which is a common side effect of many cancer treatments. Evidence is also emerging that it can have a profound effect on many central nervous system disorders such as macular degeneration,[16] Alzheimer's Disease,[17] traumatic brain injury,[18] and neuropathic pain, such as postherpetic neuralgia.[19]

[11] Stergioulas, A., et al., "Effects of low-level laser therapy and eccentric exercises in the treatment of recreational athletes with chronic Achilles tendinopathy," *American Journal of Sports Medicine* 36 no. 5 (2008): 881–887.

[12] GN, S., et al., "Radiological and biochemical effects (CTX-II, MMP-3, 8, and 13) of low-level laser therapy (LLLT) in chronic osteoarthritis in Al-Kharj, Saudi Arabia," *Lasers Medical Science* 32 no. 2 (2017): 297–303.

[13] Glazov, G., M. Yelland, and J. Emery, "Low-level laser therapy for chronic non-specific low back pain: a meta-analysis of randomised controlled trials," *Acupuncture Medicine* 34 no. 5 (2016): 328–341.

[14] Chow, R.T., et al., "Efficacy of low-level laser therapy in the management of neck pain: a systematic review and meta-analysis of randomised placebo or active-treatment controlled trials," *Lancet* 374 no. 9705 (2009): 1897 –1898.

[15] Ferreira, B., F.M. da Motta Silveira, and F.A. de Orange, "Low-level laser therapy prevents severe oral mucositis in patients submitted to hematopoietic stem cell transplantation: a randomized clinical trial," *Support Care Cancer* 24 no. 3 (2016): 1035–1042.

[16] Merry, G.F., et al., "Photobiomodulation reduces drusen volume and improves visual acuity and contrast sensitivity in dry age-related macular degeneration," *Acta Ophthalmol*, 2016.

[17] Saltmarche, A.E., et al., "Significant Improvement in Cognition in Mild to Moderately Severe Dementia Cases Treated with Transcranial Plus Intranasal Photobiomodulation: Case Series Report," *Photomedicine Laser Surgery*, 2017.

[18] Chen, Y.T., et al., "Early application of low-level laser may reduce the incidence of postherpetic neuralgia (PHN)," *Journal of the American Academy of Dermatology* 75 no. 3 (2016): 572–577.

[19] Maiman, T.H., "Stimulated Optical Radiation in Ruby," *Nature* 187 no. 4736 (1960): 493–494.

Discovery

In 1960, Ted Maiman developed the first working laser.[20] In 1967 Professor Andre Mester, a medical doctor and a scientist in Hungary wanted to find out if the laser ray might cause harm to the internal organs of mice (such as causing cancer). He shaved the hair from the abdomen of twenty mice, applied a low-intensity laser beam multiple times over many days to ten of the mice, and kept the others as an untreated control group. One of the observations was that the hair grew back more quickly in the treated group. This was the first report of the stimulating effect of low-power lasers. He also observed that with too much treatment, the hair growth could be inhibited.[21]

Nomenclature

Unfortunately, this therapy has been endowed with too many names, at least 53 different terms[22] have appeared in the literature over the last 50 years, which reduced its discoverability. A popular early term through the 1980s was Laser Biostimulation. Since the 1990s, Low-level Laser Therapy (LLLT) was in vogue. Later the marketing term Cold Laser Therapy emerged on the internet. Finally, a consensus was reached in 2014 at the joint conference of the World Association for Laser Therapy and North American Association for Laser Therapy.

---

[20] Mester, E., Szende, B., and J.G. Tota, "Effect of laser on hair growth of mice," *Kiserletes Orvostudomany* 19 (1967): 628-631.

[21] Carroll, J.D., "Pubmed fails to correctly index most LLLT/photobiomodulation research, how big is the problem?", *Lasers in Surgery and Medicine* 46 no. 4 (2014): 352-352.

[22] Anders, J.J., R.J. Lanzafame, and P.R. Arany, "Low-level light/laser therapy versus photobiomodulation therapy," *Photomedicine and Laser Surgery* 33 no. 4 (2015): 183-184.

It was agreed that Photobiomodulation (PBM) was a more suitable description of the mechanism and that when applied to patients it becomes Photobiomodulation Therapy. At the time of writing, the abbreviation for Photobiomodulation Therapy has not been discussed. Some write "PBM therapy," and others write "PBMT." Subsequently, the National Library of Medicine (USA) included Photobiomodulation as an official Medical Subject Heading (MeSH), so this is becoming the preferred medical name.

How Can One Therapy Work on So Many Challenging Medical Problems?

All the diseases mentioned above have one thing in common: oxidative stress. Most acute pathologies (injuries, degenerative diseases) feature oxidative stress (commonly called free radicals) as a cause or component of their disease process. Oxidative stress causes necrosis (cell death), starts inflammation, triggers the aging process, and activates degenerative diseases, such as cancer, Alzheimer's disease, osteoarthritis, and MS, depending on your genetic weaknesses. PBMT is very good at reducing oxidative stress.[23] It is worth understanding why light does this, because it also explains improved blood flow and tissue repair.In conclusion, I want to talk about two studies on neck pain. The first of these is "The clinical efficacy of low power laser therapy on pain and function in cervical osteoarthritis," (Özdemir 2001). All the following parameters improved in the treatment group: pain, paravertebral muscle spasm, lordosis angle (neck stoop), and the range of

---

[23] Huang, Y.Y., et al., "Low-level laser therapy (LLLT) reduces oxidative stress in primary cortical neurons in vitro," *Journal of Biophotonics*, 6 no. 10 (2016): 829-38.

neck motion and function. There was improvement in these parameters by almost 65 percent in the treatment group with virtually no change in the placebo group. The second study was on the effect of PBMT on chronic neck pain. The subjects were randomized into a double-blind study and treated 14 times over seven weeks. Measurements were done at the start and at seven and 12 weeks. These measurements used the visual analog pain scale, which is one of the gold standards of pain assessment. The pain scores reduced markedly in the treatment group. Forty percent improved greatly or by "much." Another 42 percent improved somewhat. About 17 percent were the same, and 1–2 percent were worse (Chow 2006). I am impressed with both above studies and a review and meta-analysis of neck pain and PBMT treatments (Chow 2009). I see many chronic neck pain patients, and this "Star Trek-like" treatment is the best solution that I have seen in over forty years.

Similar studies for lower-back pain and sciatica support this treatment as well. I suggest that you read chapter 35 of this book if you suffer from neck pain, lower-back pain, or any other musculoskeletal ailment. Efrati showed that HBOT diminished fibromyalgia (Efrati 2015). In the last few weeks, I learned of a study discussing cartilage formation, as assessed by MRI (personal communication). They found the treatment over an eight-week period with PBMT increased the knee cartilage thickness from 2–4 mm. This is profound. I no longer think of getting my knees, hips, or shoulders replaced. Instead, I would consider PBMT and HBOT, because both have healing effects and are also stem cell boosters. If those in combination happened to fail, then I would consider stem cell joint injection by an expert. If you follow this path, I suggest the stem cells recovered from your own fat tissue. A great review on mesenchymal stem cells' life and fate is by Eggenhofer (2014).

In this chapter, I have given you a synopsis of my personal concepts on reducing chronic pain. Chronic pain is perceived in the brain and spinal cord, which is also known as the central nervous system. I hope you can see that chronic pain solutions should similarly be brain-recovery solutions. This, coupled with the frequency of one-third to one-half of people having chronic pain, should explain why I have included this chapter.

19: The New MS (Microvascular Syndrome)

I believe we have reached a major crossroads in understanding MS. This understanding permits an entirely new realm of possibilities. It is time to ditch the word "autoimmune" when talking about MS. In forty years of searching, we have never found the "smoking gun" of autoimmune MS, which would be antibodies to myelin. Furthermore, MS affects the eyes, and yet they have no myelin. Ophthalmologists have been telling neurologists this for years. Now I would like to state that MS should stand for "microvascular syndrome" rather than "multiple sclerosis." Multiple sclerosis means "multiple scars." We have known for some time that any vascular illness is associated with more rapid disability progression in MS (Marrie et al. 2010). This is easy to understand once we accept MS as a vascular (blood vessel) illness. Further support of this is the importance of BBB (Blood Brain Barrier) which is endothelial health (Zlokovic 2008). Neurologist Dr. Swank published in 1958 that MS patients had frequent, tiny, under-the-skin hemorrhages. He suggested this predicted their associated leaky BBB (Swank 1958) and led him to develop the quite successful Swank diet for MS.

A huge epidemiological study done on people with MS (15,684 cases) and matched controls (78,420 people) lends much credence to the vascular component within MS (Capkun et al. 2015). Within the comorbidities or associated diseases they found MS patients had 3.8 times as many strokes as controls. This study was corroborated by an earlier Swedish study which revealed the high risk of cardiovascular diseases after a diagnosis of MS (Jadidi 2013). They noted nearly double the risk of heart attack, stroke, and heart failure. We should heed this concept if we have MS. Happily, anything we do to reduce our cardiovascular risk will likely slow our MS as well. This is the point I am trying to make.

The term "microvascular syndrome" was coined by Prof. Philip James of Scotland, who has published on MS since the 1980s (James 1983, 1986). A great deal of evidence in the literature supports this new concept. I will endeavor to help you understand why this concept is so useful. This new name for MS permits understanding of how the brain changes in MS. This new MS includes inflammation and blood-brain barrier injury, which everyone agrees describes MS. Microvascular syndrome also explains the CCSVI (chronic cerebrospinal venous insufficiency) component as a partial trigger for MS. Finally, neurologists frequently citing abundance of immune cells near an MS lesion as confirming autoimmunity is bogus. There are no more lymphocytes around a MS lesion than around a stroke. This is confirmed in the literature. It is also interesting to note Thom's title "Intramicroparticle nitrogen dioxide is a bubble nucleation site leading to decompression-induced neutrophil activation and vascular injury" (Thom 2013).This is consistent with the identical MRI visualized brain injury of divers' decompression injury to MS.

The MS pathology information and MRI information (Law 2004) confirm that injury occurs at the endpoint of the longest blood vessels within the brain once they become veins, venules, or micro veins, which are visible only with a micro-scope, because they are about the size of a red blood cell (seven microns). The injury and pathology changes virtually always occur around the smallest veins at the end of the longest transit distance from the heart. Of course, the farther from the heart the lower the concentration of oxygen or hypoxia. Hypoxia begets inflammation (Eltzschig 2011). The concentration of oxygen is the lowest in these small veins. This is significant, because this is where the injuries predominate because of the unhappy triad: 1) low oxygen or hypoxia, 2) slow movement of blood, and 3) the area where microemboli (small blood clot particles or fat emboli) tend to stick to the blood vessel wall (James 1983). The presence of hypoxia makes the blood vessel wall, the endothelium, especially susceptible to injury from the microemboli. The combination of these two, hypoxia and microemboli, causes blood-brain barrier (BBB) breakdown. This is really injury to the blood vessel wall or endothelium, because that is what forms the BBB. Once this barrier is broken, many toxins and even red blood cells can enter the brain. The immune system responds but primarily as a garbage clean-up operation, which is part of its function.

One clinical example of microemboli-triggering MS symptoms is Hughes syndrome, or, as it's called in North America, antiphospholipid syndrome. Many of these people do best if they stay on a drug or supplement regime to minimize these clots, which stem from an overactive fibrin (clotting) system. A second type of microemboli is fat emboli. Prof. James published this clinical example of fat microemboli triggering MS in the *Lancet* (James 1983). Finally, the micro embolus of lipopolysaccharide (LPS) is a product of leaky gut. LPS is known to be a triggering event of inflammation in the brain in a number of brain illnesses, including MS. An article in the *Annals of Neurology* (Desai 2016) describes the use of LPS to trigger an MS response in lab animals. Each of these three types of microemboli can, independently or in combination, trigger BBB injury and initiate the inflammatory cascade. Therefore, the appropriate name of MS is microvascular syndrome. An MRI study (Alexander 2015) at the University of Buffalo confirmed microparticles in relapsing-remitting and secondary progressive MS.

This inflammatory cascade consists of four items: redness, swelling, heat, and pain or loss of function. We are unable to perceive the heat or pain within the brain but are certainly aware of the redness, swelling, and loss of cognitive function. When you see unidentified bright objects (UBOs, a.k.a. white matter hyper intensities or WMHs) on an MRI of the brain, you are unable to differentiate between edema, swelling, and scarring. However, the edema is reversible once the inflammation is reversed. This accounts for the people who have some recovery from their MS brain lesions. I like the summary article on non-pharmacological approaches to ameliorate MS symptoms (Juurlink 2015). I believe the best way to treat an MS attack acutely is to use supplemental oxygen. The highest amount is delivered the fastest with HBOT. However, if this is not available, then I highly recommend the use of normal barometric pressure oxygen therapy (NBOT), which I simply call 0_2 therapy. If done optimally, this will increase circulating dissolved oxygen four to five times. You can read more about this in chapter 30.

In 2011, in the *New England Journal of Medicine*, hypoxia was described as a major trigger of inflammation by the activation of hypoxia inducible factor-1 (HIF-1) (Semenza 2011). We also know that hypoxia is the biggest trigger of reactive oxygen species (ROS) and free radical release, which injures and even kills cells. ROS release is partly treatable with antioxidants, such as coenzyme Q10, vitamin C, glutathione, and alpha lipoic acid. However, treating the initial ROS trigger of hypoxia with supplemental oxygen is even better than anti-oxidants or at least an incredible adjunct to antioxidants.

The radiology literature is quite conclusive that the UBOs or WMHs detected in MS patients are initiated by hypoxia. It seems that the only people not accepting this hypoxia premise in MS are the MS neurologists. I have a dream that one day they will accept the hypoxia concept. When I listened to vascular neurologist Dr. Alireza Minagar of Louisiana State University speak in New York at the 2016 International Society of Neurovascular Disease (ISNVD) conference, I realized we were getting closer to my dream. He talked in detail about MS in the brain. He spoke of the inflammation and blood-brain barrier breakdown found in MS. He admitted that the trigger was still not known. I was able to ask the first question after his presentation. I asked if hypoxia could be the trigger of MS. He stated that this was possible and mentioned an *Annals of Neurology* article published a few weeks previous by R.A. Desai, PhD, et al., including Dr. Kenneth J. Smith (2016). He said the article supported this possibility of hypoxia triggering MS. I was greatly cheered by his reply and bought his book at the conference. I realized his book did not have the concept of hypoxia as a trigger of MS, but I was excited to find an individual neurologist open to this principle. The only other neurologist in North America whom I know is open to this concept in MS is Dr. David Hubbard of California. His son has MS. Earlier work published by A. L. Davies of Kenneth Smith and Desai's lab showed neurological deficits caused by tissue hypoxia (Davies 2013).

Within 24 hours of the meeting in New York, I was visiting Prof. James in Dundee, Scotland. He is the one who inspired me to believe that hypoxia is indeed a significant trigger in MS. I learned this from his superb book, *Oxygen and the Brain: The Journey of Our Lifetime* (James 2014). This book is a landmark in our understanding of the critical value and importance of oxygen in all healing, especially the brain. Professor James and I soon found Desai's article in the *Annals of Neurology* and studied it in detail together (Desai 2016). Prior to this ground-breaking article, we were considering publishing about hypoxia and MS in the *Journal of Medical Hypothesis*. We did not need to do this because of the Desai and Smith article. However, we realized it is always better to have people publish well-researched information in such a significant peer-reviewed journal as the *Annals of Neurology* than to write the hypothesis ourselves. The Desai article, presented by the team of Dr. Kenneth J. Smith at the Department of Neuroinflammation and Queens Square Multiple Sclerosis Centre and the Department of Brain Repair and Rehabilitation, UCL Institute of Neurology in London, UK, elegantly described how hypoxia was a trigger in a new MS model. They went on to describe how 80 percent oxygen was a treatment of these MS lesions that were produced in their model. In earlier days, Dr. Smith had interacted back and forth over articles with Prof. James. The article was titled "Cause and Prevention of Demyelination in a Model Multiple Sclerosis Lesion." In the article's objectives, they stated that "neuropathological evidence suggests that demyelination can occur in the relative absence of lymphocytes, and with distinctive characteristics suggestive of a tissue energy deficit." Within the article, they demonstrated that this tissue energy deficit can be reversed with supplemental oxygen. I quote the final part of the discussion in this paper under Therapy: "It is striking that the demyelination can be greatly reduced, or even prevented by simply raising inspired oxygen at normobaric pressure for the first two days when the lesion is vulnerable to hypoxia. Therapeutically, it is encouraging that oxygen is easily administered and there is substantial clinical evidence that oxygen administration is generally safe, if delivered at moderate concentration and duration" (Desai 2016).

This helps confirm that hypoxia is one of the key triggers of MS. For the first time in nearly fifty years, we have a new model for the investigation of MS. Experimental autoimmune encephalomyelitis (EAE) can now be replaced as a research model of MS. An interesting sidebar here is a research article several years ago that revealed that supplemental oxygen could reverse the EAE process. Prof. James and I celebrated by going for high tea at the Gleneagles Golf Clubhouse, 2005 host of the G-8 summit. More importantly, the tea room over-looks the land previously owned by the family of John Scott Haldane. He was a giant in medicine and anaesthesia. He was well ahead of his time in using supplemental oxygen to treat carbon monoxide poisoning in coal miners and chlorine-gassed soldiers in World War I.

Why celebrate? We believe the article by Dr. Smith and his lab will help move forward this whole new paradigm for MS. This lab's article on how the lesions of MS can be triggered by hypoxia and treated by oxygen is a game changer. This research was done by a well-recognized team at the world-class Queen Square Multiple Sclerosis Centre Council in the UK. Second, it was published in a prestigious neurology journal. Finally, it was funded by the Medical Research Council, the Multiple Sclerosis Society in the United Kingdom, and the National Multiple Sclerosis Society in the United States. I suspect this is one of the most important pieces of research that these societies have ever funded. Part of our dream is being real-ized. New researchers in neuroscience and physicians training in neurology will read this article, and a shift will begin. Yes, the shift may take a generation, but we are finally started on this path.

Before leaving this discussion on the MS microvascular syndrome, I want to point out one more major fact that will interest you. Prof. James is one of the world's experts on deep-sea diving injuries. He has consulted around the world after developing major expertise in the North Sea oil development in the 1980s and 1990s. He relates that, post dive, divers frequently experience MS-like symptoms. On MRI, the UBOs are identical to those seen on an MS patients' MRIs. Often, these lesions are in exactly the same parts of the brain as MS. The accepted injury in divers is nitrogen microbubbles. Recent data suggests there are some fat microemboli components as well. Isn't this an interesting concept for all physicians, particularly MS neurologists?

Finally, you may be wondering how I tie chronic cerebrovascular venous insufficiency (CCSVI) into my hypoxia, microemboli microvascular hypothesis. This is quite easy because of a study by Dr. Ivo Petrov, of Sofia, Bulgaria (Petrov 2016). He studied the concentrations of oxygen, carbon dioxide, and oxygen saturation above and below the internal jugular vein narrowing in patients with CCSVI. He repeated this study after venous balloon angioplasty. He demonstrated that the venous blood above the relative venous blockage was hypoxic and hypercarbic (elevated in carbon dioxide). This abnormality normalized once the relative venous obstruction was treated with balloon angioplasty. This fits well with the clinical improvement of nearly two-thirds of patients who have had this venous treatment. If the venous outflow from the brain is partially blocked, commonly at the internal jugular vein valve, there are consequences. The areas that this vein drains from the brain have a relative back pressure. As a consequence, these areas with relatively higher pressure receive less of the new flow of fresh arterial oxygenated blood. This is because blood flow, like all things, follows the path of least resistance. This relative resistance is resolved by the venous balloon angioplasty. Consequently, these areas receive more fresh blood flow and more oxygen. This is why these MS individuals or Ménière's disease individuals see an improvement of their symptoms. For people with MS, this will usually be less fatigue and improved cognition, reduced sleep disturbance, and reduced headaches. My own balloon venous angioplasty by Dr. Michael Arata delivered all these benefits.

I have noted that not all my benefits from the procedure persisted. However, since then, I have discovered that supplemental oxygen can treat many of the same issues. For this reason, I have done more than 350 hyperbaric oxygen treatment (HBOT) sessions. I am fortunate to have access to a hyperbaric oxygenation treatment centre in my community. Happily, many people with MS in the last thirty years in the UK and other communities, such as Gibraltar and Jersey, have access to community-based oxygen treatment centres. Development of these centres is well described in Dr. James' book, *Oxygen and the Brain*. These centres have done more than four million treatments for people with MS. The long-term data have shown that following a series of twenty treatments, and ideally one per week thereafter, MS symptoms have dramatically stabilized, and MS progression is reduced (James 1986). The research also confirms that it is good for cognitive function, fatigue, and bladder function. More recently, I have added normal baric oxygen supplementation to my set of treatment choices. Perhaps now MS neurologists will have an easier time accepting the validity of treating CCSVI and realizing why it may help some of their MS patients.

Other Choices:

1. GFT or FMT: see chapter 33. Improved microbiome diversity will improve MS. The first pilot study suggesting this "Diet Modulation of Gut Microbiome in MS Patients" demonstrated this (Saresella 2017).
2. Cannabis is often a great help with spasticity and pain (Pryce 2012; Zajicek 2003; Wilcox 2018).

20: Headaches, Migraines, Epilepsy, and Menière's Disease

I have put these four seemingly quite different diagnoses together, because each begins as a type of depolarization or "electrical flooding" of a part of the brain. Similarly, the treatment options also share some parallels.

If you have ever had a migraine headache, you will find this chapter very informative. I have struggled with migraines for more than thirty-five years, so I have a great deal of empathy for fellow migraine sufferers. More is now understood regarding the triggers of migraines and therapies. I will endeavour to help you understand this intermittent crippling problem. My goal is to give you more choices beyond the traditional options.

A migraine headache is a chronic episodic primary headache. It is believed to be a neurovascular pain syndrome with altered brain neuron processing. This change in nerve processing includes activation of brainstem nuclei, cortical hyperexcitability, and spreading cortical depression (Iadecola 2002). In short, it affects the entire brain and primarily involves the trigeminal neurovascular system. The trigeminal is the fifth cranial nerve and supplies a major part of the face. It is a source of the horrific pain of trigeminal neuralgia. When this cranial nerve is triggered, it creates painful inflammation in the outside brain blood vessels that supply the dura mater (the fine lining around the brain just inside the skull). Symptoms of migraine headaches can last fourteen to seventy-two hours and may be severe (Bolay 2002).

Migraine headaches are the second most common headache and affect approximately 12 percent of the population at some point in their lifetime. In fact, if only one of the several migraine headache criteria is missing for the diagnosis of a migraine headache, then it is called probable migraine, and the incidence doubles to 24 percent of the population. Women have a greater incidence of migraines, with an 18 percent lifetime possibility of getting a migraine headache. One common trigger is the hormonal shifts at the time of the menstrual cycle. Once the estrogen levels fall with menopause, migraine headaches are usually quite diminished, often completely. Nearly 45 percent of migraine sufferers begin in childhood or adolescence. Often in children, these are preceded by abdominal pain, which has been called abdominal migraine. This is abdominal pain where no pathology, such as appendicitis, can be found.

I've experienced migraine headaches since my mid-twenties, and they persist today. One of my first migraine headache attacks was associated with terrible nausea and vomiting. I needed admission to hospital for three days for intravenous fluids and ongoing antinausea therapy. I eventually learned that gluten was a major trigger for me. An additional trigger is altitude and lack of sleep. When I was in my fifties, I learned that treating my jugular veins in the neck with angioplasty could dramatically reduce my headaches.

Today's research has shown that migraine headaches associated with high altitude and microgravity are similar to the clinical syndrome of cerebral venous hypertension. Classically, raised pressure within the brain (idiopathic intracranial hypertension) results in headaches. Similarly, any obstruction to venous outflow from the brain (CCSVI) also causes headaches. Also, a slight increase in central venous pressure within the chest cavity aggravates headaches. One probable cause of this altitude trigger is the role of hypoxia at altitude, which results in hypoxia-induced pulmonary vasoconstriction. This means the blood vessels within the chest get smaller when there is inadequate oxygen. As a consequence of this, the blood returning to the heart is impeded, and the central venous pressure rises. This concept is explained by H. Wilson et al. in *High Altitude Medicine and Biology* (Wilson 2011).

Another way to help you understand the importance of venous hypertension is to list the clinical syndromes that it impacts

- Idiopathic intracranial hypertension
- Obstructive sleep apnea
- Chiari malformation
- Migraine
- Traumatic brain injury involving the CSF cisterns
- Space adaptation syndrome
- Other headaches, such as exertional

At rest, the brain receives about 14 percent of the heart's five liters per minute, or approximately 700 ml per minute. Therefore, the jugular veins have to drain this same amount. Any compromise to this drainage, such as a tight shirt collar, results in greater cerebral venous pressures and raised intracranial pressure. One of my anatomy professors in medical school could not close his top shirt button without developing a headache. Hypoxia-induced headache can be used as a model for the same problem. Hence, high-altitude research suggests venous congestion, secondary to hypoxia. Similarly, obstructive sleep apnea is associated with morning headaches and irregular breathing (Cheyne-Stokes). A morning headache, present upon awakening, is a major clue of insufficient venous drainage of the brain. Wilson et al. reported a study using 3 Tesla MRI to show middle cerebral artery dilatation in hypoxia (2011). They studied seven subjects on room air, 21 percent oxygen, and then studied them again on a hypoxic mixture of 12 percent oxygen for three hours. Five of the seven individuals reported headaches on the 12 percent oxygen, and the other two noted head "fullness." This tentatively supports a mechanism of venous engorgement secondary to hypoxia.

Space Adaptation Syndrome

Two thirds of space shuttle astronauts experience space motion sickness. This is probably vestibular/balance disturbance due to fluid shifts. Many astronauts suffer headaches and the loss of peripheral vision. Again, this is believed to be due to venous engorgement, because the brain's venous outflow cannot keep pace with the inflow from the arterial system. This can even progress to facial swelling. Dr. Paolo Zamboni is studying with NASA in space to help them understand space adaptation syndrome and for him to further understand CCSVI. Overall, there is increasing interest in the role of the venous system and development of neurological disorders. Dr. Zamboni was the first to demonstrate and treat this in MS patients. Although his description of CCSVI is a hotly debated topic, it makes a great deal of sense to me. When I was treated for my own reduced venous outflow in my jugular veins, I was headache free for at least six months after angioplasty. Now I suggest and use supplemental oxygen, because it is easier to access and relatively less expensive.

One of the current recommended treatments for cluster headaches, particularly in Europe, is 20-40 minutes of breathing a high-percentage of oxygen, about 70-80 percent (Petersen 2016). I use this to treat my migraine headaches. A cluster headache, in essence, is a seventy-two-hour migraine headache. I suggest extra oxygen for any migraine headache, the sooner the better. If I happen to be home or near an oxygen hyperbaric chamber, then I will go in at two atmospheres for 40 to 60 minutes. We know that relatively high amounts of oxygen to the brain will cause a secondary vasoconstriction. It is probably this vasoconstriction that is helping to break the excessively dilated blood vessels. Vasoconstriction is how the traditional migraine treatment pills of Sumatriptan and others also work. Personally, I prefer oxygen, now that I've tried both.

Migraine Headache, Microemboli, and Possible Mini Stroke

Some researchers are now suggesting that up to half of migraine headaches with aura are triggered by microemboli (Nozari 2010). These tiny emboli can be tiny blood clots, fat emboli, or even small particles of food or bacteria from a leaky gut. Most emboli are filtered out by the lungs, as the venous blood is pumped there first. However, some micro-emboli get through. In addition, up to 25 percent of adults have a Patent Foramen Ovale (PFO). Interestingly, women have more PFOs, more migraines, and more MS. Are these connected? This means they have a small hole between the two upper chambers, or atria, of the heart. The presence of a PFO makes one more vulnerable to stroke, decompression illness, venous air embolism, migraine with aura, and perhaps even MS. There is some evidence that PFO is one contributing factor to a migraine with aura. One study showed that migraine with aura patients were twice as likely as normal to have a PFO. The normal instance of 25 percent in the regular population was elevated to 41–48 percent in the migraine with aura group. In a 2003 study of 215 subjects, researchers found a 33 percent headache prevalence prior to PFO surgical repair. This incidence of headache was more than cut in half with closure, and it was reduced by 62 percent in patients with headache without aura. Then, in 2005, Reisman et al. reported an 80 percent reduction in the number of migraine episodes per month, after PFO closure, using a transcatheter technique (2005). Studies are still ongoing, and acceptance of this possibility of PFO repair for migraine is still relatively unavailable. However, because I have migraines, I am keen to determine whether I also have a PFO. Stay tuned.

The start of a migraine is much better understood now. The first step is felt to be cortical spreading depression. Think of this as a temporary damping of electrical activity within the brain. This cortical spreading depression is felt to be triggered by a burst of serotonin or other chemical, often from the lungs. It gets to the brain through the same microemboli concept. The second possible triggering mechanism is the actual physical microemboli. This is a miniature or subclinical stroke. It is felt that when this microemboli touches the wall of the small blood vessels, the endothelium, which may be hyper responsive, this initiates the cortical spreading depression.

The next step is when the cortical spreading depression hits the many afferents (sensory components) within the trigeminal neurovascular system. This nerve is able to trigger blood vessel changes around the face, the meninges, and blood vessels all around the surface of the brain. These vessels are very pain sensitive and generate the headache.

The foregoing discussion helps us understand how headaches are triggered. Hence, we are now better prepared to prevent them. I would like to discuss six methods on how to treat migraine headaches. I expect that many of you will find all of these new, but each of these has some research to support the concept:

1. PFO closure: This can reduce migraine headaches by up to 80 percent. The first step in this path is determining whether you have a PFO. This can be done through echocardiography. A new screening tool is to use an ear probe pulse oximeter. This is exactly like the finger clip device used in ambulances, emergency rooms, and operating theatres, but it clips onto the ear instead. The ear is chosen, because it is a good approximation of blood flow and saturation in the brain. The individual does repeated Valsalva manoeuvres while the pulse oximeter is observed and recorded. A Valsalva manoeuvre is what one does when straining to pass stool. If the pulse oximeter saturation reading goes down at the appropriate time and desaturation occurs, it is likely that the person has a PFO. This occurs, because the increased pressure in the chest raises the right atrial pressure, and the flow of the right to left shunt occurs into the left atria, left ventricle, and directly to the brain. This is due to the mixing of the less-oxygenated venous blood from the body with the regular oxygenated blood, which has just returned from the lungs (Jopling 2015).

2. Homocysteine: This is a nutrition component to consider to minimize and prevent migraines. Migraine headaches may arise in part because of the disruption the neurovascular endothelium, the blood vessel lining, which is made especially sensitive due to the elevation of homocysteine. R. Lea et al. studied this with a vitamin supplement and testing of the MTHFR (677T) genotype to see if homocysteine lowering reduced migraine disability (2009). This was a randomized double-blind placebo-controlled trial of 52 patients with

migraine with aura. They found that a daily supplement of 2 mg folic acid, 25 mg vitamin B6, and 400 µg of vitamin B12 lowered the homocysteine by 39 percent, or about 4 mcmol/L. Migraine disability was reduced in the treatment group from 61 percent of patients to 30 percent after the six months. The claimant-treated group reported a decrease in frequency from four to one and a decrease in pain score from a median of six to 4.5. No changes were noted in the placebo group. When one separated out the migraine patients into the two genetic groups, the homocysteine reduction was 31.4 percent for TT carriers (these are homozygous, about 6-7 percent of population) compared to 47.7 percent for the heterozygote individuals, which are approximately 20 percent of the population. I happen to be one of these. They suggested that the TT genotype, the homozygous group, probably needs a larger dose of the three vitamins, because there was no apparent reduction in disability for this group. I refer you to chapter 6 and 7, where you can learn of the fairly inexpensive but effective way to achieve this lower homocysteine. This will also reduce your risk of heart attack, stroke, migraine headaches, and Alzheimer's disease by up to 50 percent.

3. Oxygen therapy: The supplemental oxygen recommended at one of the health units in Birmingham, UK, is a flow of 10-12 L/min supplied through an oxygen rebreathing mask for 30-40 minutes. Research on this has demonstrated that most people will be able to reverse the headache with 5 L/min flow, but a final portion of people will need 12 L/min (Cohen 2009). This can be done at home with an oxygen concentrator, which produces 94-95 percent oxygen, which is quite

adequate. If available, another choice is hyperbaric oxygen therapy at 2 atm for 40–60 minutes under pressure, breathing pure oxygen.

4. Venous angioplasty can be used to treat CCSVI, not just MS, and also headaches. This was shown in a 2018 article published in PLOS by Clive B. Beggs et al., titled "Mid-term sustained relief from headaches after balloon angioplasty of the internal jugular veins in patients with multiple sclerosis" (Beggs 2018). The venous balloon angioplasty intervention was associated with a large and sustained reduction in pain of headache scores for more than three years. I have met Dr. Beggs at a number of conferences, and he is diligent and keen to pursue and report on good science, so I am happy to include this timely headache article. I have referred three people, without MS, for this same balloon angioplasty for headache with excellent results, albeit not necessarily lasting three years.

5. Cannabis: Many studies support this age-old use of cannabis (Rhyne 2016; Sarchielli 2007).

6. Photobiomodulation therapy for headaches is still early, but studies are underway (Hamblin 2016).

Epilepsy

People with epilepsy experience recurrent seizures, because a sudden surge of electricity (depolarization) causes a temporary disturbance in the messaging systems between brain cells. Diagnosis is primarily done with EEG (electroencephalogram). Epilepsy is the fourth most common neurological problem. Any brain injury or illness, from lupus to stroke to traumatic brain injury, can increase the possibility of epilepsy.

Treatment with anti-seizure medication only works two thirds of the time. This is despite the twenty-nine different medicines available. What are the other choices for people with treatment-resistant epilepsy? The other options include brain surgery, cannabis (CBD), deep-brain stimulation, transcranial magnetic stimulation (Tergau 1999), and a ketogenic diet. My personal favourite is CBD from cannabis. More details on this can be found under the epilepsy heading in chapter 16.

Ménière's Disease

Dr. Beggs' article now permits me to segue to Ménière's Disease, which though different from headache has similar components, triggers, and even treatments. Ménière's disease affects a substantial number of people per year. For example, the incidence in Europe is 50–200 per 100,000 people per year. The disease is characterized by intermittent episodes of vertigo lasting from minutes to hours, with fluctuating senso-rineural hearing loss, tinnitus, and ear pressure sensation. I learned this from a paper at the ISNVD meeting in New York in April 2016. The paper was by D.C. Alpini, (now deceased), P.M. Bavera, and A. Cesarani, all from Milan, Italy (Alpini 2013). In this team's earlier paper in *ScienceMED*, entitled "CCSVI in Ménière's Disease. Case or Cause?" Dr. Bavera carried out 823 detailed duplex, echo-colour Doppler (ultrasounds) in normal controls and Ménière's patients (Alpini 2013). None of these patients had MS, but 70 percent of the Ménière's patients had CCSVI per the Zamboni criteria. I was fortunate to share a panel presentation with Dr. Bavera in Vancouver at the CNHS in September 2017. He is convinced that obstructive venous outflow is clinically significant in Ménière's Disease.

Therefore, we see one more neurological illness with relatively obstructed venous outflow present (CCSVI). This frequency of CCSVI is roughly the same in MS and Ménière's Disease, at 70 percent. This suggests venous balloon angioplasty may be one more treatment option in an illness that has precious few options. Similarly, I suggest a trial of twenty HBOT treatments may be of value to resolve the symptoms. Finally, if there is no access to HBOT, then 100 percent oxygen with a rebreathing mask at home or in hospital emergency can be tried for severe acute attacks. Sudden onset sensorineural hearing loss is one of the newest accepted indications by Undersea Hyperbaric Medical Society, UHMS, for a series of HBOT treatments. A trial would be indicated, as there is virtually no downside.

21: Stroke

Almost all of us know someone who has suffered a stroke (cerebrovascular accident or CVA). Over 790,000 strokes occur per year in the USA, and 600,000 of these are first-time strokes. A stroke happens every 40 seconds, and a stroke kills someone every four minutes! These numbers tell us prevention is key, and the best investigation and treatment can help prevent a second stroke. Similarly, most of us lose hope once we hear the word "stroke." Why? Because until recently, giving up hope was almost all we had to offer. In the 1990s, the "decade of the brain," we began to have hope for rapid diagnosis and treatment of stroke. It was found that clot-busting drugs, initially streptokinase and then TPA (tissue plasminogen activator) helped dissolve the blood clot causing the stroke. If given within a four-hour window, nearly complete recovery might occur. This clot-busting for stroke was following the clot-busting for heart attack or MI (myocardial infarction). I became aware of this stroke treatment when I helped start the Centre of Excellence for Stroke Research in Saskatoon at the University of Saskatchewan. We received a $1-million grant from the Heart and Stroke Foundation to start the center. Stroke neurologist Dr. A. Shuaib was my close colleague and friend when we teamed up with two other clinicians and four basic science researchers to research stroke with cell culture, animal studies, patients, and epidemiology (population studies). Dr. Shuaib has gone on to help make this a significant subspecialty within neurology. Today, he works at the University of Alberta. He is my mentor and guide in clinical stroke and taught me a great deal. I thank him for that.

My other basic scientists/neuroscientists of the time were Leif Hertz, MD, astrocyte and neuron cell culture expert; Bernie Juurlink, neuroanatomist and cell biologist; and Jim Thornhill, neurophysiologist. Today, I am fortunate to still be able to call on the expertise of Bernie Juurlink, as he retired to Vancouver Island, near where I live. He has written extensively on lifestyle change to reduce inflammation and oxidative stress (Juurlink 2010). My early training with these colleagues prepared me well for when I was diagnosed with MS in 1996. You will already have read about neurovascular disease, especially venous issues with MS and arterial and venous with traumatic brain injury and even Alzheimer's. I wanted you to understand how these brain problems are linked to blood flow and oxygen delivery, just as they are in stroke. Similarly, treatment options are available for stroke that can help the above and also help stroke victims. There is no longer a need to semi-abandon stroke victims, which is almost all we did in the early 1980s, treating the stroke ward like a vegetable patch—feed and water daily only. I regret this, but it was the pattern of the time.

To whet your appetite, I want to present a case of stroke in a man who, for several years, has made a remarkable comeback from six hours of care per day to less than two. This is very powerful and is a testimony to this fellow and his brother for not giving up and always looking for new opportunities for recovery—just like I do!

Gregory's Journey: Stroke-bleeding and Embolic (clot)

My [Gregory's] health crisis began when I suffered a severe cerebral bleed on the left side of my brain on December 18, 2013, at age 59.

Though I was less than five minutes away from the hospital when the stroke began, it resulted in my right arm and leg being completely pelagic. Little did I realize this was the beginning of a long road to only partial recovery.

Though I can give the exact date of my stroke, I suffered for many years prior with deceptively subtle symptoms. Symptoms that, as time went on, became more severe. Unfortunately, like multitudes of diseases, the primary symptom was constant fatigue and skin rashes, indicating liver toxicity and dysfunction.

After arriving at the hospital, a brain scan was performed, revealing the size and location of the cerebral bleed. I spent 21 days in hospital, during which I began doing basic physiotherapy almost immediately. Upon discharge, my brother, Vincent, became my full-time care provider. After acquiring the basic equipment— hospital bed, wheelchair, shower bench, and so on—we were ready to begin my in-home physiotherapy program. Fortunately, we were able to hire our friend, Josh, who had a wide range of experience in working with clients afflicted with mental and physical challenges. Josh agreed to work with me three days a week for three- to four-hour intervals. It was a tough and painful beginning, but within two months, Josh succeeded in helping me re-train and re-activate my right arm as well as stand up and take small steps with my pelagic right leg. This by itself exceeded the expectations of the physicians and therapists who helped oversee my case during my stay in hospital. Though I had utilized herbs and a generally healthy diet and lifestyle decades prior to my stroke, Josh boosted my diet big time. He accomplished this by implementing a raw food diet, a back-to-basics dietary lifestyle that his wife, Jody, had used for years to help control her Crohn's Disease. This entailed blending ideas from the Mediterranean and Paleo diets. This transformed my diet to being 85 percent raw organic fruits, nuts, seeds, and vegetables. To concentrate and improve absorption, we used a Green Star machine to make power-packed juice from the raw fruits and vegetables as well as to make blended smoothies using raw eggs, goat milk, and a variety of fruit and other ingredients, such as chia seeds and yogurt. All this, along with Josh's consistent physio program, which included visits to our local pool and gym, gave my body the energy it needed to do what each human body is so masterfully designed to do: heal itself.

After nine months of Josh's program, I had exceeded expectations for my recovery, but pieces of the puzzle were still missing. It was then Josh suggested we contact Dr. John Cline, an MD in Nanaimo who practiced integrative medicine. Dr. Cline's contribution in diagnosing the primary cause of my stroke and related health challenges was immeasurable. Through proper testing, Dr. Cline determined I had hemochromatosis, a genetic mutation that causes your body to over-absorb iron. To deal with this excess iron, the body oxidizes it into ferritin and stores it, usually in the heart, liver, and pancreas. If left untreated, the excess ferritin causes problems for these key organs, leading to serious health issues and death. To manage this disease, one simply has to go through a series of one-pint phlebotomies (blood draws). This forces the body to replace the blood and utilize the excess stored ferritin. This lowers the ferritin to a safe, normal level, and it is maintained there by doing a phlebotomy once or twice a year depending on one's iron intake. This was a major piece in the puzzle of recovery for me.

I continued on my path of recovery by doing a series of intravenous chelation treatments using EDTA and DMPS under Dr. Cline's care. These treatments are designed to flush out toxic metals that, depending on their levels, can be a major roadblock in one's overall health and well-being. Detoxifying our bodies because of our exposure to mercury, lead, and myriad other *human-made toxic chemicals is undoubtedly one of the biggest challenges today. In conjunction with Dr. Cline's chelation treatments, I began doing coffee and herbal enemas. Adding this to my regime has also played a supreme role in my recovery by reducing pain and facilitating my body's detoxification process. It was then, in December 2015, that Dr. Cline suggested we contact Dr. Code in regard to trying hyperbaric oxygen therapy. Dr. Code lived only 15 minutes away from my home near Duncan, BC, and was working with Andrew Paterson, a commercial diver. Using the hyperbaric oxygen tanks on his farm, Dr. Code and Andrew have succeeded in providing many people easy access to this simple, foundational therapy, which has been used safely and effectively for decades. Oxygen is life and is a foundational pillar in helping the body recover its natural vitality and balance. Breathing pure oxygen in a pressurized tank allows the body to absorb and utilize oxygen more efficiently, which enhances the healing process in a natural way. Of all the puzzle pieces I have discovered thus far, hyperbaric oxygen is the one from which I have derived the most benefit.*

Ironically, at the same time as I began my hyperbaric therapy, Josh, with Dr. Code's help, discovered a new treatment for healing called "Thor Laser." After training in Thor's Laser treatment protocols, Josh procured a portable Thor Laser unit and later a Thor Laser pod bed.

Adding Thor Laser treatments provided another key component to my recovery puzzle, especially since the HBOT and Thor Laser work well together. I can attest to this firsthand, having done 175 HBOT sessions in conjunction with over 160 Thor Laser treatments during the past two years.

Though I still have more than a few hills to climb, I have stabilized my health issues. I genuinely feel better and have more energy and vitality. I am also pain-free and medication free. I believe that is a result of consistently using all these invaluable tools, including a raw-food diet, chelation, coffee enemas, hyperbaric oxygen treatments, Thor Laser, and exercise. I feel blessed to having been exposed to these techniques, which allow my body to continue its recovery to vital health.

Regardless of what condition one may have, I believe answers are out there. Viable, effective choices are possible, but you must seek them, research them with science and empirical evidence, and give yourself the opportunity to discover what works for you.

Stroke research has taught us a great deal. The vast majority, 85 percent, of strokes are embolic, where a piece of tissue, usually a clot or plaque, is carried from the carotid artery (20 percent), the heart (20 percent), or elsewhere in the body, when its origin is unknown, and called cryptogenic stroke. A much smaller number of CVAs (cerebrovascular accidents), about 15 percent, are due to bleeding, often from a berry aneurysm. These latter types often need neurosurgical intervention or interventional radiology, and quickly, as many sufferers die quickly. I will not focus on this group, but I will say that if they survive the initial injury, many of the brain recovery interventions will help their quality of life too.

Stroke prevention is key and the same risk factors of preventing other cardiovascular diseases, MI, MS (Levine 2016), Alzheimer's, and vascular dementia will help a great deal. This starts with:

1. Stopping cigarette smoking
2. Optimizing blood homocysteine levels
3. Controlling blood sugar
4. Optimizing blood-clotting status
5. Controlling blood pressure, hopefully with diet, and lifestyle, especially exercise. If needed, good blood-pressure-lowering medication can be important too.

I will not address blood cholesterol here, because I don't believe this path is nearly as helpful as it is frequently suggested, with the statin protocol.

To begin, let us consider vascular health, especially health of the arteries, as these are considered first. However, remember at least 1–3 percent of strokes are venous in origin. All arteries and veins suffer the same diet and lifestyle injuries, so this is where most of us should begin. The regular term for this is "atherosclerosis" or, in lay terms, "hardening of the arteries," which does not include the veins, although it should. These vessels all share a cellular lining called endothelium. Endothelial health is the secret to a long life and a functioning brain.

The journal *Stroke* presents a comprehensive discussion (Meschia 2014). In the United States, approximately 800,000 people per year experience a stroke. For 610,000 of those, it is their first stroke. Twenty-six percent of people over age 65 remain dependent in their activities after six months, and 46 percent have cognitive deficits. More than half of the people view a major stroke as worse than death. Prevention is key, as reperfusion therapies are not as optimal as we would like. Primary prevention is important, because 76 percent of strokes are a first-time event.

Ten modifiable risk factors can prevent 90 percent of embolic and hemorrhagic stroke. These factors are aligned with the American Heart Association's "Life's Simple" campaign for ideal cardiovascular health. Independent stroke predictors include age, elevated systolic blood pressure, elevated blood pressure, diabetes, smoking, known cardiovascular disease (e.g., myocardial infarct), atrial fibrillation, and left ventricle hypertrophy (enlargement and thickening) on EKG (electrocardiogram) of the heart. Some scoring systems omit smoking but include marital status, impaired expiratory flow (impaired breathing out), physical disability, depression score, serum creatine (kidney function), and "time to walk fifteen feet." There appears to be no positive association between total cholesterol and stroke mortality. You can find an online risk calculator at http://my.americanheart.org/cvriskcalculator.

The risks for stroke cited in the literature also include:
- Low birth weight (difficult to change!)

- Ethnicity—increased risk if African American, Hispanic/Latino American, and even Native American
- Family history—increased risk by approximately 30 percent, and even higher for women
- Brain aneurysms—increased risk by 8 percent if one has polycystic kidney disease (autosomal dominant) and 7 percent if one has Ehlers-Danlos Type IV (vascular Ehlers-Danlos)

Modifiable risk factors are well documented. These include:

- Physical inactivity: If active, the risk of stroke can be decreased by 25-30 percent. Some physical activity is better than none. The minimum beneficial activity is 150 minutes per week of fast walking or 75 minutes per week running or equivalent. I prefer interval time on an elliptical, twenty minutes a day.
- Diet: Reduced salt in the diet seems to be somewhat effective in decreasing stroke incidence in African Americans. A high intake of fruits and vegetables provides the greatest protection against stroke. Aim for nine to 10 servings of fruits and vegetables per day. Ketchup and French fries are not the best choices. A Mediterranean Diet is also helpful, especially if it is high in nuts (walnuts, hazelnuts, almonds) and extra virgin olive oil. The DASH (Dietary Approach to Stop Hypertension) diet, which promotes a high intake of fruits and vegetables, has also been recommended for lowering blood pressure and stroke prevention and is a good starting place.
- Folate supplement: Documented to reduce stroke and heart attack by lowering homocysteine (see Supplements chapter 6) (Sepe 2007; Wang 2007).

Obesity and diabetes are both risk factors for stroke and heart disease. More than half of Americans aged 65 or older have at least pre-diabetes. Metabolic syndrome is another grouping that signals a higher risk of stroke.

Atrial fibrillation increases the risk of stroke by four to five times, so if your pulse is irregular, see your family physician or osteopathic doctor. Atrial fibrillation means something other than the regular sino-atrial node are sending electrical impulses. This happens erratically, so on exam the pulse can be irregularly irregular. This is easily confirmed on an EKG rhythm strip (a run of a few seconds on the EKG paper).

The next question regarding atrial fibrillation is, what's triggering it? The most common trigger in young males is from excessive alcohol intake. Once alcohol is ruled out, other investigations include an echo or ultrasound of the heart. This can determine if a valve problem is present. If so, hopefully this can be repaired. Regardless of whether you have a valve problem, anticoagulation is recommended. This is needed as soon as possible, because the quivering or fibrillating atria can readily send off a clot or thrombus. This is what causes 40 percent of strokes. If anticoagulation is not possible medically, sometimes the cardiologist will suggest closure of the left atrial appendage. This is done through a catheter that "ties off" this small pocket, which is the most common area for clots to form when atrial fibrillation is present.

Other cardiac conditions that increase your risk of stroke include:

1. Acute heart attack or myocardial infarction (MI).
2. Cardiomyopathy, which is a non-functioning part of the heart muscle. This may be due to a local loss of oxygen supply or ischemia (such as an MI), or it may be non-ischemic cardiomyopathy, often from a virus (coxsackie B) infection or prolonged alcohol abuse.
3. Patent foramen ovale (PFO), which is when the opening or hole between the heart's upper chambers or atria fails to close. This is present in 20–25 percent of the

population. Examples of when this becomes a possible risk factor is in divers or individuals parachuting from high above the earth (40,000–70,000 feet), migraine headaches, and possibly MS (the new MS, Microvascular Syndrome) (Jersey 2010). The presence of this PFO reduces the lungs' ability to act as a filter of small clots or particles leaking through a leaky gut or even from a tiny fat embolus or plaque. Tiny fat emboli can be formed from a minimal soft tissue injury. Research suggests if you carefully and optimally select which patients to treat with closure, you will reduce their stroke risk, migraine headaches, and, I suggest, MS attacks.

4. Valvular heart disease. This occurs when one of the four valves, especially the mitral valve between the left atrium and left ventricle, is injured or malfunctioning. This can increase turbulence and secondary clot formation (remember Virchow's triad). The clot then travels to the brain, and a stroke results.

5. Cardiac tumours. Here either a piece of a tumour or a clot formed secondary to the blood turbulence and stasis travels to the brain and causes a stroke.

6. Aortic atherosclerosis. This is disease of the aorta's vessel wall with plaque and/or clot of this huge vessel leaving the heart and supplying the entire body. If a clot leaves this area and travels to the brain, it will cause a stroke or at least a TIA (transient ischemic attack, a mini stroke, of less than twenty-four hours' duration).

Forty per cent of all strokes can be attributed to the above six conditions. Asymptomatic (silent) carotid artery stenosis can result in plaque and clots. This condition accounts for about 20 percent of embolic strokes. The narrowing or stenosis usually occurs at the bifurcation or splitting of the common carotid artery into the internal and external carotid arteries.

This occurs on each side of the neck, because the carotid arteries are immediately beside the internal jugular veins.

Stroke Treatment

I am delighted to be writing about what to do for stroke victims. For too long, we have told patients, "You will receive six weeks of rehabilitation, and all the recovery you will achieve will be in the first two years." Now we have an enhanced understanding of brain recovery and neuroplasticity and other modalities that we know will help people. However, in most cases, your neurologist and personal physician will not be aware of these alternatives. They may even say the therapies I suggest are a waste of money or provide "false hope." I assure you this is not the case.

Stroke is described as loss of blood supply and oxygen and nutrients to a region of the brain. It is inferred that all these cells die in a few minutes or at least within three to five hours. This is the time window suggested to begin a clot-dissolving or clot-busting drug in embolic or non-bleeding but not hemorrhagic strokes. Studies in neuroscience have shown that most of these injured cells are still alive but are not functioning, hence, the term "idling neurons." This suggests these cells are getting enough oxygen to survive but not the higher amount for energy production to permit function. Brain and heart cells need more energy and, therefore, more oxygen than other cells. If we provide more oxygen to these cells by HBOT, NBOT, or PBMT, then most of these cells can regain function.

In addition, the brain can heal or create new tiny blood vessels, providing a new source of oxygen and nutrients. This can also permit recovery of idling neurons. Over several weeks of relative hypoxia, new small blood vessels (capillaries, venules, and arterioles) will increase by up to 50 percent. The body provides stem cells locally but can be helped further by HBOT and/or PBMT. HBOT is the most tried and true to date, but PBMT is showing considerable early promise. Each therapy can increase circulating stem cells by six to eight times (Thom 2006; Hamblin 2016).

My recommendations for someone who has suffered a new stroke or "brain attack" are as follows.

1. Begin use of 100-percent oxygen rebreathing mask immediately and continue for three days, followed by nasal prongs at 5 L/min. This is sometimes termed NBOT, NormoBaric Oxygen Therapy. I prefer 0_2 therapy as a term.

2. Get to a major hospital, so an urgent MRI can rule out a bleeding or hemorrhagic stroke. If indicated and within the appropriate time window (3-4.5 hours), the neurologist or emergency physician will order a clot-busting drug (e.g., TPA, tissue plasminogen activator).

3. Begin oxygen therapy, including HBOT, as soon as possible. If HBOT is not available, continue oxygen-rebreathing mask for two to five days or even longer. This will deliver 60-70 percent oxygen only, but this can boost the circulating dissolved oxygen by four or five times that of room air, which provides 21 percent oxygen.

4. If you begin HBOT, start daily treatments for one hour at 1.5 atm for 20-40 treatments. If there is no response in the first five days, increase the pressure to 1.75 atm and continue the protocol. This 1.75 percent atm seems to be the sweet spot for stroke recovery and is my own personal preference.

5. All rehabilitative efforts, both active and passive, can begin as soon as possible. The patient's airway must be protected at all times, so they do not sustain aspiration

pneumonia from loss of throat and swallowing due to neurological injury.

6. If available, begin PBMT on the region of the brain affected by the stroke. It is a useful adjunct to oxygen therapy, but oxygen therapy is paramount.

If you suffer a bleeding or hemorrhagic stroke, which it is 15 percent of the time, you need a neurosurgical consultation as soon as possible to determine optional surgical intervention. Once you are stable, HBOT can be started. Continue oxygen therapy by mask throughout, full oxygen for three days, then nasal prongs at 5 L/min.

Neurosurgical care is critical, because in most cases, the injured brain will swell. The brain is inside a bone shell. If swelling becomes excessive, death may be preventable by a neurosurgeon. In the many neurosurgical cases I have been part of, as either the anesthesiologist or intensive care physician, I have always been impressed with the neurosurgeon's wisdom and intervention. They understand the relative urgency of each scenario.

Once the critical care features are dealt with, remember the ongoing oxygen therapy and optimal nutrition to assist healing. In addition, rehabilitation and exercise, including vibration treatment, will increase the speed of mobility and walking recovery. The exercise will increase the brain-derived neurotropic factor (BDNF) protein, which will increase brain healing. If seizures are an issue, then continued oxygen with HBOT can help. Another assist for seizures might be the use of high CBD with little or no THC. In the last year, I learned of one patient treated in a Vancouver hospital with high CBD for seizures after a severe and major bleeding stroke. I applaud the openness of the neurologist and epileptologist (medical specialist in epilepsy) in using cannabis as a safe intervention in this case.

22: Traumatic Brain Injury, CTE, Cerebral Palsy, and PTSD

Traumatic brain injury (TBI) occurs when an external force injures the brain (Shalev 2017). Cerebral palsy (CP) occurs when there is a generalized or localized lack of oxygen injury. In this way, CP and TBI are one and the same. TBI can result in physical, cognitive, social, emotional, and behavioural symptoms. The result can range from complete recovery to permanent disability and even death. The most common causes are falls, especially in the very young and the elderly, motor vehicle accidents, and violence. Traumatic brain injury is a major cause of death and disability worldwide, especially in children and young adults, particularly males. In this chapter, I discuss such injuries and the increased risk of repetitive traumatic brain injuries. I include a discussion of the relatively common, up to one third of players, NFL injury: chronic traumatic encephalopathy (CTE). In addition, I discuss some of the new MRI techniques helping us see residual injury, which heretofore have been called "normal." Finally, I talk about solutions to assist people afflicted with such injuries, who deserve much more than being told, "We can no longer help you," or, "You will just have to live with it." Too often this has been told to

TBI, CP, CTE, and PTSD patients, whether they are athletes, soldiers, and/or victims of motor vehicle accidents.

Traumatic Brain Injury

Traumatic brain injury is defined as damage to the brain from an external mechanical force, such as acceleration or deceleration, impact, such as blast waves, or penetrating injury. Brain function is temporarily or permanently impaired, and structural damage may or may not be seen with an MRI. A few years ago, I was impressed to see that high-quality MRI (3 or 7 Tesla) can demonstrate this, even in patients who were previously described as normal MRI. Until recently, many of these people were told they were imagining their symptoms, because there was nothing visible on their MRI. These high-quality MRIs reveal an incredible pruning of blood vessels after traumatic brain injury. Imagine a tree with all its leaves and small branches stripped away by a hurricane or a tornado. This loss of blood vessels and, therefore, loss of oxygen supply causes hypoxia in the previously well-supplied areas of the brain secondary to the forces of trauma.

Nearly 40 percent of all deaths from acute injuries in the USA are a result of TBI. TBI is a leading cause of death in young people. Each year 200,000 TBI victims need hospitalization, and a much larger number, nearly 2 million, individuals sustain a mild TBI or concussion requiring contact with a physician. This is a huge loss of at least one day of work or of continued disability. The majority of soldiers and many hockey and football players sustain these injuries but are given no solutions other than rest, if that. Multiple TBIs, or the mild episodes called concussions, are particularly hard on the brain. Explosions from IEDs (improvised explosive device) are especially common in modern war zones. Consequently, I routinely ask my war veteran clients about TBI, loss of consciousness, or concussions. Almost all those who served overseas admit to such injuries.

Men are twice as likely to sustain a traumatic brain injury. In women, I find that horseback riding and motor vehicle accidents tend to be the most common events precipitating a TBI. Unfortunately, women often have a more difficult time recovering from a TBI. Is this perhaps due to slightly smaller blood vessels, which means recovery of adequate flow takes a little longer? In the United States, motor vehicle accidents are the leading cause of traumatic brain injury. In the United Kingdom, motor vehicle accidents are number three after falls and assaults. Firearms are number three in the United States. Seatbelts and bicycle helmets have helped considerably, but TBIs from gunshots have increased in the last few years. Finally, alcohol is a major factor in many TBIs and is often an associated factor.

Primary injury

Traumatic brain injury results from an outside force applied to the skull, injuring the brain. Obvious injuries are skull fractures, bleeds, or hematomas inside the skull and penetrating injuries, such as bullets. Less obvious are blows that move the brain against the skull and the reverse process or contra-coup injury, when it suddenly moves back to its original position. The brain is injured in both events. The brain is a lot like a bowl of jelly floating inside a closed space. When a blow is sustained, a tear in the blood vessels, a.k.a. "pruning," occurs. Think of the tree of blood vessels losing many of its small branches as a tree would lose its leaves and branches in a hurricane. Secondary to this pruning is a lack of fresh blood containing oxygen and thus hypoxia in these areas. The hypoxia triggers inflammation, of which swelling is one of the components. This swelling, or edema, inside the skull can be so severe that it is lethal. Also, subsequent swelling impinges on the blood vessels and worsens the hypoxia, inflammation, and overall injury. In many ways, this parallels a severe stroke, particularly the bleeding type.

Secondary Injury

This is the injury caused by the cellular damage created by the initial period. The secondary injury results from damaged cells releasing a number of neurochemical mediators, particularly the excitatory amino acids, such as glutamate. I believe the biggest trigger is the hypoxia from the torn vessels as well as the red blood cells leaking into the area, which are high in iron. This iron presence is a major trigger of oxidation, and release of reactive oxygen species causes significant damage. The hypoxia and secondary swelling of inflammation increases the distance that the dissolved oxygen must travel from its release from the hemoglobin molecule inside the blood vessels. This greater distance aggravates the hypoxia of any adjacent brain cells, because the oxygen concentration continues to fall the further it must diffuse or travel.

I hope you are picking up a common theme here regarding the need for oxygen. Lack of oxygen results in further damage to the tissues. In fact, deaths due to severe traumatic brain injury can be reduced by half simply through the use of supplemental oxygen. The best way to do this is hyperbaric oxygen treatment (HBOT). Alternatively, a 100-percent re-breathing mask is especially useful if HBOT is not available.

This increased oxygen must begin as soon as possible after the injury and for several hours per day for several days thereafter. The more severe the injury, including coma, the more days of use should be continued.

The pictures or images of traumatic brain injury are best done with MRI. However, a CT scan is the next-best option. I vividly remember special MRIs shown by Dr. Mark Haacke, PhD, of Wayne State University at the first meeting of the Canadian Neurovascular Health Society in 2011. He stated that many regular MRIs of traumatic brain injury are called normal, and yet the patient is told they are fine and that they are malingering. This is usually untrue. If MRIs are done at a higher Tesla and using other techniques, the images will reveal the pruning that I spoke of earlier. These brains are definitely not normal. Remember, the brain is two percent of our body but needs twenty percent of our body's oxygen. You can learn more about oxygen supplementation in the chapter about hyperbaric oxygen treatment or, if such treatment is unavailable, the alternatives in the chapter on oxygen and cognition. Now I would like to present a personal story of one of my clients that illustrates the benefits of oxygen therapy even some years after the injury.

Mona's Story

Case Study: Hyperbaric Oxygen Therapy and Traumatic Brain Injury
Gender: Female
Age: 58 years
First injury: 1998 (moderate traumatic brain injury)
Second injury: 2014 (mild traumatic brain injury) and many physical damages

Non-smoker, non-drinker, and non-drug user (includes prescription pain medications or OTC drugs)

December 2016: eleven 60-minute sessions HBOT at 1.5 atm

After my first session, I stepped out of the chamber and struggled with my equilibrium and getting my legs to work. I had to sit on the edge of the chamber to steady myself. Walking back the one kilometre to the Airbnb was very disconcerting, as I was struggling to keep my balance and to focus, to make my muscles work. By the time I arrived, I was exhausted and went directly to bed.

After my fifth session, 70 percent of my pain was gone. My titanium knee was clunking because of the gap left from the reduction in swelling. My other knee was actually able to straighten, something it had been unable to do since the accident in 2014.

Since the accident in 1998, changing gears and multi-tasking have been non-existent in my life. Hence, sending out Christmas cards has been arduous, time consuming, and fatiguing. Since the accident in 2014, I had not sent out any cards. After the fifth session, I was able to sit down and get 40 cards ready for the mail. I was astounded, and I was not fatigued! The cobwebs that once made it difficult to move about in my brain were gone for the first time in eighteen years.

At the end of the 11 sessions, my speech was clearer, faster, and there was a return of my long-gone wicked sense of humour. I felt like I was finally being reunited with my long-lost self. It was so good to be back in my body.

I did not have one PTSD episode during the first session, which is amazing, as I was having them once or twice a day prior to my first session of HBOT.

I was finally able to wake up with minimal pain and not having an entire body ache. My skin looked brighter and more alive, almost like a mini facelift, and my once-clogged lymphatic system was clear.

However, the most amazing experience happened when I arrived home. I was able to have my first conversation with my dad in over two years. My dad has onset dementia, which means he has difficulty carrying on a conversation or thinking of what to say, and I, prior to the HBOT, was in the same boat. Hence, our conversations were painful, strained, and left neither of us wanting to do it again. However, I was able to carry on the conversation, and we talked for over 45 minutes. It felt so glorious!

On the sixth day after I returned home, I noticed a degradation of my cognitive function and energy, and the cobwebs were returning. I had a couple of very sad days. I did not want to slide back, especially after I knew what I could feel like. I had no desire to return to my previous self. The pain was returning, and I was back to every step being excruciating. Lying in bed was once again uncomfortable to downright painful. I wanted to keep the feeling that I had when I returned from the eleven sessions so badly. I felt like a junkie looking for a fix. I was desperate.

January 2017: twelve 90-minute sessions HBOT at 1.75 atm

After my third session, I was back to where I was at the end of my first HBOT session. I was so thrilled. Pain gone, brain clear, less fatigue, and I was getting "chatty and flirty." Wonderful long-lost feelings regained after such a long time.

The seventh session had me recalling events from forty years back for no apparent reason. It was like the cobwebs were removed, and old thoughts and memories resurfaced. Some of this was unpleasant, as it was like opening the floodgates. I was walking to my chiro appointment and, out of the blue, I stopped and thought of Rene (an old friend and amazing hairdresser). Then I saw his shop, right where it was when I left the island many years ago.

Over the past 18HBOT sessions, I had been walking right by with no recognition.

The ninth session had me welcoming home another old friend: my intuition! I was once again picking up on energy and feeling it! I do not have words to describe how glorious that was. I felt vibrant and alive. My sparkling eyes were back with a vengeance. I was teasing, not only able to pick up on subtle nuances but also responding in a timely manner for the first time in 18 years. Cooking was getting easier too, as I was able to multi-task to a certain extent.

The tenth session was amazing physically. My posture became more upright, and for the first time in over two years, the rotation three dimensionally in my pelvis finally released and straightened. I could finally use my arms without pain. Trying to repair these physical constraints over the past two years had cost me countless dollars; my farm status, because of my inability to use my body; and my self-esteem and created the need for saddle modifications, weed-control modifications, and the list keeps growing.

After my eleventh session, I had an amazing evening! Not only because of the people I was with but because I managed in a noisy environment. I didn't miss a beat in the conversation and was even able to "find" the names of people I was running into that I hadn't seen for a very long time. And, drum roll please, I was not exhausted at the end of the evening.

After the twelfth session, I was catching a flight home, and for the first time since the first accident, I did not need help finding my way around the airport. I knew where to go.

Seven days passed since my last HBOT, and I had no degradation. I still had not had a PTSD episode. I was able to rake and shovel without pain, and I was back to walking for two and a half hours with the dogs—and no pain! I was also experiencing an amazing decrease in fatigue.

Fifteen days passed, and pain returned, making every step excruciating.

*Twenty days passed, and I started to decline cognitively and
had my first PTSD episode since I started HBOT. Glimpses of
the fatigue were also returning. I was 14 days away from my
next scheduled HBOT, which felt like eternity. When my sparkle
energy dived, I felt lost.*

February 2017: seventeen 90-minute sessions HBOT at 1.75 atm

*I arrived at an amazing birthday supper with friends and then
went to a Pink Floyd tribute concert. Prior to that evening, when
I was asked whether I liked Pink Floyd, I had no idea, as I was
aware of the name but nothing else. Once they started playing, I
found myself recognizing not only the songs but also the lyrics.
I also had flashbacks to what I was doing at the moment I first
heard their songs over 40 years ago. This is something I had not
been able to do since my first Moderate TBI in 1998.*

*My first HBOT session in February left me in the same con-
dition as my first HBOT session in December. Discombobulated.
Exhausted. Difficulty getting my brain to work. Slept deeply and
awoke feeling peaceful and very quiet on a cellular level.*

*After the fifth session, my inflammation and pain decreased
substantially once again. After the eighth session, I was pain free.
My body was responding much better to the chiropractic treatments as well. Clearly, for me to have a good quality of life, HBOT
has to remain a part of my daily routine.*

*The changes from this round of HBOT have been life alter-
ing. I am back driving with no fatigue, no hesitation, no problem
judging time or distance, and, most importantly, not doing stupid,
impulsive things. Being able to drive is a huge freedom.*

*The change between my horses and me has me smiling from ear
to ear. Prior to my first brain injury in 1998, I was an amazing
horse person, connected in every sense. After the first brain injury, I
lost the connectedness and the timing. As a result, my relationship*

with horses changed. I felt the disconnect, and so did they. Of course, me being me, with no quit in me, I just kept plugging along like an ant. I even managed to train an awesome horse or two, but there was no connection. It felt empty. When I had my second brain injury in 2014, I also developed PTSD, and the effects of this on my relationship with my horses was disastrous. My horses would run to the far end of the pasture if I opened the house door. I have no words to express how abandoned I felt. No matter how hard I tried to calm that energy inside, the horses still picked it up. Gemini became a worried, uncomfortable horse. Riding was a chore and no longer fun, and the disconnect seemed miles wide. I actually thought my horse days were over. Enter HBOT.

No more PTSD, physical and emotional energy returned, spiritual energy soaring off the charts, no pain, and better mobility. I took Gemini to a Heather Nelson Liberty clinic in March 2017, and words cannot convey the magic I felt when my connectedness returned.

Finally, toward the end of the day, it was my turn for my private lesson. I was tired from watching all day, and I had not done Liberty before, so I had no idea of what to expect. I took Gemini into the ring and allowed him to move off and do some exploring, which he did. Then I asked him to come to me, which he did. We started by doing inside and outside circles, which he did but with some attitude. I sent him off again, and this time when he came back, he was willing. Heather had me take him in a figure eight around barrels, and then she had me send him on his own. He made it all look easy. Then Heather gave me the obstacle maze to do. Gemini, being the tank he is, with lots of forward movement, meant we kind of crashed through it. So, I really focused on our second attempt. I mean really focused. I got Gemini to the opening, and I sent all my energy down my whip, the tip of which I placed on the ground a few feet in front of him. Mentally, I was saying, put your head down, and just follow the whip. Gemini lowered his head, and, in that moment, I felt *the connection. As I dragged the whip, Gemini followed exactly where the whip went. Once we got out of the maze, the connectedness was so strong, I was able to send him out at quite a distance to do circles or around the barrels. To be able to feel this after not having it for nineteen years was profound and so beautiful. The next day, I was the first student ever in Heather's Liberty classes to ride. I was bareback with Gemini's halter on and a rope draped around his neck, but I was riding with no reins or control, using only my body to direct Gemini. At first I was worried about falling off. Then I just focused on what Heather was telling me to do. It was an amazing experience that had me grinning from ear to ear. Bareback again after 19 years!*

With all that HBOT has done for me, I have now purchased my own chamber, so I never have to worry about degradation. I will still travel to the island to have three weeks' worth of HBOT at 1.75 atm once a year, as my home chamber is only capable of 1.3 atm.

Endocannabinoids and Traumatic Brain Injury (TBI) and Cerebral Palsy (CP)

TBI triggers the release of harmful mediators, such as the amino acid glutamate. One of the body's main protective mechanisms is triggered, the endogenous cannabinoid (eCB) system. Endogenous cannabinoids are markedly increased in response to pathogenic events, especially trauma and hypoxia. Considerable research now show eCBs are part of the brain's repair mechanism (Shohami 2011). These repair mechanisms use cannabinoid receptor pathways to control neuronal survival and repair. The levels of 2-AG are significantly elevated after TBI. In studies of mice with TBI, 2-AG was administered. The 2-AG decreased brain edema and inflammation, reduced injury, and improved clinical recovery. An interesting article relates cannabinoids and perinatal brain injury, effectively a type of Cerebral Palsy (Fernandez-Lopes 2013).

I realize it is early days for these human clinical trials, but this must be considered as data starts to support the use of cannabis in TBI (Shohami 2011; Mechoulam 2002; Nguyen 2014). None of our current drugs used in TBI are helpful. In fact, steroids are now contraindicated. In addition, there are virtually no downsides or side effects to this new choice of cannabis in TBI. However, it is prudent to use mostly CBD or a product containing 1:1 of CBD to THC. Excess THC will muddy the waters of assessment, especially in the cannabis-naïve person.

PBMT is another possibility in TBI. At present, this would be in the chronic phase after hospitalization. One day, I believe we will use PBMT in the acute phase as a useful adjunct.

TBI is an aggravating or triggering factor in almost all brain problems. Optimal attention to TBI and repeated concussions is tantamount in preventing many neurodegenerative diseases, such as MS, Parkinson's, and Alzheimer's.

Before ending, I must emphasize that although eCB and PBMT are showing future promise, the most critical recovery option is oxygen. Oxygen therapy must be used acutely in all TBI and concussions (Stoller 2015). If a sports player had his or her "bell rung," oxygen will help the athlete's brain recover better and faster. Therefore, I suggest oxygen concentrators or a supply of oxygen be available at hockey rinks, football or soccer fields, and at equestrian or motocross events. We only get one brain, and transplants are not an option!

Chronic Traumatic Encephalopathy (CTE)

I just finished reading the book *Concussion* (2015) by Jean Laskas. This book was recently released as a movie starring Will Smith. The book and the movie will grab and disturb you whether you are an NFL football fan or not. The book describes CTE (chronic traumatic encephalopathy). CTE is more common than previously believed and is found in at least one third of retired pro football players. It causes dramatic memory loss, outbursts of anger and violence, and early dementia, even in people in their late thirties and forties.

If you look at the entire brain with the naked eye, you will see nothing of note. However, if you look at a microscopic slice through the brain, you see tiny bleeding spots. If you look at a prepared microscopic brain slice, you will see a huge number of neural fibril tangles. These are called Tau proteins. These types of proteins are also seen in Alzheimer's disease, which is the number one cause of dementia.

The CTE diagnosis is discussed at www.thebraintrust-foundation.org. The website supports good science and the football players' perspective of brain injury. It was started to support the work of Dr. Bennet Omalu. He is a brilliant neuropathologist who initially discovered CTE in the brain of Mike Webster, formerly of the Pittsburgh Steelers. Mike Webster was chosen for the Pro Bowl 10 times and earned four Super Bowl rings playing centre for the Steelers. Before his death, his brain illness caused him to be occasionally violent, extremely forgetful, and a completely changed husband and father. It cost him his marriage and eventually his life.

Dr. Omalu, in conjunction with two of his senior colleagues, published the first recorded case of CTE in neurosurgery (Omalu 2005). Football player Terry Long, a receiver for the Pittsburgh Steelers, died prematurely of CTE. His case was also submitted for publication in *Neurosurgery* (Omalu 2006) by Dr. Omalu and others. A third case of CTE was documented but the politics of medicine and confrontation with the NFL blocked this third case from being published.This occurred partly to block the third case report as this would make a "series" and mean more in the published literature.

The movie adaptation of *Concussion* outlines how NFL owners and medical professionals continually denied the occurrence of CTE. It portrayed how the football players affected by CTE learned to commit suicide by gunshot wound to the chest in order to preserve their brain for the study of CTE. You will learn from the movie and the book that the NFL has worked hard to cover things up and even committed fraud and lied to the press. However, the cat is partly out of the bag. The issue of CTE will not be denied once many people see the movie. The results have been so dramatic in the United States, that a year or so ago, there was a 10 percent reduction in young boys starting to play tackle football under the Pop Warner system. A recent commentary can be found in *JAMA Neurology* (Kaup 2017).

You may note a partial parallel with my MS discussion in chapter 20. In that chapter, I discussed how 14 percent of MS patients have microvascular bleeds. This was determined by a prospective study of 100 patients with 100 controls by Dr. M. Haacke and his colleagues at Wayne State University. It is possible that at least some of the injury that starts CTE is also from microvascular bleeds.

When I spoke of MS, I also spoke of neck strap muscles potentially blocking venous flow, with a secondary potential retrograde hydraulic injury back into the veins of the brain. This problem is likely aggravated if there is a partial block of the vein valves of the internal jugular vein and the valves of this vein and the heart. Now think of a football lineman at college or pro level. These fellows have almost no neck, because their neck strap muscles are so highly developed by intense fitness programs. Perhaps a significant part of the CTE is aggravated by a component of the chronic cerebrospinal venous insufficiency. My intent is to review this concept with wiser more experienced brain experts. Perhaps early diagnosis and treatment of vein-flow variations can prevent CTE in more people. Alternatively, it may tell us who is at the highest risk of this particular brain injury.

It is possible that CTE is a much more progressed type of traumatic brain injury. If so, we should look at commonalities in prevention, diagnosis, and treatment. Soon Dr. Paolo Zamboni's NASA research will provide a reproducible, accurate, non-invasive measure of neck veins using readily available ultrasound. Then we can prospectively solve some of these questions.

When I attended my first International Society of Neurovascular Disease conference in Bologna, Italy, in 2011, I learned more about neurovascular brain injury. The keynote speaker was Prof. Berislav Zlokovic of Rochester, New York. He spoke about Alzheimer's disease as having two stages of injury. The first injury is vascular. He did not say whether this injury was venous or arterial. I suspect it can be either or both. Certainly, vascular dementia is 30-40 percent of all dementia and is a strong second in the incidence of dementia problems. Therefore, the sum of Alzheimer's and vascular dementia, 80-85 percent, makes a powerful case for careful investigation of any vascular predecessor to this devastating illness. Dementia is destroying people's lives, their families, and overtaxing our medical system. Dementia in North America has reached the breaking point. It will destroy the health care system as we know it.

Treatment already exists for vascular brain injury, including TBI and CP. This is, quite simply, oxygen therapy. I refer you to my chapter on oxygen therapy with hyperbaric oxygen. If interested, you should also read the excellent book *Oxygen and the Brain* by Dr. Philip B James, as mentioned earlier.

Hypoxia causes inflammation, and this has been reported in several recent articles in the *New England Journal of Medicine* (Eltzschig 2011). If one relieves or reverses the hypoxia, then one may be able to reverse the inflammation. This same information is the cornerstone of injury in Alzheimer's, traumatic brain injury, and even stroke. Currently, Dr. David Harrison, MD, FRCPC, is doing a double-blind controlled trial on the treatment of mature strokes with hyperbaric oxygen in Vancouver, BC. After reviewing the literature, he is reasonably hopeful that his results will move us further along the path of HBOT for brain injury. In addition, in New Orleans, Dr. Paul Harch has published papers on the success of treating traumatic brain injury with oxygen therapy (Harch 2009, 2012). He has done most of the studies on young men injured during military service in the Middle East.

The United States Military had researched HBOT for traumatic brain injury, but HBOT was not commonly used for treatment. However, the Pentagon has recently agreed to fund HBOT for TBI and PTSD for members of the armed forces. This truly indicates a change of policy as a result of evidence-based medicine.

Today the reality of TBI is becoming better known, especially by informed parents. A personal example related to TBI was when we strongly recommended a bike helmet for our middle child, then eleven years of age. He was not impressed. This changed when he slipped and fell during a training run, banged his head, was dazed, amnestic, and had a headache. He always wore a helmet after that! A second example is my interventional radiologist colleague in California. After seeing the movie *Concussion*, he insisted that his fourteen-year-old son not play high school football. He was right—even though his son may not yet appreciate it.

Pentagon Funds Treatments of TBI and PTSD

H.R.2810 - 115th Congress (2017–2018): National Defense Authorization Act for Fiscal Year 2018

SEC. 703. PROVISION OF HYPERBARIC OXYGEN THERAPY FOR CERTAIN MEMBERS OF THE ARMED FORCES.

(a) HBOT Treatment.—

(1) IN GENERAL.—Chapter 55 of title 10, United States Code, is amended by inserting after section 1074n the following new section:

> **"§ 1074o. Provision of hyperbaric oxygen therapy for certain members** *HBOT*

"(a) In General.—The Secretary may furnish hyperbaric oxygen therapy available at a military medical treatment facility to a covered member if such therapy is prescribed by a physician to treat post-traumatic stress disorder or traumatic brain injury.

"(b) Covered Member Defined.—In this section, the term 'covered member' means a member of the armed forces who is—

"(1) serving on active duty; and

"(2) diagnosed with post-traumatic stress disorder or traumatic brain injury.".

(2) CLERICAL AMENDMENT.—The table of sections at the beginning of such chapter is amended by inserting after the item relating to section 1074n the following new item:

"1074o. Provision of hyperbaric oxygen therapy for certain members.".

(b) Effective Date.—The amendments made by subsection (a) shall take effect 90 days after the date of the enactment of this Act.

https://www.congress.gov/bill/115th-congress/house-bill/2810/text#toc-HFB5D79CF9C0440259226C24FB7F369B1

PTSD

I believe that PTSD occurs in much the same way as "windup" occurs in chronic pain. Windup is the phenomenon to describe how repeated and frequent perceptions of pain "burns" a new and persistent pathway from the pain site to the brain. The result is the brain perceives pain even after the source of the pain is healed. A great example is post-herpetic neuralgia, which is pain after a shingles attack. In this case, 5 percent of people with shingles have such severe and recurring pain for several weeks that the pain continues to recur intermittently or continuously even after the skin has healed. The same happens with phantom limb pain. I suggest that major emotional pain may trigger a similar "burned-in" pathway. Consequently, almost anything can trigger an episode any time thereafter. I suspect PTSD is a similar occurrence within the brain. The traumatic experience can be recurrent as in multiple rape or sexual abuse episodes or a single event, such as an explosion. I suggest the same windup or imprinting occurs in the same part of the brain. In many ways, PTSD is similar to a stroke or TBI. A sudden cataclysmic event triggers glutamate, an excitatory neurotransmitter, to be released in excess, and the event perception persists over the long term. PTSD is characterized by the persistence of intense reactions to reminders of a traumatic event, altered mood, a sense of imminent threat, disturbed sleep, and hypervigilance. "One way of thinking about PTSD is an overactivation of the fear system that can't be inhibited, can't be normally modulated," per Dr. Kerry Ressler of Emory University in Atlanta in 2017 (Jovanovic 2010). In other words, the PTSD brain can't get out of "overdrive," which can come on suddenly and with no warning. Effects can be dramatic and emotionally crippling to individuals with severe consequences for loved ones as well.

Psychotherapy can often help but not always. Antidepressants are often used but, frankly, are rarely helpful. Instead, I suggest the treatment for PTSD, TBI, and stroke can also be similar. Evidence confirms that PTSD will respond to HBOT, cannabis (Oneil 2017; Neumeister 2013; Das 2013; Greer 2014), and PBMT. This is incredibly important, because most folks who suffer from PTSD do so through no fault of their own but are instead victims of being in the wrong place at the wrong time. Family members have told Sue Sisley, an Arizona psychiatrist, that cannabis has given them their spouse or their father back. Although cannabis does not remove bad memories, it allows one to not fixate on such memories. Medical cannabis seems to support the endocannabinoid system and may permit a more normal recovery. The CBDs of cannabis also increase brain-derived neurotropic factor (BDNF), which enhances neuron interconnections and even new neurons. I believe this helps the brain heal itself or at least helps the brain's neuroplasticity toward recovery.

O_2 therapy protocols can be found at the end of chapters 21 (Stroke) and 30 (Oxygen and Cognitive Function).

23: Alzheimer's, Vascular, and Other Dementias

In this chapter, I begin with some simple tools to determine if you or your loved one are having cognitive challenges. This is no reason to "do nothing" until you have a confirmed diagnosis before changing your diet and lifestyle. In fact, nothing could be further from the truth.

Please do not believe that a new Alzheimer's drug is on the horizon. All pharmaceutical companies have abandoned their neuroscience research track. Of the 244 experimental Alzheimer drugs tested from 2000 to 2010, exactly one—memantine—was approved. Memantine effects are modest at best. The long-term use of Aricept has shown it works for only for a few months at most. Aricept is a cholinesterase inhibitor. Thus, it makes more acetylcholine available at cholinergic synapses, where nerve cells interact.

Finally, Alzheimer's is the only one of the 10 top causes of death for which there is no effective treatment. In this chapter, you will learn what you can do to change the above grim statement. Yes, there is light, at the end of the tunnel. The only caveat is the sooner you embrace the changes, the better your chances. As in all illnesses, if you are end-stage, there are few, if any, options left to reverse Alzheimer's.

Alzheimer's is the most common type of dementia and is currently deemed to be incurable. This is from a 2017 review in *Nature*, where they discuss Alzheimer's from a systemic view (Wang 2017). This means discussing not just brain issues but the entire body's well-being. This makes sense to me, as the earliest changes of Alzheimer's are changes of circulation, reducing blood flow and, therefore, reducing oxygen and nutrients to the brain cells. Most of these changes are reversible with diet and lifestyle (Ornish 1990).

In his book *The End of Alzheimer's,* Dr. D. Bredesen has written, "Alzheimer's disease can be prevented, and in many cases its associated cognitive decline can be reversed." His book includes the science that supports his conclusions (Bredesen 2017). In addition, it is a practical, easy-to-use, step-by-step manual to prevent and reverse cognitive decline of early Alzheimer's. In 2014, he published a study reporting the reversal of cognitive decline in nine out of ten patients. He named his protocol ReCODE, which stands for Reversal in Aging of Cognitive Decline.

Here are ten suggestions that may help you decide if you have Alzheimer's or other dementia in early stages.

1. Memory loss that disrupts daily life: One of the most common signs of Alzheimer's is memory loss, especially forgetting recently learned information. Other signs include forgetting dates for events, asking for the same information over and over, an increased need to rely on memory aids (e.g., reminder notes or electronic devices), or relying on family members for help with things you used to handle on their own. A typical age-related change is sometimes forgetting names or appointments but remembering them later.

2. Challenges in planning or solving problems: Some people may experience changes in their ability to develop a follow-up plan or work with numbers. They may have

trouble following a familiar recipe or keeping track of monthly bills. They may have difficulty concentrating and take much longer to do things than they did before. A typical age-related change is making occasional errors when balancing a cheque book.

3. Difficulty in completing familiar tasks at home, at work, or during leisure activities: People with Alzheimer's often find it hard to complete daily tasks. Sometimes, people may have trouble driving to a familiar location, managing a budget at work, or remembering the rules of a favourite game. A typical age-related change is occasionally needing help in using the settings on a microwave or recording a television show.

4. Confusion with time or place: People with Alzheimer's can lose track of dates, seasons, and the passage of time. They may have trouble understanding something if it is not happening immediately. Sometimes, they may forget where they are or how they got there. A typical age-related change is getting confused about the day of the week but figuring it out later.

5. Trouble understanding visual images and spatial relationships: For some people, vision problems is a sign of Alzheimer's. They may have difficulty reading, judging distance, and determining colour or contrast, which may cause problems with driving. A typical age-related change is vision problems related to cataracts.

6. New problems with words and speaking or writing: People with Alzheimer's may have trouble following or joining conversations. They may stop in the middle of a conversation and have no idea how to continue, or they may repeat themselves. They may struggle with vocabulary, have problems finding the right word, or call things by the wrong name. An example is calling a watch a

"hand clock." A typical age-related change is sometimes having trouble finding the right word.

7. Misplacing things and losing the ability to retrace steps: People with Alzheimer's disease may put things in unusual places. They may lose things and be unable to go back over their steps to find them again. Sometimes, they may accuse others of stealing. This may occur more frequently over time. A typical age-related change is misplacing things from time to time and having difficulty retracing steps to find them.

8. Decreased or poor judgment: People with Alzheimer's may experience changes in judgment or decision-making. For example, they may use poor judgment when dealing with money, giving large amounts to telemarketers. They may pay less attention to grooming or keeping themselves clean. A typical age-related change is making an occasional bad decision.

9. Withdrawal from work or social activities: People with Alzheimer's may start to remove themselves from hobbies, social activities, work projects, or sports. They may have trouble keeping up with a favourite sports team or remembering how to complete a favourite hobby. They may also avoid being social because of the changes they have experienced. A typical age-related change is sometimes feeling weary of work, family, and social obligations.

10. Changes in mood and personality: People with Alzheimer's can become confused, suspicious, depressed, fearful, or anxious. They may be easily upset at home, at work, with friends, or in places where they are out of their comfort zone. A typical age-related change is developing specific ways of doing things and becoming irritable when a routine is disrupted.

What should you do if you notice some of the above signs? Use these signs as early detection to get the maximum benefit from available treatments, so you have more time to plan for the future, locate care and support services for you and your loved ones, and participate in building the right care team and social support. Explore www.alz.org. This website is sponsored by the Alzheimer's Association, and they have a 24/7 helpline that you can call at 1-800-272-3900. They have helpful suggestions and list all the drugs that work in about half of all people for six to twelve months.

My personal suggestion is to focus heavily on exercise, stimulating activities, and developing a support team for the caregiver. Access to care is becoming increasingly difficult everywhere in the world. Consequently, more family members and loved ones are required to provide care. Supporting the caregiver's health is particularly important, because if he or she becomes incapacitated mentally, physically, or emotionally, the patient must immediately go into care.

Next, I discuss some of the reversible components of cognitive problems. It is important to address these, as this may well slow the onset of the Alzheimer's disease itself. You can find a discussion of mild to moderate and severe Alzheimer's at www.emedicine.medscape.com. I will include some of these here to expedite your understanding.

First, mild Alzheimer's demonstrates the following signs:
- Memory loss
- Confusion about the location of familiar places
- Taking longer to accomplish normal daily tasks
- Trouble handling money and paying bills
- Compromised judgment often leading to bad decisions
- Loss of spontaneity and sense of initiative
- Mood and personality changes
- Increased anxiety

Moderate-stage Alzheimer's is suggested when the following signs appear:

- Increased memory loss and confusion with a shortened attention span
- Problems recognizing friends and family members
- Difficulty with language
- Problems with reading, writing, and working with numbers
- Difficulty organizing thoughts and thinking logically
- Inability to learn new things or to cope with new or unexpected situations
- Restlessness, agitation, tearfulness, and wandering, especially in the late afternoon or at night
- Repetitive statements or movements
- Occasional muscle twitches
- Hallucinations, delusions, suspiciousness or paranoia, irritability, loss of impulse control shown through behaviours, such as undressing at inappropriate times or places or using vulgar language
- Perceptual motor problems, such as trouble getting out of the chair or setting the table

Severe-stage Alzheimer's has progressed to the following:

- Cannot recognize family or loved ones and cannot communicate effectively
- Completely dependent on others for care
- Weight loss
- Seizures
- Skin infections
- Difficulty swallowing
- Groaning, moaning, or grunting
- Increased sleep
- Lack of bowel and bladder control

When individuals suddenly deteriorate in their mental function, including many or all of the above signs and symptoms, then it is important they be evaluated by an experienced clinician. This evaluation will typically include ruling out recent infection, such as a urinary tract infection, and possibly even an MRI to rule out a chronic subdural hematoma or normal pressure hydrocephalus. Each of these conditions is potentially treatable and will hopefully resolve some of the symptoms. It is up to the clinician to evaluate this sudden change in condition. It is important to include the possibility of drugs or drug interactions contributing to the sudden change.

The two most important nutrient components to address when cognitive problems are present are thyroid deficiency and some vitamin deficiencies. Low thyroid hormone can certainly present with cognitive problems and depression. (Each of these are well addressed in their respective chapters in this book.) The other important item to address can be determined by measuring the serum homocysteine. This is available in most regular labs, because it is also used as an assessment for cardiovascular risks. It is important that you learn your actual number, because you will probably like to have a number lower than the typical cardiovascular disease number. Excellent research in the United Kingdom has revealed that if homocysteine can be kept below seven, then the likelihood of Alzheimer's is cut in half. I know of nothing else that is this significant.

If the homocysteine is greater than seven, then I strongly recommend supplementation with vitamin B6, vitamin B12, and methyl folate. We now know the serum homocysteine is indicative to how well the body is handling toxins through one important pathway. There is a genetic variation among people that is called the methylenetetrahydrofolate reductase (MTHFR). MTHFR is the rate-limiting enzyme in the methyl cycle, and it is encoded by the MTHFR gene. This enzyme plays a role in the processing of amino acids, which are the building blocks of proteins. It enables the body to take homocysteine to its final step of the important amino acid cysteine.

Approximately 5-6 percent of the population is homozygous for this genetic variation, and they will need much more supplementation of the three vitamins mentioned above. In addition, they may have problems with sleep and anxiety. Approximately 25 percent of the population is heterozygous for this variation, and they will also benefit from supplementation.

The MTHFR gene can be tested for at 23andMe or a number of other selected laboratories, including Great Plains Labs. I have sent many patients for investigations at this lab, and they are excellent in their follow up and quality of work. In addition, I travelled to Kansas City to do their three-day training session in optimal lab evaluation. Optimizing your serum homocysteine will have distinct benefits to your heart health and blood vessel health. If you can optimize your serum homocysteine with the help of your health care practitioner, then you probably do not need to spend the extra money on your personal genetics.

The other group that may benefit from some vitamin supplementation are those with malabsorption problems. This includes people diagnosed with celiac or non-celiac gluten sensitivity. Non-celiac gluten sensitivity is believed to be about 10 percent of the population and maybe even as high as 30 percent. Unfortunately, it is the brain and other neurological tissues that can function poorly or not at all in the presence of gluten. The other significant group with malabsorption problems is those people diagnosed with inflammatory bowel disease or inflammatory bowel syndrome (IBS). In general, if the gut is unhealthy, particular vitamins, especially B12 and D, are at risk. Both are critical for optimal brain function.

Gut bacteria may play a role in Alzheimer's. This research was done at Lund University in Sweden and reported in *Scientific Reports* in February 2017 (Harach 2017). It shows that intestinal bacteria can accelerate the development of Alzheimer's disease. Exactly how our gut microbiota is composed depends on which bacteria we receive at birth, our genes, and our diet. This study shows there is a direct causal link between gut bacteria and Alzheimer's disease. They are beginning to research ways to prevent the disease and delay the onset. A further example is "Obesity and gut's dysbiosis promote neuroinflammation, cognitive impairment and vulnerability to Alzheimer's disease" (Daulatzai 2014). This research made me consider the possibility of a Gut Flora Transplant,GFT, also known as fecal microbiota transplant,FMT, as described in chapter 34 of this book. Supportive evidence of low-grade brain infection was also found and reported (Pisa 2017).

One other important area to address in someone with reduced cognitive function, where Alzheimer's is being considered, is the function of the mitochondria or energy production within the brain cells. As discussed, brain neurons require a huge amount of energy to function optimally. One of the other names that has been talked about with Alzheimer's is type 3 diabetes mellitus. There is considerable evidence that in these patients, glucose is unable to enter the brain cells and, therefore, they are lacking this energy substrate to produce ATP or energy packets. Some people dramatically respond to medium-chain triglycerides, which can be bought in a formulation at the pharmacy or ingested by using coconut oil several times a day. If this is ineffective over a period of eight to twelve weeks, review the chapter on mitochondrial function (chapter 7), because other subtle components might be assisted by supplementation.

One more avenue that I would explore if I were developing early signs of Alzheimer's or other dementia is oxygen supplementation. One of the aggravating features with early Alzheimer's is lack of energy within neurons. Adding extra oxygen is the second way to potentially provide more energy formation within the mitochondria of the neurons. This is something that you can undertake on your own safely and for relatively minimal cost. If you want to approach this optimally, then I recommend 20–40 treatments of hyperbaric oxygen at between 1.5–2.0 atm. This is the amount of pressure used and is not dramatically different from what you experience in a jet plane flying at 35,0000 feet and pressurized to 8,500 feet. People vary for the sweet spot, so I recommend that you start at 1.5 atm for five days. If there is no improvement, then increase to 1.75 atm for another five days. If there is still no improvement, increase to 2.0 atm for the remaining treatments. It is well documented that the vasoconstriction that may occur by going above 2.0 atm may diminish the dissolved oxygen bathing the neurons in the brain. My sweet spot seems to be 1.75 atm. I do this for one hour at depth at least once a week, as I have had recurrent cognitive problems for more than twenty years with my MS. In the last three years, I have done more than 350 hyperbaric oxygenation treatments. I believe this has been a great assist for my cluster headaches and my cognitive function. I particularly wanted my cognitive function optimal for the writing of this book. In addition to hyperbaric treatments, I routinely use pillow oxygen at night. For further details, read chapter 30 of this book.

Another avenue to consider is use of cannabis and the endocannabinoid system for Alzheimer's. First, it takes the edge off Alzheimer's (Campbell 2009). Second, it helps block the inflammatory response of amyloid proteotoxicity (Currais 2016). Third, there is a molecular link between cannabis components and Alzheimer's (Eubanks 2006). Finally, cannabinoids may be able to prevent Alzheimer's (Ramirez 2005).

Finally, I must again inform you of the recently published book by neurologist researcher Dale Bredesen, MD, *The End of Alzheimer's* (Bredesen 2017). This well-written book talks of three types of Alzheimer's and the best therapies for them, all of which fall into the integrative medicine practitioner's expertise. This reinforces to me that we are on the right track. So, take heart!

24: Parkinson's Disease

I first learned about Parkinson's disease at the University of Saskatchewan, where neurologist Ali Rajput is one of the pioneers of the study of Parkinson's. I was naïve in my early twenties and thought of Parkinson's as an old person's disease. However, in 1996, when I was diagnosed with MS, one of my close medical school friends, P.L., was diagnosed with Parkinson's disease at the same age. I still remember his neurologist asking him to write "Mary had a Little Lamb." After P.L. wrote it in ever-smaller letters, he was diagnosed with Parkinson's disease. He had several other signs, but once he demonstrated micrographia, the diagnosis was confirmed.

In this chapter, I describe some of the basics about Parkinson's disease, including some of the principles about treating it or preventing it and some of the interventions that may prove useful. This brain illness is being diagnosed more and more commonly, and over one million people in North America have the diagnosis. Regular medical progress and pharmaceutical treatment of Parkinson's has progressed slowly. Consequently, many people suffer severely as their illness progresses and the regular treatment of L-dopa often stops helping.

In 1998, Parkinson's disease jumped into the public consciousness when Canadian actor Michael J. Fox openly talked about his diagnosis. He was still a young man, perhaps best known for the movie *Back to the Future* and the TV series *Spin City*. His book, *Lucky Man* (Fox 2002), is quite inspirational, as he discusses his journey with this chronic illness.

Substantia Nigra and Parkinson's Disease

Parkinson's disease is a slow progression of illness that affects movement, muscle control, and balance. Part of the disease process develops as cells are destroyed in certain parts of the brain, particularly the crescent-shaped cell mass known as the substantia nigra. Nerve cells in the substantia nigra send out fibres to tissues located on both sides of the brain. These cells release essential neurotransmitters that help control movement and coordination. Substantia nigra is Latin for "black substance." The substantia nigra area appears darker because of the high concentrations of neural melanin dopaminergic neurons. Parkinson's disease is characterized by the death of dopaminergic neurons in the substantia nigra pars compacta. The substantia nigra is an important player in brain function, especially with items such as eye movement, motor planning, reward seeking, learning, and addiction. The substantia nigra also serves as a major source of GABAergic inhibition of various brain targets. The pars compacta is believed to regulate the sleep-wake cycle, which is consistent with Parkinson's symptoms, such as insomnia and REM sleep disturbance.

Parkinson's disease is partly due to the death of dopaminergic neurons in the pars compacta. Blood-brain barrier dysfunction is part of this (Kortekaas 2005). The major symptoms include tremor, akinesia, bradykinesia, and stiffness. Other symptoms include changes to posture, fatigue, sleep changes, and depression. Akinesia is the ability to initiate voluntary movements. Bradykinesia is the slowness of initiation of voluntary movements. The four key symptoms of Parkinson's disease are bradykinesia, tremor, rigidity, and postural instability.

Other neurological conditions that can produce tremor include MS, stroke, chronic kidney disease, and TBI. Additional sources of tremor include a diagnosis of Parkinson's but also can be secondary to drugs, such as amphetamines, cocaine, caffeine, corticosteroids, SSRIs, or alcohol, mercury poisoning or withdrawal of such drugs, such as alcohol and benzodiazepines. Tremors are also aggravated by lack of sleep, lack of particular B vitamins, and excess stress. Especially critical are deficiencies of magnesium and thiamine,vitamin B1. Alcohol also potentiates GABAergic transmission. In Parkinson's disease, the typical tremor is worse at rest and often decreases if the patient is distracted.

A simple way of considering Parkinson's disease is a lack of dopamine because of the death or injury of the dopaminergic-producing neurons. Typically, once an individual is diagnosed with Parkinson's, they have lost 50–80 percent of their dopaminergic neurons. Often if they have a distinct tremor, they are started on L-dopa or some variation thereof. This provides increased dopamine to the critical parts of the brain and often helps symptoms. However, it can worsen symptoms, and debate continues as to whether it may actually aggravate the illness, making its progress more rapid. I suggest you defer L-dopa until all other avenues have been tried.

Low-level Pesticide Exposure Linked to Parkinson's Disease

A considerable body of evidence indicates that environmental toxins can initiate and/or aggravate Parkinson's disease.

Organochlorine insecticides are one problem in triggering or aggravating Parkinson's (Corrigan 2000). Another example of how this occurs is a fungicide called benomyl. This compound was banned by the United States' EPA (Environmental Protection Agency) after it was found to be a potential carcinogen. Benomyl blocks an important enzyme called aldehyde dehydrogenase (ALDH). This enzyme is able to change aldehydes, which are toxic to dopamine cells, into less-toxic compounds. A recent study on eleven similar pesticides showed that, even at low concentrations of exposure, they have a detrimental effect on dopaminergic cells. In addition, there is a common genetic variant among humans and this enzyme, where the increase of Parkinson's disease is increased six-fold. These individuals are especially sensitive to the effects of the ALDH-blocking effects of pesticides. The following pesticides are known to create a risk of Parkinson's, if there is prolonged occupational exposure: permethrin, beta-HCH, the herbicides paraquat and 2,4-D, and the fungicide maneb. In 2009, the US Department of Veterans Affairs added Parkinson's disease to the list of diseases associated with exposure to agent orange.

Unfortunately, many of these herbicide and pesticide agents are now being approved to treat super weeds. An example is the 2–2.5-meter-tall red root pigweed. This weed is now resistant to Roundup, despite using large amounts. As a consequence, the chemical companies are asking for addition of 2,4-D and agent orange. Tragically, this is being seriously considered. Independent research reveals that chronic exposure to organophosphate pesticides also increases the risk of developing Parkinson's. Two of these are paraquat and rotenone. Both of these are lipophilic (fat loving), and this makes them resistant to breaking down in water. In addition, they accumulate in your fat and, unfortunately, both cross the blood-brain barrier.

Hence, you need to avoid pesticide exposure home, in your community, and in the food you (reduce your risk of Parkinson's by reducing your (all types of environmental toxins. Furthermore, av trial solvents, such as TCE, a common degreasing ἁ ., ἀιια dry cleaning chemicals, as these have also been linked to Parkinson's. Finally, make sure your silver amalgam dental fillings are removed. These are more than 50 percent mercury. Mercury causes cell membranes to leak and inhibits key enzymes that your body needs for energy production and removal of toxins. Mercury toxicity is also known to worsen chronic brain illnesses, including MS, Parkinson's, and probably Alzheimer's as well (Houston 2011).

Drug Considerations

When we talk about drugs used frequently today that may be linked to Parkinson's disease, number one on the list is a statin. Experts within the cardiovascular literature have stated that the side effects of statin drugs are far greater than any potential for prevention of heart disease. Dr. Chand, deputy chairman of the British Medical Association, suggested that it was high time that statins were avoided in the low cardiovascular risk population and should, at most, only be given to people with existing heart disease. It was well stated by Dr. Xuemei Huang, professor of neurology at Penn State College of medicine in Pennsylvania: "If we blanket prescribe statins to people, we would be creating a huge population of people with neurological problems" (Huang 2015). An unstated concept is that cholesterol is important for brain recovery and healing. By keeping it low, we are not doing anyone any favours. This includes not reducing their risk of heart attack. Finally,

...enever a statin is prescribed, it is recommended that the individual also be started on coenzyme Q10 (CoQ10). This is recommended, because the statin blocks cholesterol before the formation of the body's CoQ10. CoQ10 is recognized to be helpful in minimizing Parkinson's, so whenever we prescribe a statin, we must automatically recommend a CoQ10 supplement. I suggest 200 mg three times a day. I recently saw in consultation a 70-year-old man with 20 years of Parkinson's disease. I was distressed to learn that he had been on statins several years because of a stroke but had never been recommended to be on CoQ10. I did my best to alter his approach and said I would prefer statins to be discontinued for several months to see if his severe Parkinson's improved.

The Gut and Parkinson's Disease

In December 2014, Tilip Scheperjans MD, PhD, and colleagues from the University of Helsinki Finland, examined the intestinal contents of 72 people with Parkinson's disease and 72 people without Parkinson's disease (Scheperjans 2014). They found that people with Parkinson's disease had lesser amounts of a certain bacteria called Prevotella. In addition, this particular bacteria varied among the subgroups of those with Parkinson's disease with differing motor symptoms. In Dr. Scheperjans' study, Prevotella was present in Parkinson's patients but in lower amounts. This bacteria is key in the formation of thiamine and folate. It also helps maintain the intestinal barrier to minimize the absorption of environmental toxins. If we are unable to tolerate environmental toxins, then we are more subject to the injuries they can create. Parkinson's disease is one of the key diseases amongst this group. Dr. Scheperjans and his team also found that in patients with more severe postural instability and gait difficulty but less tremor, the bacterium Enterobacteriaceae was present at higher levels. I want to credit the Michael J. Fox foundation for Parkinson's research for this information, as displayed by Rachel Dolhun on her blog (Dolhun 2018).

Parkinson's disease has a clear effect on our gut. Nearly 80 percent of Parkinson's patients suffer from constipation. This can be present for up to twenty years before the diagnosis is reached. Also, alpha-synuclein, a protein that clumps in the brains of everyone with Parkinson's, has also been found within the nerves controlling the intestines and, therefore, outside the brain. Is it possible that this abnormal protein triggers constipation years prior to Parkinson's ? Later, when the bacteria and illness spreads to the brain, does it cause motor symptoms there? Finally, these researchers believe the gut's normal bacteria might affect the functioning of the gut nerves, which could, in turn, affect the nerves of the brain. An example of this is that the majority of neuron signals go up to the brain via the vagus nerve. As an anaesthesiologist, I thought the majority of vagus nerve traffic went from the brain to the heart and gut. However, now that I'm better informed, I have been corrected! Much of the interaction of the gut-brain axis probably communicates or travels through the vagus nerve.

Further research by Dr. Elizabeth Svensson et al. was published in *Neurology* in an article entitled "Vagotomy and subsequent risk of Parkinson's disease" (Svensson 2015). "Vagotomy" means cutting of the vagus nerve surgically. They compared patients who had had a complete vagotomy with the general population. Risk of Parkinson's disease was reduced in those who had a complete vagotomy, and this included a twenty-year follow up. At the end of the paper, they discussed their conclusion: "full truncal vagotomy is associated with the decreased risk for subsequent Parkinson's disease, suggesting that the vagal nerve may be critically involved in the pathogenesis of Parkinson's disease." I interpret the above as suggesting that Parkinson's disease begins in the gut. The gut-brain axis is now the accepted new norm. Within this accepted norm, the superhighway connecting the gut and the brain is the vagus nerve. Much of the traffic from the gut to the brain can include bacteria, which are able to travel via this nerve as well as through the bloodstream. Now let us focus on the microbiota data as the next piece of the puzzle.

"Both the enteric nervous system and the dorsal motor nucleus of the vagus are affected by Lewy body pathology at early stages of PD (Parkinson's Disease). This early involvement provides insights into the pathophysiology of gastrointestinal dysmotility in this disorder and may constitute an important step in the beginning (pathogenesis) of Lewy body disease."(Cersosimo 2008)

"Much of the presently available data suggest that the primary PD process is the major factor in the etiology of gut dysfunction in this patient population. This may be mediated by both central and peripheral mechanisms. Involvement of the dorsal motor nucleus of the vagus might produce dysfunction of muscles controlling deglutition and esophageal motility, thereby leading to drooling, dysphagia, and gastroesophageal reflux" (Edwards 1992).

"In conclusion, we here provide the first experimental evidence that different α-synuclein forms can propagate from the gut to the brain, and that microtubule-associated transport is involved in the translocation of aggregated α-synuclein in neurons. These data represent not only the first demonstration of abnormal intestinal permeability in PD subjects but also the first correlation of increased intestinal permeability in PD with intestinal α-synuclein, the hallmark of PD" (Holmqvist 2014).

Gut Microbiota Regulate Motor Deficits and Neural Inflammation

The last few years have revealed that intestinal microbiota influence neurodevelopment, modulate behaviour, and contribute to neurological disorders. However, an actual functional link between gut bacteria and neurodegenerative diseases was unexplored until recently. T.R. Sampson wrote "Gut Microbiota Regulate Motor Deficits and Neuroinflammation in a Model of Parkinson's Disease" (Sampson 2016). One of the components of Parkinson's is the aggregation of the protein alpha-synuclein. The research model revealed that this aggregation happens first in the gut. They reported that gut microbiota are required for motor deficits, microglia activation, and alpha-synuclein pathology. They also learned that antibiotic treatment would reduce this microbial recolonization, which changed pathophysiology in adult animals. Later in the study, they found that oral administration of specific microbial metabolites to germ-free mice promoted neural inflammation and motor symptoms. In fact, when they took microbiota from Parkinson's disease-affected patients, they found it worsened the physical impairments when compared to microbiota transplants from healthy human donors. These findings reveal that bacteria regulate disorders in mice. They suggest that alterations in the human microbiota represents a risk factor for Parkinson's disease.

The above landmark paper by Sampson suggests that we must increasingly focus on the health of the gut microbiota. In simple terms, we must avoid antibiotics or antibiotic-containing foods as much as possible. Notable among these is glyphosate or Roundup. It was patented as an antibiotic by Monsanto in 2010. Therefore, if you eat a food that was harvested with Roundup, it is concentrated in the seed, and you are taking in an antibiotic. In North America, Roundup is used on the vast majority of wheat, potatoes, sweet potatoes, and sugar. In addition to the problem of the antibiotic action, Roundup dramatic reduces the liver's ability to detoxify, due to the direct injury to the P450 enzyme pathway. The consequence of this is that the liver is unable to break down any toxins taken in. So, they cause much more injury, not only to the gut microbiota but also to all cells, including the neurons in the brain.

We must do everything we can to protect our health, because these changes probably occur twenty to thirty years before the development of the illness, whether Parkinson's or Alzheimer's. Everyone should learn how to protect their health. In the future, there may be some advantage to faecal microbial transplant (FMT, or GFT, gut flora transplant) to rescue those with injured microbiota. See chapter 33 for the discussion on GFT. In fact, I have already referred one patient with the suggestion of early Parkinson's on his MRI to have a FMT (GFT) at the Taymount Clinic in the UK.

Healthy Lifestyle Choices to Reduce Your Risk of Parkinson's Disease

Currently, we are unable to cure Parkinson's disease, so prevention or slowing its progression is critical. An interesting human study with PET (Positron Emission Tomography) revealed "Blood-Brain Barrier dysfunction in parkinsonian midbrain in vivo" that injured BBB is a causative mechanism in Parkinson's. This concept and the previous discussion helps me recommend organic whole foods. Ideally, as mentioned, you should eat 50 different foods per week as one of the best ways to enhance your microbiota diversity. Supplemental nutrients are another possibility. I do regular supplementation, which is known to help prevent Parkinson's as well as control my MS. These include vitamin D, Omega-3 oils containing EPA and DHA, CoQ10, green tea, and alpha-lipoic acid. Epidemiologic studies have continued to suggest that vitamin D deficiency is a factor in the development of Parkinson's disease. I recommend supplementing your vitamin D until your serum vitamin D 25-OH is at least 100 nmol/L, which is 40 ng/ml in USA units.

Other Possibilities to Help Control Parkinson's

Exercise

Exercise, particularly vigorous walking, can have a dramatic benefit in slowing Parkinson's progression. I first learned of this in *The Brain's Way of Healing* (Doidge 2015) by Norman Doidge, MD. He went to South Africa to meet a gentleman with Parkinson's by the name of John Pepper. John sent an email letter to Dr. Doidge in September 2008. The following is a component of that letter, which I have taken from Dr. Doidge's book:

> I live in South Africa and about Parkinson's disease since 1968. I do a lot of exercise and have learned to use my conscious brain to control the movements, which are normally controlled by the subconscious brain. I wrote a book about my experience, but it has been rejected by the medical profession without looking into my case, because I no longer looked like a Parkinson's disease sufferer. I no longer take Parkinson's disease medication, although I still have

most of the symptoms. I walk 15 miles per week, in three sessions of 5 miles. The glial-derived neurotrophic factor produced in the brain appears to have restored the damaged cells. However, they do not cure the cause of Parkinson's disease, and if I stop exercising, I go backward . . . I am sure that I can help many newly diagnosed patients, if I can encourage them to do serious regular exercise. Please let me know your thoughts on this matter.

Dr. Doidge discusses this case in detail over 68 pages. It has convinced me, because John Pepper gives many examples of other Parkinson's disease patients who have had success with his recommendation. I believe this is an excellent example of neuroplasticity. We know that exercise enhances brain-derived neurotrophic factor (BDNF). We also know that consistent and repetitive exercise is a superb way to rebuild and enhance important pathways within the brain. I realize this is easier to talk about than it is to do, but, frankly, you have nothing to lose and many things to gain. Everyone can afford this, and you do not need the blessing of your physician, because there are no harmful downsides. If you improve enough, you might consider tapering off your medications, with your physician's assistance.

Hyperbaric Oxygen Therapy (HBOT) at modest pressures 1.3 – 2.0 atmospheres absolute

Hypoxia is probably one of the triggering factors for the injury that occurs in the substantia nigra. Certainly, the lack of energy from reduced mitochondrial function is an accepted component of Parkinson's disease. 0-2 therapy is a route that

I would pursue, because there is virtually no downside, and it has significant benefits. A study in Moscow by the neurology department headed by Prof. V. Ya Neretin used HBOT to treat sixty-four patients suffering from Parkinson's disease and diverse causes (Neretin 1989). Each of them had eight to 12 different sessions at 1.3–2.0 atm. The exposure time to oxygen was forty to sixty minutes. Fifty-five of the sixty-four patients noted a marked beneficial effect. The best results occurred in patients under sixty-five years and with a history of diagnosis within the last five years. It worked best in people with rigidity problems and less well in people with tremor problems. There is also a case study by ML Hoggard et al in California (Hoggard 2015). A 72-year-old man with Parkinson's disease had been diagnosed for 18 months and was on Sinemet (L-Dopa), 10/100, with three doses three times a day. He was treated at 1.9 atm for one hour, 5 times a week for 5 weeks. Sophisticated testing showed a 10 percent improvement in his right hand and a 32 percent improvement in his left (nondominant) hand. He was able to discontinue all his Sinemet medication. This was particularly surprising and impressed the physicians. It is probable because many of the cells, which were not working adequately within the substantia nigra, recovered to a degree. HBOT is known to increase stem cells in circulation eight times (Thom 2006).

Cannabis

Several articles reveal a potential role for cannabis in Parkinson's (Carroll 2004; Lotan 2014; Dawson 2002; McSherry 2005; Venderová 2004). The key principle is to start low with primarily a CBD dominant with some THC. Once stabilized for two to four weeks, try for three months to determine if beneficial. These diagnoses begin slowly and often improve slowly too. This means a trial of three to six months may be needed to show improvement.

Photobiomodulation Therapy (PBMT)

More details are available in chapter 35. The easiest reference is Hamblin (2016). Of special note here is the newly created LED (light emitting diode) helmet by Thor Laser in 2018. The helmet has resulted in a dramatic improvement in one significantly impaired Parkinson's patient. This patient was relatively immobile, and had limited facial expressions (the mask of Parkinson's). After several days of treatment, this patient had increased mobility and was smiling with more normal facial expressions. This is a promising technology that requires further research.

25: Chronic Mold, Lyme, and CIRS

I have seen a number of clients with this challenging diagnosis and treatment requirements. Only upon discussion with my integrative medicine colleague, Dr. K. Johnson, did I decide to include the topic in this book. This inclusion was further enhanced by Dr. Dale Bredesen's book *The End of Alzheimer's* (2017). He includes type 3 Alzheimer's as inhalational (mold) or chronic Lyme infection based. Finally, an excellent interview by Dr. Jill Carnahan on her website, www.jillcarnahan.com, helped my resolve to broach this tough topic. I do not have all the answers, but by looking at Dr. Carnahan's website and www.survivingmold.com, you can begin to find answers. The latter website lists clinicians certified in chronic inflammatory response syndrome (CIRS) protocol. This resource is critical if you fail to find a CIRS-informed clinician near you or online. Karen D. Johnson, MD, who is listed as being in Hawaii, hails from Canada and has been a colleague of mine since our time as classmates in medical school. The list of practitioners on the website includes a Canadian, Bruce Hoffman, MD, in Alberta. Each of the people certified have completed Shoemaker's training and two essays on CIRS and evidence-based medicine. With her consent, I have included Dr. Johnson's essay below.

Diagnosis and Treatment of Chronic Inflammatory Response Syndrome—CIRS

Karen D. Johnson MD, ABOIM, IFMCP

Have you been sick for a long time without any improvement in spite of multiple medical visits to different clinicians and a multitude of tests and treatments? You may have CIRS.

CIRS, as the name implies, is a chronic illness. It is a cluster of symptoms that affect multiple systems in the body. It was first described by Dr. Ritchie Shoemaker, who continues to do extensive research on diagnosing, treating and understanding the syndrome down to a genomic level.[25] CIRS is caused by exposure to a biological agent (biotoxin) in your environment that your body cannot clear in part because of your genetics. The biotoxin can be exposure to:

1. Mold from a water-damaged building (WDB, CIRS-WDB). Up to 50 percent of buildings in the US have a history of water damage

2. Lyme or co-infections from a tick bite (CIRS-LYME), resulting in inability to clear the biotoxin after antibiotic treatment

3. Exposure to a dinoflagellate such as *Pfiesteria* or *Ciguatera*. This can occur after eating tropical reef fish contaminated with Ciguatoxin or exposure to infected fish or water

4. Exposure to blue-green algae (Cylindrospermopsis or Microcystis) in infected waterways

---

[25] "Surviving Mold—What is CIRS," Surviving Mold, December 2014, http://www.survivingmold.com/news/2014/12/what-is-cirs/. Ryan, J.C., Wu, Q., Shoemaker, R.C., "Transcriptomic signatures in whole blood of patients who acquire a chronic inflammatory response syndrome (CIRS) following an exposure to the marine toxin ciguatoxin," *BMC Medical Genomics* 8, no. 15 (April 2015), https://www.ncbi.nlm.nih.gov/pubmed/25889530.

5. Bite from recluse spider.

Returning to the genetics I mentioned above, you may ask, why am I sick and nobody else that lives or works in the WDB is sick? Why did I not get better after I was treated with antibiotics for Lyme and other people who were treated are not still sick?

This is explained by your HLA (human leukocyte antigen) profile. Each person has an individual profile that allows our immune system to recognize or not recognize biotoxins. Some people can be mold sensitive, some can be Lyme sensitive, and some can have multiple sensitivities. Each individual profile indicates whether your body can efficiently clear that biotoxin or not clear it. Approximately one quarter of the population is susceptible to mold toxins. A blood test or cheek swab can determine your HLA profile.

There are two main components to our immune system. The innate immune system is what we were born with. It is the initial defense against foreign invaders. When confronted with an invader, the immune system releases signals to the body that there is danger. The body responds quickly producing chemicals as the first line of defense to destroy the invader. This is nonspecific and could be compared to dumping "bleach" on the invader. These chemicals (not really bleach) are what make us feel so ill when we are coming down with something. It is usually not the bug itself that makes us feel this way but the host response to the illness.

The second part of the immune system is the adaptive immune system. This is a much more precise system and rather than dumping bleach everywhere, produces antibodies to specifically remove the invader. It takes time for our body to make antibodies specific to the invader and therefore we have the innate immune system as the frontline of defense.

Some people lack the ability to make antibodies against certain biotoxins. This is what I was referring to above with

HLA types that cannot recognize certain biotoxins. If this happens, the toxins cannot be removed by the adaptive immune system and persist in our body. Our body does have a backup plan which is not very efficient. Our liver secretes the biotoxin into the bile, which is dumped into the gut; however, these biotoxins are tiny, and 95 percent of them are quickly reabsorbed in the gut. This is compounded if our problem is mold toxicity from a WDB, and we have ongoing exposure.

So, what happens? The innate immune system continues to do its job in the only way it knows how, keeps dumping "bleach" on the problem, and the person becomes increasingly ill with time.[26]

How Do You Know If You Have CIRS?

Dr. Shoemaker has specific case criteria for CIRS diagnosis. These include:

1. An exposure history that includes one of the following: living or working in a WDB, history of a tick bite, onset of symptoms after becoming ill from eating reef fish, or exposure to blue algae or dinoflagellates. Exposure to a WDB can be verified by presence of visible mold growth, musty smells, or a positive ERMI (Environmental Relative Moldiness Index). An ERMI is a test done on the building in question by obtaining dust samples that are evaluated for the presence of mold fragments or spores. ERMI testing can be ordered from www.mycometrics.com or www.envirobiomics.com.

---

[26] Rawat, M.A. Al-Sadi, "Modulation of Intestinal Epithelial Junction Permeability: MMP-9," *Inflammatory Bowel Diseases* (February 2017), http://journals.lww.com/ibdjournal/Abstract/2017/02001/P_272_MMP_9_ Modulation_of_Intestinal_Epithelial.275.aspx.

2. Your symptoms cannot be explained as the result of any other illness. This includes taking a complete health history and doing a thorough physical exam.
3. You need to have multiple symptoms in multiple systems of your body to be diagnosed with CIRS. Dr. Shoemaker has developed the following symptom chart to evaluate patients for multisystem, multi-symptom illness.

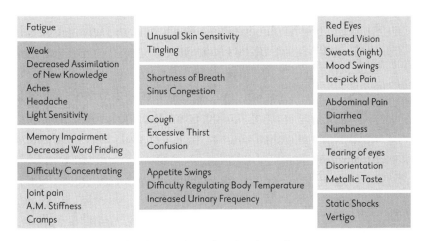

Fatigue		Red Eyes
	Unusual Skin Sensitivity	Blurred Vision
Weak	Tingling	Sweats (night)
Decreased Assimilation of New Knowledge		Mood Swings
Aches	Shortness of Breath	Ice-pick Pain
Headache	Sinus Congestion	
Light Sensitivity		Abdominal Pain
	Cough	Diarrhea
Memory Impairment	Excessive Thirst	Numbness
Decreased Word Finding	Confusion	
		Tearing of eyes
Difficulty Concentrating	Appetite Swings	Disorientation
	Difficulty Regulating Body Temperature	Metallic Taste
Joint pain	Increased Urinary Frequency	
A.M. Stiffness		Static Shocks
Cramps		Vertigo

Used with permission of Ritchie Shoemaker MD

You need at least one symptom in at least six of the thirteen symptom clusters to be considered for CIRS. Eight of thirteen symptom clusters indicates a high probability of CIRS.

If these criteria are met, additional testing will be done.

A simple additional test includes visual contrast sensitivity testing. This test is done in my office and is not the same as a vision test to assess your near and far vision but is a test that measures your ability to discern contrast. Visual contrast perception is impaired in a significant number of people with CIRS as a result of the effect the biotoxin has on reducing blood flow around the optic nerve.

Lab tests are then ordered. Most people have had extensive lab tests done already, however, tests for CIRS look at how your immune system is responding to a biotoxin. The tests can indicate if your immune system is being overstimulated. Standard lab tests are typically normal in CIRS and if abnormal usually are the result of some other problem.

Five of the following lab tests ordered need to be abnormal to diagnose CIRS.

1. HLA haplotype determination (as discussed above): Twenty-four percent of the population have an HLA type that makes them susceptible to CIRS-WDB. However, having the haplotype does not mean you will get CIRS. You still need the exposure. Ninety-five percent of people with CIRS have a susceptible haplotype.

2. MSH (alpha melanocyte-stimulating hormone) level: This is a protein released from the hypothalamus and pituitary gland in the brain. It controls melatonin and hormone levels, including sex hormones and cortisol. MSH affects mucus membrane integrity (leaky gut), regulates our immune system, and controls inflammation. If MSH is low, many symptoms will be experienced, including headache, brain fog, chronic fatigue, sleep disruption, and chronic pain. Chronic pain can be a major symptom with CIRS and results from reduction in our natural endorphin production in addition to the inflammatory effects of cytokines (signaling molecules that result from stimulation of the innate immune system). Normal MSH range is 35–81 pg/ml.

3. MMP-9 (Matrix Metalloproteinase-9): Its release is triggered by the innate immune system. MMP-9 contributes to increased permeability (leaky membranes) by dissolving a protein in tissue to allow molecules to pass more readily out of blood vessels, into joints, the lungs, nerves, and the brain. This is needed in an acute injury to get the fighting power to the site of injury but is dangerous long term, as there will be ongoing delivery

of inflammatory compounds into the above tissues. Normal MMP-9 range is 85–332 ng/ml

4. TGF-beta-1 (Transforming Growth Factor beta-1) is a conductor of our immune system.[27] If TGF-beta is in the normal range, it keeps the balance between the side of our immune system that needs to be alert to fight an intruder (pathogenic T cells) but yet not be so active that our immune system attacks our own tissue. This control is managed by beneficial T regulatory cells (T-reg) and T helper cells. When there is imbalance and deficiency of T-reg cells, autoimmune disease can develop. Elevated TGF-beta not only signals our body to keep making cells to fight the intruder, but these same cells have a positive feedback and stimulate the production of more TGF-beta. High levels of TGF-beta can lead to remodeling of tissue in the lungs, leading to shortness of breath and asthma-like symptoms. Other organs in the body, such as the liver, heart, and kidneys, can also be affected. The normal level of TGF-beta-1 is under 2380 pg/ml.

5. ADH (anti-diuretic hormone) and osmolality-ADH assists in controlling the salt and water balance in our body. In a normal situation, if we are dehydrated, ADH output increases to prevent diuresis (urination), and this will conserve fluid. ADH is produced in the brain and stored in the pituitary gland. Its release is controlled by MSH. The dysregulation in normal production of MSH affects ADH levels. This results in headaches, increased thirst, frequent urination and, if severe enough, our body tries to sweat out the excess salt, resulting in increased susceptibility to static shocks from the sodium present

---

[27] Noack, Miossec, "Th17 and regulatory T-cell balance in autoimmune and inflammatory disease," *Autoimmunity Reviews* (June 2014), www.sciencedirect.com/science/article/pii/S1568997214000081.

on the skin. Normal range ADH: 1–13.3 pg/ml; osmolality: 280–300 mOsmol.

6. VEGF (vascular endothelial growth factor): VEGF is produced by the body to stimulate the growth of new blood vessels. Initially, VEGF levels rise due to decreased blood flow to the tissue as the result of cytokines attracting sticky substances to the lining of blood vessels, causing white blood cells to become trapped and blocking the blood vessel. There is, however, a subsequent decline in VEGF as a result of prolonged elevation of TGF-beta-1. Unfortunately, the blockage in the blood vessels persists, worsening an already compromised blood flow to the tissue. Normal range VEGF: 31–86 pg/ml.

7. C4a and C3a: These are split products of the complement system. They are anaphylatoxins (cause allergic reaction). Biotoxins stimulate the immune system to produce these substances. Complement split products can result in swelling, histamine release, contraction of smooth muscles, and essentially all the symptoms of an allergic reaction. High levels result in increased symptoms. To produce C3a, a microbial cell membrane must be present. This requires looking for an infective agent. Lyme is one infection that needs to be considered with elevation of C3a. Normal range C4a: less than 2830 ng/ml. Normal range C3a: less than 940 ng/ml.

8. VIP (vasoactive intestinal peptide) is made in the gut, pancreas, and brain. It helps reduce the inflammatory response by regulating the immune response. Treatment with this substance can restore many of the imbalances and symptoms seen with CIRS. Normal range VIP: 23–63 pg/ml.[28]

---

[28] Ganea, D., Hooper, K.M., and Kong, W., "The neuropeptide vasoactive intestinal peptide: direct effects on immune cells and involvement in

9. Cortisol and ACTH levels: MSH controls the release of ACTH from the pituitary gland. ACTH is released in response to stress and stimulates the adrenal to produce cortisol. There is an initial rise in cortisol in CIRS; however, as the stress of the illness persists, dysregulation is seen in both levels of ACTH and cortisol. Normal range: ACTH: 8–37 pg/ml. AM Cortisol: 4.3–21 ug/dl.

10. MARCoNS (multiple antibiotic resistant coagulase negative staphylococcus): MARCoNS is frequently cultured from the back of the nose in people with CIRS. It does not usually cause symptoms and is not to be confused with MRSA. It is not an infection in the true sense of the word; however, it turns on further damaging cytokines. Low MSH predisposes one to development of MARCoNS by impairing mucosal immune function. MARCoNS can then interfere with production of MSH, compounding the problem. MARCoNS can reside in biofilm, which protects it from our own natural defenses and from antibiotics. MARCoNS can also affect genetics by controlling which genes are turned on or off. Culture for MARCoNS is obtained by taking a 2–3-inch-deep nasal culture and sending it for API Staph culture. Normal result: negative culture.

Additional lab tests that also can be abnormal in CIRS include:

1. Leptin: a hormone produced by the fat cells. Leptin controls our appetite and allows our fat cells to be burned for energy. Leptin attaches to the leptin receptor in the hypothalamus of the brain and is responsible for controlling the production of MSH and beta endorphin (a substance that is our natural pain reliever). Cytokines

---

inflammatory and autoimmune diseases," *Acta Physiologica* (Nov. 24, 2014), http://onlinelibrary.wiley.com/doi/10.1111/apha.12427/full.

cross the blood-brain barrier and bind to receptors, preventing leptin from binding. The body tries to compensate by producing more leptin. This cycle can result in weight gain and an inability to lose body fat despite dieting and exercise. Normal range: Women: 1.1–27.5 ng/ml; men: 0.5–13.8 ng/ml.

2. Von Willebrand's disease: This can be acquired as a result of an elevated C4a level in CIRS. It results in easy bleeding, particularly nosebleeds. This complication is rare. Testing involves a von Willebrand's panel, and normal results indicate absence of the disease.

3. Screening for presence of autoimmune antibodies: Several antibodies can be abnormal as a result of elevated TGF-beta-1. Two examples are anti-gliadin antibodies, which, if present, result in gluten sensitivity and anti-cardiolipin antibodies, which can cause clotting disorders.

4. CD4+CD25++T-regs: These are immune cells with specific markers on the cell surface. These cells increase as MSH levels rise and indicate an improving immune system. Low levels of T-regs increase the chance of allergy and autoimmunity. The levels of these cells can monitor progress of treatment. CD4+ CD25++ levels should be greater than 18 percent

5. Hormone testing: Testosterone levels may be low as a result of decreased production of LH (luteinizing hormone) and FSH (follicle-stimulating hormone) from the pituitary. Testosterone levels fall even further as a result of increased aromatase levels in CIRS. Aromatase is an enzyme that converts testosterone to estrogen. Testosterone levels may be low and estrogen levels elevated with symptoms of testosterone deficiency and estrogen excess in men and women. Testing includes

DHEA-S, testosterone, and estradiol levels. Normal levels vary for sex and age.

6. PAX Gene testing is being developed by Dr. Shoemaker to further understand the effect of the biotoxin on our genes and the response to treatment at a genetic level to further assist in diagnosis and treatment.[29]

Additional Screening

NeuroQuant Cranial MRI: An MRI of the brain that is interpreted with a software program called NeuroQuant. NeuroQuant measures the volume of different areas of the brain. This can be quite helpful as a diagnostic tool, because the abnormalities seen with CIRS-WDB are different from CIRS-LYME.

People with CIRS-WDB will have shrinkage (atrophy) of an area called the caudate nucleus accompanied by swelling in other areas. CIRS-LYME, however results in atrophy of the putamen. This test can also monitor progress of treatment. NeuroQuant is also being used in the Bredesen protocol to monitor patients with cognitive impairment. This is an excellent flowchart Dr. Shoemaker developed to understand the course of CIRS.

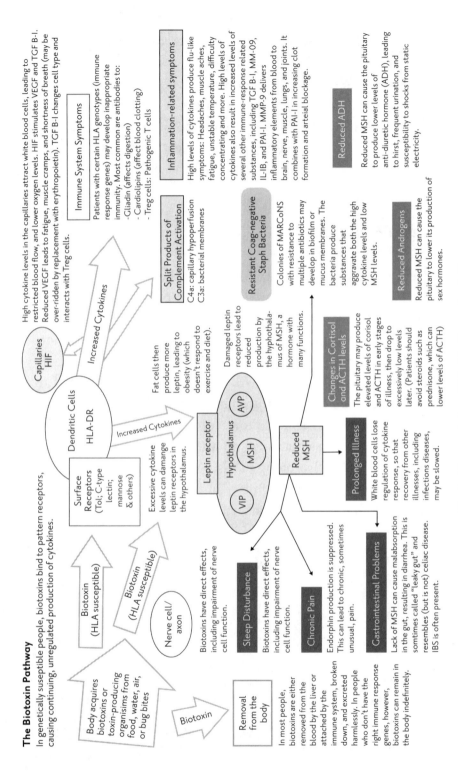

The Biotoxin Pathway

In genetically susceptible people, biotoxins bind to pattern receptors, causing continuing, unregulated production of cytokines.

High cytokine levels in the capillaries attract white blood cells, leading to restricted blood flow, and lower oxygen levels. HIF stimulates VEGF and TGF B-I. Reduced VEGF leads to fatigue, muscle cramps, and shortness of breath (may be over-ridden by replacement with erythropoietin). TGF B-I changes cell type and interacts with Treg cells.

Immune System Symptoms

Patients with certain HLA genotypes (immune response genes) may develop inappropriate immunity. Most common are antibodies to:
- Gliadin (affects digestion)
- Cardiolipins (affect blood clotting)
- Treg cells: Pathogenic T cells

Inflammation-related symptoms

High levels of cytokines produce flu-like symptoms: Headaches, muscle aches, fatigue, unstable temperature, difficulty concentrating and more. High levels of cytokines also result in increased levels of several other immune-response related substances, including TGF B-I, MM-09, IL-IB, and PAI-I. MMP-9 delivers inflammatory elements from blood to brain, nerve, muscle, lungs, and joints. It combines with PAI-I in increasing clot formation and arteial blockage.

Split Products of Complement Activation

C4a: capillary hypoperfusion
C3a: bacterial membranes

Capillaries HIF

Increased Cytokines

Dendritic Cells HLA-DR

Increased Cytokines

Surface Receptors (Tol; C-type lectin; mannose & others)

Excessive cytokine levels can damage leptin receptors in the hypothalamus.

Leptin receptor

Hypothalamus

AVP

MSH

VIP

Damaged leptin receptors lead to reduced production by the hypothalamus of MSH, a hormone with many functions.

Fat cells then produce more leptin, leading to obesity (which doesn't respond to exercise and diet).

Resistant Coag-negative Staph Bacteria

Colonies of MARCoNS with resistance to multiple antibiotics may develop in biofilm or mucus membranes. The bacteria produce substances that aggravate both the high cytokine levels and low MSH levels.

Reduced ADH

Reduced MSH can cause the pituitary to produce lower levels of anti-diuretic hormone (ADH), leading to thirst, frequent urination, and susceptibility to shocks from static electricity.

Reduced Androgens

Reduced MSH can cause the pituitary to lower its production of sex hormones.

Changes in Cortisol and ACTH levels

The pituitary may produce elevated levels of corisol and ACTH in early stages of illness, then drop to excessively low levels later. (Patients should avoid steroids such as prednisone, which can lower levels of ACTH)

Reduced MSH

Prolonged Illness

White blood cells lose regulation of cytokine response, so that recovery from other illnesses, including infections diseases, may be slowed.

Biotoxin (HLA susceptible)

Biotoxin (HLA susceptible)

Nerve cell/ axon

Biotoxins have direct effects, including impairment of nerve cell function.

Sleep Disturbance

Biotoxins have direct effects, including impairment of nerve cell function.

Chronic Pain

Endorphin production is suppressed. This can lead to chronic, sometimes unusual, pain.

Gastrointestinal Problems

Lack of MSH can cause malabsorption in the gut, resulting in diarrhea. This is somtimes called "leaky gut" and resembles (but is not) celiac disease. IBS is often present.

Body acquires biotoxins or toxin-producing organisims from food, water, air, or bug bites.

Removal from the body

Biotoxin

In most people, biotoxins are either removed from the blood by the liver or attached by the immune system, broken down, and excreted harmlessly. In people who don't have the right immune response genes, however, biotoxins can remain in the body indefinitely.

Used with permission of Ritchie Shoemaker MD

Treatment – Yes, There Is Hope!

Treatment is stepwise, starting at the bottom of the pyramid and moving up. Skipping steps will not assist in more rapid recovery and may actually interfere with recovery.

Dr. Shoemaker uses this treatment pyramid in correcting abnormalities in CIRS.

At each step, retesting of VCS and innate immune markers, such as MMP-9, C4a, TGF-beta-1, CD4+ CD25++ T-regs, and any previous abnormalities can be monitored to assess progress.

1. The first step is removal from exposure. This applies primarily to CIRS-WDB. This is the most difficult for patients for multiple reasons, including cost and attachment to personal items. ERMI testing is indicated to determine where exposure is occurring. The workplace may need to also be tested. Symptomatic improvement will not occur if ongoing exposure to the biotoxin continues. The professional assistance of an indoor environmental professional

Treatment Steps

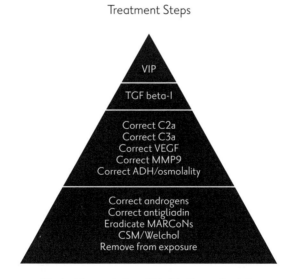

Used with permission of Ritchie Shoemaker MD

(IEP) is strongly recommended to assist in evaluation and remediation.[30] The affected person should not occupy the affected building during remediation. Repeat testing, either with ERMI or HERTSMI-2 (Health Effects Roster of Type Specific Formers of Mycotoxins and Inflammagens, see www.mycometrics.com or www.envirobiomics.com) is required before re-entering the affected building. Inflammagens are chemicals that trigger an inflammatory response in the body.

2. Removal of biotoxins: If you have CIRS-WDB, you *do not* have mold growing in your body. Instead, you have toxins from mold exposure. You *do not* need antifungal medications to treat this illness.[31] Cholestyramine (CSM) is a drug that is approved for lowering cholesterol and is being used off label in this treatment application (which means it does not have FDA approval to treat this condition). CSM has a positive charge and structure that attracts the negatively charged biotoxins present in the bile. The biotoxins are irreversibly bound and eliminated in the stool. CSM is not absorbed; however, it does have side effects of constipation, gas, and bloating. The dose is 4 grams in 6 oz of water followed by another 6 oz of water, 4 times daily, 30 minutes before meals. It can bind to prescription meds and supplements, which should be taken one hour prior to CSM or two hours after. Constipation must be avoided. Dietary

---

[30] Berndtson, K., et al., "Medically sound remediation of water damaged buildings in cases of CIRS," *Surviving* Mold, January 2016, https://www.survivingmold.com/docs/MEDICAL_CONSENSUS_1_19_2016_INDOOR_AIR_KB_FINAL.pdf.

[31] Shoemaker, R.C., House, D., Ryan, J.C., "Structural brain abnormalities in patients with inflammatory illness acquired following exposure to water damaged buildings: A volumetric MRI study using NeuroQuant," *Neurotoxicology* 45 (September 2014): 18–26, https://www.ncbi.nlm.nih.gov/pubmed/24946038.

fibre, magnesium, and other bowel stimulants may be required to prevent constipation. An alternative treatment is a prescription drug, Welchol (625 mg and dosed 2 tablets three times daily with meals). This drug is also FDA approved to treat elevated cholesterol. Welchol is only 25 percent as effective as CSM as a binder; however, it causes fewer GI side effects. It is also much more expensive. Some people become ill with binders. This is likely the result of their mobilization of more cytokines, especially MMP-9. Side effects can be reduced with high-dose (3-4 grams) omega-3 supplementation daily starting 1 week before starting CSM. Treatment with binders is continued until VCS test results are normal, symptoms are the same as controls, and lab results have normalized. A low-amylose diet is helpful in reducing insulin levels, reducing inflammation, and assisting in weight loss.[32] This diet is recommended along with CSM.

3. Eradication of MARCoNS: If MARCoNS testing by API staph swab is positive, it needs to be treated after one month of treatment with CSM. Treatment consists compounded nasal spray containing 25 ppm colloidal silver/EDTA 0.5% with mucolox, 2 sprays to each nostril tid for 30 days. The treatment for MARCoNS previously used BEG nasal spray, however increasing lack of response to treatment has been seen and is attributed to previous use of antifungals. Repeat culture needs to be done post treatment. If the culture remains positive, other family members, cats or dogs may be the source of re-infection.

---

[32] Maier, K., "The No-Amylose Diet," *Livestrong.com*, August 2013, http://www.livestrong.com/article/335261-the-no-amylose-diet/#ixzz18n8hXyTi/.

4. A gluten-free diet should be followed if gluten antibodies are present. This diet should be followed for a minimum of three months. Retesting should be done, and if antibodies are still positive, the likelihood of celiac disease needs to be considered. Eliminating gluten also reduces amylose in your diet. Many people are gluten sensitive as a result of leaky gut, and most feel better eliminating gluten even if testing is negative. A no-risk trial is worth it.

   It is important to allow healing to occur on many levels. The food we eat provides information to our cells that can be good or bad depending on our choices. Avoiding toxic exposure reduces the overall toxic burden in the body. Eat organic food whenever possible. Pay attention to what you eat, the air you breathe, and what you put on your skin.

5. Correction of hormone levels: This is done carefully with the addition of DHEA. Estrogen and DHEA-S levels need to be monitored while on treatment. DHEA will be discontinued when levels return to normal. DHEA is a hormone that is converted to testosterone. Less conversion to estrogen occurs with DHEA than with testosterone supplementation. If testosterone is given directly, it can be converted to estrogen, worsening the imbalance in men and women. This imbalance will resolve once the underlying overstimulation of the immune system is corrected.

6. Correct ADH/osmolality: DDAVP is a prescription form of ADH and can be used cautiously 0.2 mg every other night for 2 weeks. This, again, is off-label use. Daily weights and monitoring blood pressure and for edema needs to be done while on treatment. ADH/osmolality and electrolyte levels need to be retested two weeks after starting treatment.

7. Correct elevated MMP-9: This involves reducing inflammation with a low-amylose diet and 3–4 grams of omega-3 daily for one month. If there is no improvement, Actos 45 mg daily for 10 days can be used. Actos reduces insulin resistance and inflammation. Its use has lost favor because of a black box warning by the FDA of developing bladder cancer with long-term use of over one year. As a result of these concerns, current treatment protocol involves the use of VIP nasal spray to correct MMP-9 elevation.

8. Correct VEGF: Treatment with a low-amylose diet and high-dose omega-3 supplementation should be continued if VEGF abnormalities persist. The final step in treatment with VIP nasal spray will also address this.

9. Correct elevated C3a: The underlying cause needs to be addressed first. If it is due to Lyme, this needs to be treated. Autoimmune diseases, such as lupus, also result in elevated C3a. After the underlying cause has been addressed, inflammation and C3a levels are reduced with high-dose (80 mg) statins. Pre-treatment with CoQ10 200 mg daily starting 10 days before the statin reduces the risk of side effects. Muscle pain, fatigue, and elevation of liver enzymes can occur with high-dose statins.

10. Correct elevated C4a with VIP nasal spray 50 mcg/0.1 ml: one spray in alternating nostrils 4 times daily for minimum duration of 4 months. When symptoms improve, and lab values normalize, dosage can be reduced to 50 mcg twice daily for 1 month. Before VIP can be used, the following requirements must be met: VCS testing must be normal, MARCoNS testing negative, lipase level normal and ERMI less than 2 or HERTSMI-2 less than or equal to 10. The first dose should be administered in the office and the patient

monitored with pre and post labs. If no adverse reaction occurs, lipase, C4a, TGF-beta-1, MMP-9, and any abnormal labs should be checked in 1 month. VIP needs to be discontinued if lipase elevates or abdominal pain or rash develops.

11. Correct elevated TGF-beta-1: Losartan (a drug to lower blood pressure) produces a degradation product that lowers TGF-beta. Dosage is 12.5 mg daily and increased to 25 mg twice a day if tolerated. If a person already has low blood pressure, it may not be tolerated, and VIP nasal spray, with the above directions and guidelines, can be substituted. Note that other blood pressure medications do not have the same effect as Losartan. There are anecdotal reports Bilberry 1000 mg three times daily can also result in lowering of TGF beta-1 and in view of excellent safety profile it is worth considering if losartan cannot be used due to concerns of hypotension.

12. Correct low VIP: If recovery has not yet occurred, VIP nasal spray should be continued with the above guidelines and dosage. VIP nasal spray has many beneficial effects. VIP downregulates cytokines, raises VEGF, CD4+ CD25++ T-regs, restores circadian rhythm (sleep), regulates auto-immunity, restores normal hormone levels by down-regulating aromatase, increases endorphins, improves exercise tolerance, and has been shown to normalize genomics. VIP can also help people with multiple chemical sensitivities by down-regulating olfactory-driven neurons.

Avoiding re-exposure is critical; however, sometimes it is unavoidable. People do not want to live in terror of travelling outside their "safe bubble." If re-exposure occurs, identifying the source is beneficial to prevent repeated exposure.

Retest VCS and lab markers and, if abnormal, retreat with CSM/Welchol. Continue up the pyramid until symptoms resolve and markers are back in the normal range. People who have had CIRS have a tendency to become "sicker quicker" upon re-exposure. Prevention is best.

CIRS is a very misunderstood disease at best and denied by many at worst. Thanks to the research and dedication of Dr. Shoemaker, who followed the evidence, there is now clinical validation supported by thousands of cases for the diagnosis and treatment of CIRS.

It is important to understand the pathway the biotoxin takes in our body, which results in a cascade of symptoms. This understanding provides the knowledge of how and why these treatment steps are taken to reverse the disease.

This diagnosis is not made easily. As outlined above, multiple criteria must be met. The diagnosis is then validated with numerous tests that analyze the effect of the biotoxin on multiple systems. Tests range from VCS testing; multiple lab tests, including determining genetic susceptibility; MRI volumetric imaging; and now Dr. Shoemaker is on the cutting edge with his genomic research. This will "personalize" diagnosis and treatment by understanding what the biotoxin is doing in your body at a cellular/genetic level.

This is an exciting frontier to be part of. For me, it provides an important piece to the puzzle of chronic illness.

26: Mental Health: ADHD, Depression, Anxiety, Schizophrenia, and Autism Spectrum Disorder

If you look around you in a large crowd in either Canada or the United States, you will find that at least ten percent of these people are on an antidepressant medication. If you look at a group of women in their forties and fifties, then one in four will be on antidepressants. Signs of clinical depression include malaise, inner agitation, fatigue, low libido, poor memory, irritability, sleep problems, persistent stress, and a general feeling of being flat, overwhelmed, and even trapped. Currently, 14 percent of Caucasian males are taking an anti-depressant medication. At this rate, by 2020, the diagnosis of depression will take over from heart disease as a major cause of disability worldwide.

Thirty to 40 years ago, we were told that depression was a chemical imbalance in the brain. This has never been proven. Any up-to-date psychiatrist would admit this is not the case. In reality, depression is inflammation of the brain. Hence, the fairly recent *Time* magazine article with the famous cover of the brain on fire. Almost all brain illnesses are actually excess inflammation. Most of the time, the triggering problem comes from an inflamed, irritable, and leaky gut. For years drug companies told us that their antidepressants (i.e., Zoloft, Prozac) were critical for depression recovery. Well, the emperor has no clothes, because these agents do not actually help. Yes, they make us feel different but not with their touted mechanism. In addition, we know that 70–80 percent of serotonin production in our body is produced in our gastrointestinal tract. Similarly, 50 percent of our dopamine production is also from the gut.

Current research has confirmed that depression is in the same category of excess inflammation as Parkinson's, MS, and Alzheimer's (Brogan 2017). If you give people drugs that raise their inflammatory cytokines, they get depressed almost immediately. An example is interferon, which is used in the treatment of MS and hepatitis C. In this chapter, you will learn of lab investigations that can show biological reasons for many mental health problems.

Our current diet is also pro-inflammatory. This is especially the case if you eat the SAD (Standard American Diet), which is the typical Western diet. This diet is high in refined carbohydrates and trans fats and low in fruits and vegetables. This can be measured to some degree by measuring C-reactive protein. Elevated C-reactive protein, a known cardiac risk factor, is a lab measurement that confirms an increase in the body's inflammation. A lot of research in the United Kingdom has recently determined that even modestly elevated C-reactive protein can double the risk of getting Alzheimer's disease. In addition, C-reactive protein elevation in ALS (Amyotrophic Lateral Sclerosis) also called Lou Gehrig's disease, signifies more rapid decline (Lunetta et al. 2017).

Another lab measurement, elevated blood sugar, is a signal of ongoing elevated inflammation. We have known for some time that a spike in blood sugar causes a spike in insulin, which causes a spike in inflammation. Type 2 diabetics are more at risk for Alzheimer's and mood disorders. The final laboratory measurements I would like to mention are serum homocysteine (reviewed elsewhere under supplements) and LPS or lipopolysaccharide. LPS is known to be a by-product of an unhealthy gastrointestinal tract and is a dramatic trigger of more inflammation throughout the body in the presence of a leaky gut.

Once again, we are reminded that a leaky gut and a leaky blood-brain barrier usually predispose us to ADHD, depression, schizophrenia, autism spectrum disorder, and eventually dementia. Evidence continues to mount that anything that negatively impacts our gut microbiome (e.g., bacteria, fungi, parasites, and viruses) does the same thing to our brain and mental health. This includes drugs like antibiotics, corticosteroids, and chemotherapy, including monoclonal drugs like Humera.

However, there is also a bright side. If we change our diet to reduce the problem foods, then our gut can begin to recover (Kaplan 2015). In addition, we can add probiotics, the friendly bacteria, and prebiotics, the food for the friendly, useful bacteria within our gastrointestinal tract. My favourite supplements are vitamin D and fish oils. Other supplements that have been useful include the Chinese herbs berberine and goldenseal and more regular supplements, such as curcumin, green tea extracts, probiotics, prebiotics, and fermented foods. Sorry, beer, wine, and spirits do not count! You can also see improved mood with single or broad-spectrum micronutrients (Popper 2014).

An overstressed body and brain also damages the gut lining and your gut microbiome. Elevated serum cortisol can alter the mixture of bacteria within the gut and worsen leaky gut. The probiotic Bifidobacterium infantis is particularly useful in reversing the downside of this excess stress. Bimuno is a prebiotic that enhances the growth of our own Bifidus. This is even better than a Bifidus probiotic, because it enhances our own strains, which are more "wild" and likely to stay attached to our gut lining. In addition, cortisol levels are tied to our circadian rhythm. This explains why insomnia is a frequent component of mood disorders, including depression. Gut bacteria can stimulate some cytokines, such as TNF-alpha and some interleukins. When these cytokines, produced in appropriate amounts and times, are combined with the optimal cortisol, they induce a deep, non-REM sleep. This sleep is the most restorative of any sleep. Dr. David Perlmutter, a neurologist, states in his book, *Brain Maker*, "balance the gut, break through the insomnia" (Perlmutter 2015).

Now that you understand the link between gut health and depression and mental health, I have a simple suggestion. Virtually every discussion point about depression can be applied to anxiety problems. Of course, depression and anxiety go hand in hand with some people. Certainly, they are related psychologically. In addition, they share many symptoms, such as abdominal pain, nausea, diarrhea, constipation, bloating, and even headache.

Lab Investigations

If you need objective data toward confirming that your anxiety, depression, schizophrenia, or autism spectrum disorder are related to your gut issues, this can be measured. I speak of the Organic Acid Test (OAT) available at Great Plains Laboratory (GPL). The early OAT was developed by William Shaw, PhD, at the Centers for Disease Control (CDC). He has supervised large departments of endocrinology, nutritional biochemistry, toxicology, and immunology. After six years within CDC, he started the Great Plains Lab. Dr. Shaw has written multiple books and sponsored eight annual conferences on Integrative

Medicine for Mental Health (IMMH). These are fantastic conferences with current and leading-edge information. IMMH supports a whole-body approach to mental health disorders. These meetings educate practitioners about how to help their patients regain mental wellness through the use of individualized metabolic testing, nutritional therapies, and dietary interventions. Relevant lab analysis is used to treat underlying biomedical issues, which may include nutritional deficiencies, food allergies, infections, toxicities, and genetic disorders

Dr. Shaw did his PhD in biochemistry and human physiology. He is board certified by the American Board of Clinical Chemistry in the fields of clinical chemistry and toxicology. Dr. Shaw is a dedicated, altruistic, and brilliant individual who has gathered a superb team around him at GPL. In addition, they conduct training seminars around the world to advance and spread their wisdom and resources. Finally, they have a nutritional supplement company with many needed, but hard-to-locate supplements. This company is run by the knowledgeable Lori Knowles-Jimenez and her team at New Beginnings Nutritionals in Lenexa, KS. See www.nbnus.net, where I access lithium orotate for many clients.

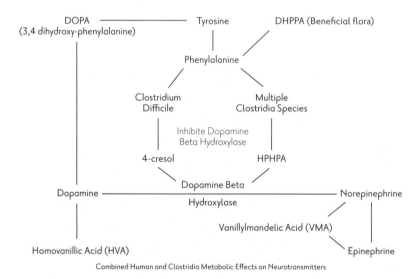

Combined Human and Clostridia Metabolic Effects on Neurotransmitters

The OAT is a simple urine test that provides a great deal of information. First, it reveals dysbiosis, overgrowth of yeast, or Clostridium difficile or other Clostridium bacteria strains. In addition, the OAT can measure the breakdown products of tryptophan and serotonin. See the above flow diagram from the OAT brochure of GPL. These measurements are helpful in understanding the body's levels of these proteins. Tryptophan is the key precursor to serotonin. On occasion, most of the tryptophan is broken down into kynurenine by enzymes, primarily in the gastrointestinal tract. This occurs when a particular group of bacteria is in excess of normal. When this occurs, the OAT reveals high levels of kynurenine, which corresponds to low tryptophan levels. One probiotic, Bifidobacterium infantis, has been shown to interfere with the breakdown of tryptophan into kynurenine. Thus, this probiotic has also been shown to lower kynurenine as well as calm the stress response. Further interventions are possible with the excellent advice that comes with most of the test results. Many of these are based on the urine results of HPAHA and 4-p-cresol. Treatment of abnormality in these can dramatically improve neurobehavioral function in both schizophrenia and autism patients. Initial treatment beyond diet control is use of either antibiotic vancomycin or metronidazole. The pulsing of these agents permits longer use, which assists in reduction of many strains of clostridia and their spores. These spores can create a flare after antibiotics are completed, as these spores are quite resistant to antibiotics until they come out of the spore phase.

Psychosis story with a happy ending:

I want to tell you a story of a young man with an initial diagnosis of psychosis and possible schizophrenia. This story has a happy ending. WR is a 25 year old young man who saw me first in 2018. He had recently been missing for two days and ended up being picked up by the police and legally committed to a mental hospital. He said everything was about electrical waves and music waves. He stated to me that he was very dialled in to the north-south compass and the axis has swung 60 degrees from true north. He was creating with his right and left to control chaos.

According to both parents, he was smashing the home bathroom with a hammer the evening before I saw him. He was temporarily settled some with an anti-psychotic drug injection (this calms dopamine excess). He was also being given pure CBD cannabis. At no time had he taken THC cannabis.

He was then tested with the organic acid test (OAT test) of his urine at Great Plains Laboratory. His results revealed that he had five times the upper normal level of HPHPA. This compound is produced when there is an overgrowth of particular Clostridium strains. It impacts the body by reducing its ability to change dopamine to norepinephrine. The consequences are dopamine excess behaviour which can include delusions and even violence.

When I saw him, he had delusional thoughts as mentioned above and was intermittently in a near catatonic state. Once I had received the lab results, I started him on antibiotics which included metronidazole and vancomycin. Within two weeks, when I saw him again, he was a changed man. He was no longer in a near catatonic state, had considerable insight about himself, was no longer delusional, and had a normal sparkle back in his eyes. His parents went from frightened and devastated to relieved and overjoyed. They felt they had their son back. His mother asked me to include the concept in this book "that you should never lose hope and keep looking for new therapies, even though your general practitioner and psychiatrist may not have anything more to offer other than regular drug therapy."

GPL has a host of other lab investigations that specialize in the diagnosis and treatment of mental health disorders, mitochondrial disorders, neurological diseases, chronic health issues, and immune diseases. Therefore, the next time your clinician says nothing more can be done other than medication, look to the references in the literature and books by excellent authors like Kelly Brogan (2017), James Greenblatt (2016), Kurt Woeller (2012, 2016), David Perlmutter (2016), and William Shaw (2010).

To help your understanding, I will now tell you about a case history. Elizabeth was a 53-year-old woman who came to see me for problems with depression. She had been on an antidepressant medication for fifteen years and was moderately obese despite her efforts at exercise. Her diagnosis of depression had been confirmed by a psychiatrist who had added a further medication with minimal improvement.

Elizabeth was born by C-section and was not breastfed. She had repeated ear infections as a child, which were treated by antibiotics. As a young teen, she had repeated urinary tract infections, also treated with antibiotics. These recurrent infections resolved after ureter urologic surgery. She also tended to bloat after eating with frequent constipation. Her laboratory studies revealed low vitamin D, elevated C-reactive protein, slightly elevated TSH at 3.5, and a hemoglobin of A1c of 6.1. Follow-up assessment revealed elevated thyroid antibodies consistent with a diagnosis of Hashimoto's thyroiditis. I recommended that she be completely gluten-free for three months and that she read *Brain Maker* by Dr. David Perlmutter and/or *Wheat Belly* by Dr. William Davis. I also suggested many of her troubles were gut triggered. Disturbance of her gut health may have started in relative sequence with her birth by caesarean, no breastfeeding, and multiple antibiotics.

As these events progressed, the lining of the gastrointestinal tract became swollen and inflamed with subsequent leaky gut. This helped to precipitate her probable gluten sensitivity, weight gain, somewhat elevated blood sugar, and probably the onset of Hashimoto's thyroiditis. Then I had her start supplements such, as vitamin D (4000 IU per day), fish oil (3,000 mg of EPA plus DHA in combination), and 100 billion units of a 10- or 12-strain probiotic. I also prescribed Armor (desiccated natural thyroid hormone) 30 mg each morning.

Elizabeth saw me two months later and was a vibrant and much happier woman. She was free of constipation, had lost 15 pounds, and was four inches smaller around her middle. Of her own accord, she had been off all her antidepressants for four weeks. Her brain was clear, work was enjoyable once again, and sleep had improved. Her depression had disappeared. Finally, she thought she had her life back under control and was very grateful for that.

Cannabis

This is another choice. It is well reviewed by Walsh (2017) and Hill (2015). Other articles include schizophrenia (Foti 2010). Once again, CBD is the best choice.

Section Six
Interventions

27: Integrative Medicine/ Functional Medicine and Evidence-Based Medicine

Integrative Medicine is the term most accepted by most regular MDs to denote a broad-based approach to health care. Admittedly, it is not accepted by all physicians, but an increasing number of laypeople are interested in this wider approach to health recovery. Before Integrative Medicine, the term was Complementary and Alternative Medicine. I soon learned that most physicians felt that there was no alternative to themselves. Complementary and Alternative Medicine was a description in the early 1990s. Largely due to the efforts of Dr. Andrew Weil at the University of Arizona, the term Integrative Medicine has gained credibility. I feel very fortunate to have studied under Dr. Andrew Weil from 2006 to 2008. I was in the fifth class of some eighty MDs, DOs (Doctor of Osteopathy) and a few nurse practitioners. Our class was a broad spectrum of family practitioners, pediatricians, oncologists, radiation oncologists, internal medicine specialists, with a few surgeons, anesthesiologists and psychiatrists. While most of the program was done online, we met together for a week in Tucson three different times. We all found it very exciting to interact with others of a similar mindset.

Since then, the Integrative Medicine program at the University of Arizona has had several thousand graduates who are starting to make a significant difference in many medical schools, particularly in the United States and Canada. This is exciting to see. One half of the current family medicine residents in training at a nearby medical school are also registered in the University of Arizona Integrative Medicine program this year. That is a huge leap forward compared with 10 years ago, when the same medical school showed little or no interest in my integrative medicine skills.

A parallel program that has developed is Functional Medicine, which was initiated by Dr. Jeff Bland and others. This program is open to the same students as listed previously but also includes naturopathic doctors, osteopaths, chiropractors, registered dietitians, and pharmacists. This inclusiveness, I believe, has been a great boon to the interaction of these professions, but I suspect it has somewhat reduced acceptance by the medical schools and their academic institutions. Both Functional Medicine and Integrative Medicine have a graduate exam. However, at this point, Integrative Medicine is the only one with a recognized specialty board exam in the United States. To me, Functional Medicine emphasizes the underlying trigger or problem. It peels away the layers to determine what triggered the problem in the first place. I believe both programs are important and hope that one day there will be an open acceptance of both pathways by regular medicine. However, I will not hold my breath!

As I write this chapter, we are building an integrative health society in our community to encompass most of the treatment modalities that I endorse in this book. This facility will be primarily one site with adjunct campuses but all within a ten-kilometre radius. Practitioners will include physicians, naturopaths, physiotherapists, nutritionists, kinesiologists, and the technical support personnel for hyperbaric oxygen medicine (HBOT), photobiomodulation (PBMT), gut flora transplant (GFT) therapists (also called FMT), and vibrational exercise machines. Our goal is to become a destination for recovery with multiple modalities that can occur simultaneously over four weeks. In many cases, this will be a jump start toward optimal recovery and wellness. We also hope to have access to clinicians experienced in Dr. Ritchie Shoemaker's CIRS (chronic inflammation reaction syndrome) treatment program. This program can often help people suffering from chronic mould, chronic Lyme disease, and early Alzheimer's disease, as per Dr. Dale Bredesen, MD, who recently wrote the excellent book, *The End of Alzheimer's* (Bredesen 2017). At present, we would refer to respected online people, such as Dr. Karen Johnson, who contributed evidence-based medicine in this chapter as well as the chapter on CIRS.

Many patients will choose one or more of the above modalities in their journey to regain full or optimal health. Only a few patients will slog slowly away on the journey to wellness. Most will become discouraged. However, if many of these people can achieve a boost or jumpstart in the recovery process, more will succeed. Most of these clients are exhausted physically, mentally and emotionally by the time they have experienced most of what regular medicine specialists have to offer. Many of these people have low energy initially due to mitochondrial dysfunction, leaky gut, or unrecognized brain injury. Unfortunately, our current system relies on piecemeal efforts from a series of specialists annually. I have nicknamed this the "specialist merry-go-round." It is exhausting and demoralizing and is rarely successful in these complex cases.

Our new Genoa Integrative Health and Wellness Centre is designed to accommodate people seeking multiple recovery components. See www.genoalasertherapy.com. The goal is to permit individuals to access all of these modalities simultaneously over a period of one month. This will permit a tremendous synergy between the modalities and increase the possibility of success. At present, two of these modalities are available in parts of the world. One of these is the Better Being Hospital in Bangkok, initiated by Dr. Torsak (www. betterbeingthailand.com). I was fortunate to be able to visit his facility in early 2018. The recently established Cleveland Clinic Integrative Medicine Clinic under Dr. Mark Hyman is another such facility. I applaud their efforts and am pleased to see them being successful. In some ways, I see ours as a Canadian option with slightly different approaches and expertise. I don't know of any place where all of these relatively new interventions are possible.

I hope that the other chapters in this book help you understand the complex chronic health problems that can often be solved with an Integrative/Functional Medicine approach. For example, Dr. Dale Bredesen's success with Alzheimer's and Dr. Ritchie Shoemaker's success with mold toxicity and chronic Lyme are superb examples of the possibilities. Similarly, I believe that the new MS is now mostly treatable or at least preventable from progression in the majority of cases. It's time that individuals stand up to be counted and look at new solutions of their volition instead of waiting one or two generations for change to occur. Even though the literature supports these new changes, acceptance into regular practice will take at least twenty years. Most of us are unable or unwilling to wait that long. It is up to sick individuals, with the assistance of their family or friends, to consider new ways of healing the body.

Whenever one talks of new or different treatment or investigation models, the term "evidence-based medicine" is brought up to squelch them. However, I refer you to a superb book, *Tarnished Gold: The Sickness of Evidence-based Medicine* by Steve Hickey, PhD, and Hilary Roberts, PhD. I was

fortunate to hear Dr. Hickey speak at an orthomolecular conference and love his book (Hickey 2011).

Below is an essay by a colleague and classmate of mine,
Karen D. Johnson, republished with her permission, which
sums up my thoughts succinctly.

What Is Evidence-Based Medicine?

Karen D. Johnson, MD

Evidence-based medicine (EBM) is a philosophy of medical
practice and education, originally promoted in the 1970s by
David Sacket and Brian Ames to instruct clinicians on how
to best use clinical journals. The term EBM first appeared
in print in 1991, in the ACP Journal Club, and was coined by
Gordon Guyatt.[33]

There are various, overlapping, established definitions to
the seemingly innocent question, "What's EBM?" They range
from short, "EBM is the integration of best research evidence with clinical expertise and patient values"[34] or "EBM is
nothing more than a process of life-long, self-directed learning in which caring for patients creates the need for clinically
important information about diagnosis, prognosis, therapy,
and other clinical and health care issues,"[35] to long:

---

[33] "Evidence-based medicine," ACP Journal Club. 1991 March–April; 114: A16.
doi:10.7326/ACPJC-1991- 114-2-A16.

[34] Sackett, D.L., et al., *Evidence Based Medicine: How to Practice and Teach
EBM* Edinburgh: Churchill Livingstone, 2010.

[35] Evidence Based Medicine Working Group, "Evidence-based medicine.
A new approach to teaching the practice of medicine," *JAMA* 268 (1992):
2420–2425.

Evidence-based medicine (EBM) is the conscientious, explicit, judicious and reasonable use of modern, best evidence in making decisions about the care of individual patients. EBM integrates clinical experience and patient values with the best available research information. It is a movement which aims to increase the use of high-quality clinical research in clinical decision making. EBM requires new skills of the clinician, including efficient literature-searching, and the application of formal rules of evidence in evaluating the clinical literature. The practice of evidence-based medicine is a process of lifelong, self-directed, problem-based learning in which caring for one's patients creates the need for clinically important information about diagnosis, prognosis, therapy and other clinical and health care issues. It is not "cookbook" with recipes, but its good application brings cost-effective and better health care. The key difference between evidence-based medicine and traditional medicine is not that EBM considers the evidence while the latter does not. Both take evidence into account; however, EBM demands better evidence than has traditionally been used. One of the greatest achievements of evidence-based medicine has been the development of systematic reviews and meta-analyses, methods by which researchers identify multiple studies on a topic, separate the best ones and then critically analyse them to come up with a summary of the best available evidence. The EBM-oriented clinicians of tomorrow have three tasks: a) to use evidence summaries in clinical practice; b) to help develop and update selected systematic reviews or evidence-based guidelines in their area of expertise; and c) to enrol patients in studies of treatment, diagnosis and prognosis on which medical practice is based.[36]

The EBM process commonly involves:
1. Developing focused questions
2. Efficiently determining the best evidence to answer the questions
3. Critically appraising the evidence for validity and usefulness
4. Clinical practice application
5. Evaluating evidence performance in clinical application

EBM was created as a response to the information overload generated from the explosion of technological databases, such as MEDLINE. There were simply not enough hours in the day to read all the applicable research in various disciplines, so EBM developed algorithms for using search engines in the literature, such as adding methodology terms and clinical filters along with subject terms to optimize retrieval. However, this information overload still haunts medicine, given the very slow rate of the adoption of new clinical research, often taking an average of seventeen years for new evidence-based findings to reach clinical practice.[37]

Returning to the five steps in the EBM process:
1. Asking the right question is the first step. The PICO model for clinical questions is commonly employed, which asks the following: what is the kind of Patient,

---

36   "Evidence Based Medicine - New Approaches and Challenges," *Acta Informatica Medica* 16 no. 4 (2008): 219–225. Published online Dec. 2008 doi: 10.5455/aim.2008.16.219-225.

37   Balas, E.A., Boren S.A., "Managing clinical knowledge for health care improvement"; "Managing clinical knowledge for health care improvement," in Bemmel J., McCray A.T., editors. *Yearbook of Medical Informatics 2000: Patient-Centered Systems.* Stuttgart, Germany: Schattauer Verlagsgesellschaft mbH, 2000: 65–70J.

population or problem? What is the main Intervention or prognostic factor? What Compares with the intervention? And what is the desired Outcome?

2. "Best" evidence is arguably the biggest problem. EBM searches the evidence depending on the type of question being asked, whether it's therapy, diagnosis, prognosis, aetiology/harm, prevention, or quality improvement.

   EBM then tries to qualify the evidence into five decreasingly useful levels: Level 1, randomized controlled trials (deemed the best). Level 2a, evidence from cohort or case-control analytic studies. Level 2b, observational evidence from multiple time series. Level 3, the consensus of professional authoritarian opinions. And Level 4, anecdotal experience (obviously not the most useful).

3. Appraising evidence has many handicaps: the perfect evidence may not be available to answer your question, or the duration of a study may be inadequate, but the biggest problems are the biases of many publications favouring big pharma or special interest groups. This is so bad that

[a]s EBM became more influential, it was also hijacked to serve agendas different from what it originally aimed for. Influential randomised trials are largely done by and for the benefit of the industry. Meta-analyses and guidelines have become a factory, mostly also serving vested interests. National and federal research funds are funnelled almost exclusively to research with little relevance to health outcomes. We have supported the growth of principal investigators who excel primarily as managers absorbing more money. Diagnosis and prognosis research and efforts to individualise

treatment have fueled recurrent spurious promises. Risk factor epidemiology has excelled in salami-sliced data-dredged articles with gift authorship and has become adept at dictating policy from spurious evidence.[38]

A more fundamental problem with evidence is exposed in the ACTA definition of EBM mentioned earlier in the phrase: "[T]he application of formal rules of evidence . . ." This dogmatically relies on the scientism of the scientific method. Scientism is the claim that the scientific method allows humanity to gain privileged insight into the structural processes of nature. Unfortunately, the notions that scientific evidence corresponds to reality and that the scientific method is the only way to investigate nature have both been refuted.[39] The scientific method is the best tool in the toolbox, but it's not the only tool. Humans somehow progressed, fumbling around without the scientific method before Galileo, and many died trying.

4. Applying findings to one's clinical practice may be easy or difficult. EBM was not intended to be a cookbook, though there are critics that claim EBM may have cookbook dangers.[40] Clinicians may lazily use EBM guidelines to the patient's detriment. Clinicians can become complacent in their clinical approach and feel that if they follow the EBM guidelines they're golden.

---

[38] Ioannidis, P., MD, DSc, *Journal of Clinical Epidemiology* vol. 73 (May 2016): 82–86.

[39] For more on the pitfalls of the scientific method, I refer you to the classic, *Science in a Free Society* by physicist/philosopher Paul Feyerabend (London: Verso Books, 1978).

[40] "Evidence-Based Medicine or Cookbook Medicine? Addressing Concerns over the Standardization of Care," *Sociology Compass* 8 no. 6 (June 2014): 823–836, doi: 10.1111/soc4.12184.

Of course, this fails to adhere to integrating clinical expertise which is part of EBM.

In some clinical environments, practitioners may have problems with their peers, insurance companies, or the hospital administration for deviating from their standard of care. Insurers endorse old recommendations that have proven to be unnecessary and even harmful. Insurers and government regulators fall behind the evidence, perpetuating out-of-date knowledge.

5. Evaluating the performance of your evidence is commonly done with pre-and post-treatment test results. It may be important to assess at frequent intervals as to whether or not any of the four steps discussed above need improvement.

EBM is a useful reminder that physicians must pay attention to cutting-edge research and challenge the status quo. It's also convenient that there are institutions, like the Centre for Evidence-Based Medicine (University of Oxford) that assist one's continuing education along these lines. Yet in standardizing and teaching a definitive EBM paradigm, these institutions ironically run the risk of turning EBM into a status quo of its own.

28: Other Important Health Care Practices: Chiropractic Care, Naturopathy, Massage Therapy, and Homeopathy

Optimal health is like happiness—it is an individual journey that starts within. Unfortunately, conventional medicine has wrapped itself up in "standards of practice," "recipes," or "cookbooks" of care solutions, making individual care solutions by your physician at risk of investigation or even loss of his or her license. This is a powerful hammer used by licensing bodies and even hospitals. We have become so focused on protecting patients from the inevitable 1-3 percent of unreliable practitioners that all creativity of new modes of care is virtually eliminated. Until recently, this put at risk physicians interested in Complementary and Alternative Medicine, Integrative Medicine, or Functional Medicine. Gradually, this is shifting, but a price has been exacted against the early pioneers.

NUCCA and Chiropractic Treatment

Patients are thinking individuals too, and many have realized that their physician may not offer them all solutions. Similarly, many physicians have made light of any group not under their control. My parents figured this out early and used chiropractors for their neck and back pain problems. Hence, in my teens, when I had back pain, I saw a chiropractor for relief of a football injury. Then, during medical school, I knew an orthopedic surgeon who was first a chiropractor. He was praised by the much-published and experienced orthopedic surgeon Dr. Kirkaldy-Willis, head of the Department of Orthopedics. This was a rare event in Canada at that time.

Meanwhile, the "evidence-based" critique of chiropractors persists with its own rules. "Prescribed pubmed journals" do not include any of the quality journals of chiropractic medicine. This becomes a self-fulfilling prophecy, as regular medicine states there is no evidence of chiropractic value, but they will not credit valuable journals outside their own pubmed groups.

Dr. Ralph Gregory was a visionary and gifted chiropractic healer. His lifetime work was the relationship between the upper cervical spine (neck) and its profound influence on the function of the brain and spinal cord. Dr. Gregory developed a healing technique now known as NUCCA (National Upper Cervical Chiropractic Association). In 1941, Dr. Gregory teamed up with Dr. John Francis Grostic, and the development of the NUCCA upper cervical procedure began. Together, they developed a more biomechanically accurate system of upper cervical subluxation correction. The majority of the subluxation (misalignment) occurs at the atlas, which is C-1, the highest vertebrae on which the skull sits. The NUCCA mission statement includes "Maximizing the human potential associated with the reduction (optimal placement) of the Atlas Subluxation Complex (ASC)."

NUCCA has been studied as a treatment for migraine headaches. I am a believer in NUCCA, because it helped my migraines. In my health journey, I met Dr. Charles Woodfield, Dr. Gordon Hasick, and Dr. Shawn Thomas, all NUCCA practitioners. Dr. Woodfield is a significant researcher and is retired from clinical practice. Dr. Hasick is very experienced and is one of the main trainers of other NUCCA practitioners. NUCCA practitioners are a specialized group of chiropractors who, with gentle manipulation, optimize the alignment of C-1 and C-2. This permits optimal alignment of the entire spine and body. Dr. Thomas is an experienced NUCCA chiropractor who I see every six weeks in follow-up.

Published studies have confirmed NUCCA can lower elevated blood pressure by 10-15 percent and maintain this by follow-up treatment every eight to twelve weeks. If this works, I prefer it over a lifetime of medication.

I would like to highlight a study done in Calgary recently. The study was done by an experienced neuro-imaging radiologist headache neurologist, Dr. Werner Becker, and NUCCA chiropractors, including Dr. Gordon Hasick's study (Woodfield 2015). Eleven patients with long-term headaches resistant to all regular treatments and medications for migraine were studied. The study included comprehensive MRIs and X-rays, and NUCCA treatment was performed in a double-blind crossover design. The outcome was remarkable in that there was a reduced number of headache days. In five out of eleven patients, an increase in brain compliance was confirmed by MRI following atlas vertebrae realignment.

I have met both NUCCA practitioners and the neurologist involved in the study. The neurologist and I were both speaking at a chronic pain conference in Alberta just after the study was published. Dr. Becker confided to me that he had no idea how he was going to be able to stand up in front of an audience of neurologists to talk about the study's success. I understood. Almost all neurologists degrade chiropractors, stating that neck manipulation triggers strokes. This is utter nonsense but is a tenaciously held belief based on extremely rare case report data. The less than 1 in 10,000 incidences of stroke with manipulation is likely to be a stroke already in progress at the time of chiropractic manipulation. Counter this with the 1 percent risk of stroke as an acceptable risk with carotid or coronary (heart) angiography.

My own NUCCA practitioners, Dr. Hasick and Dr. Thomas, have both helped control my migraines. I believe they have also minimized my MS progression for over six years. I am very grateful and suggest NUCCA to most of my migraine, TBI, and MS patients. I can only encourage you to optimize your upper cervical spine, including atlas alignment via NUCCA. If you have sustained a concussion, a significant blow to the head, or whiplash injury, then misalignment has occurred. Your recovery from headaches, neck and back pain, and hypertension are likely all to benefit from NUCCA intervention. See www.nucca.org for a list of qualified NUCCA practitioners near you.

A useful adjunct to NUCCA is craniosacral therapy (CST). My NUCCA doctors suggested this to me. My wife and I see a gifted physiotherapist who trained in CST over twenty years ago. CST is gentle but significant manipulation of sacral, spinal, and cranial sutures (interconnections between bones). This enhances cerebrospinal fluid flow and blood flow through the body and is synergistic with NUCCA therapy. I realize this is counter-intuitive to the dogma that once skull sutures fuse, there is not further mobility. I suggest this dogma is an oversimplification for lazy, non-thinking medical students. If you want further objective information about NUCCA, look at Mandolesi's X-ray assessment of C1-C2 misalignment parameters in MS and CCSVI patients (Mandolesi 2015).

Massage Therapy

Massage therapy is another useful adjunct to whole-body wellness. Not only does this technique optimize muscle, ligament, and tendon health, it also helps fascia. The fascia exists throughout the musculoskeletal system. It holds us together and helps energy flow smoothly. When this flow is hampered by surgical or traumatic injury, all body components suffer.

From two years post diagnosis with MS until now, a period of some twenty years, I have had massage therapy every week or two. This has been incredibly helpful in restoring my walking mobility. We underestimate the body's interconnectedness at our peril. Fortunately, almost everyone has access to this modality, so use it. Similarly, yoga, chi gong, and Tai Chi are also about body restoration and maintenance. These can also be exceedingly helpful. Although I have not used these as much as the other treatments, they are still on my to-do list. We must determine our individual path. Simply, remember that many pieces of the puzzle exist, and there are no silver bullets. I suggest you use the resources available with a variety of modalities until you reach a successful outcome.

Naturopathic Medicine

Naturopathic medicine is a distinct primary health care system that blends modern scientific knowledge with traditional and natural forms of medicine. It includes diagnosis, treatment, and prevention using botanical medicine, clinical nutrition, hydrotherapy, homeopathy, traditional Chinese medicine, acupuncture, lifestyle counselling, health promotion, and disease prevention. I have spoken at naturopathic conferences and find them excellent colleagues, well versed in their field. I have included three chapters by Dr. Teri Jaklin, ND in this book because of her expertise.

In addition, many naturopaths and chiropractors are studying Functional Medicine alongside medical doctors and osteopathic doctors. It is brilliant that we are working more together, and I hope the earlier silos of non-interaction continue to tumble. It behooves you to find a health care practitioner who works with you and educates you on how to optimize your health. Often this will include one or more of these alternative and complementary practitioners.

Homeopathy

In 2016, I completed a course in clinical homeopathy held over nine weekends in Vancouver, BC. I received my diploma in homeopathy through the Center for Education and Development of Clinical Homeopathy (CEDH) upon passing the exam. What is homeopathy? "Homeo" means the study of similar, and "pathy" means what one feels. This is based on the concept initially written by Hippocrates in 400 BC. He stated, "By similar things a disease is produced and through the application of the like, is cured." Most of the early work in modern-day homeopathy was done by German physician Dr. Christian Samuel Hahnemann

The Homeopathic Dilution Process

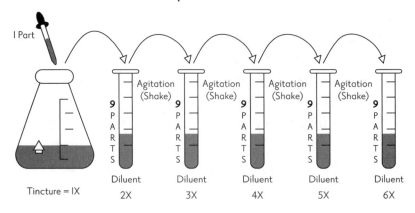

Process of attenuation (agutation) completed between diluents

(1755–1843). He stated that a substance capable of causing certain symptoms in healthy people was also capable of curing similar symptoms in sick people when given in highly diluted amounts. What are homeopathic medicines? They are ultra-diluted extracts of plants, minerals, and other substances of nature.

The highly diluted amount of homeopathic remedies can have a concentration approaching that of Avogadro's number, which is 6.02 to the twenty-third power. This has been one of the criticisms of homeopathy. Critics suggest that the amounts are so dilute, there cannot be any molecules left, and, therefore, nothing will work on the receptors in the body. This is where the lack of understanding or acceptance of things that are outside our regular purview become a problem. As an anesthesiologist, I was initially skeptical for the same reasons, as I was heavily trained in pharmacology. However, once carfentanil was developed in the 1980s, with the potency in the same range of Avogadro's number, I realized my skepticism was not really warranted and led me to study homeopathy.

The Center for Education and Development of Clinical Homeopathy (CEDH) was founded in 1972. Since then, it has trained more than 3,000 physicians in over 22 countries. Currently, in the United States, training courses are held in New York, Philadelphia, Fort Lauderdale, Chicago, San Francisco, Los Angeles, and Puerto Rico. In Canada, courses are held in Vancouver and Toronto. For information on training, go to www.cedhusa.org.

The World Health Organization (WHO) has cited homeopathy as one of the systems of traditional medicine that should be integrated worldwide with conventional medicine to provide adequate global health care. This is a traditional WHO medicine strategy that developed from 2000 to 2005. Currently, homeopathy is used by 300 million patients and 400,000 health care providers worldwide. Studies done in Europe reveal that two thirds of French physicians use some homeopathy in their practice. The major foci of homeopathy at present is on ear, nose, and throat, respiratory, and gynecologic illnesses. Homeopathy is also used as an adjunct in cancer chemotherapy and radiation therapy. This is mostly for control of side effects, permitting larger doses of chemotherapy, radiation, and prolonged intervention with standardized protocols.

My major mentor in homeopathy is Robert C. Dumont, MS, MD, who is a Pediatric Integrative Medicine specialist at the Raby Institute for Integrative Medicine at Northwestern University in Chicago. He recently gave a talk on homeopathy at the Canadian Neurovascular Health Society meeting in Ottawa in October 2016. The title of his talk was "Homeopathy: an untapped source for treatment of MS and other neurovascular disorders." I credit much of the information in my presentation to him and to my training in homeopathy at CEDH. Homeopathic medicine has been in use for more than 200 years and is practiced worldwide, especially in Europe and India. Many medical conditions, including chronic conditions, can be effectively treated or their symptoms ameliorated, by homeopathic medicine. These agents can be used alone or alongside conventional drugs. They have the advantage of being safe, non-toxic, and without adverse effects or drug interactions.

One of the interesting articles referenced by Dr. Dumont was "Homeopathy in Multiple Sclerosis." This was published in 2003 in *Complementary Therapeutic Nurse Midwifery* (Whitmarsh 2003). The article was written by T.E. Whitmarsh, who discussed the experience at the Glasgow Homeopathic Hospital. This hospital has approximately 100 admissions each year of people with MS. Of the different therapeutic modalities employed, they found the homeopathic approach provided the most benefit in MS. They felt this was because homeopathy is a whole-person approach and allows for complete individualization of treatment. Therefore, it is able to take into account many of the minutia of an individual's lifetime.

In his Integrative Medicine Clinic, Dr. Dumont routinely uses homeopathy in many of the disorders he treats. These include irritable bowel syndrome, cyclic vomiting syndrome, post-pertussis cough, gastric reflux, dysmenorrhea, chronic and recurrent sinusitis or otitis media, chronic recurrent upper and respiratory infections, chemo-induced nausea, osteoarthritis and rheumatoid arthritis, elimination of abdominal adhesions, chronic headaches, eczema and dermatitis, ADHD, and autism. My goal is to continue to learn more about homeopathy and use it for my family and my patients' health.

Homeopathic preparations are always dilutions done to varying degrees. The figure below illustrates this and how the dilutions go beyond Avogadro's number. In the United States, homeopathic medicine has been regulated by the FDA as a medicine since 1938. In Canada, homeopathic regulation comes under the Natural Health Products Directorate. Each homeopathic medicine has an identification number with the prefix HM (homeopathic medicine). Recently, the

Health Products Directorate changed its name to the Natural and Non-prescription Health Products Directorate. This name change is due to the expanded mandate given to it by Health Canada. Now it includes information on licensed natural health products, such as vitamin and mineral supplements, Chinese or Ayurvedic medicines, omega-3 and essential fatty acids, probiotics, and homeopathic medicines. Since the change in name and mandate, it also includes other items, such as toothpastes, antiperspirants, shampoos, facial products, and mouthwashes. You can verify a particular homeopathic product licensed in Canada by looking up its name and number on this database. The primary homeopathic company I use in Canada is Boiron, which is based in Montreal but has its international headquarters in France.

A similar identification method exists in Europe for homeopathic medicines. The European Committee for Homeopathy (ECH) represents all medical doctors with an additional qualification in homeopathy. The ECH is organized in forty associations in twenty-five European countries and has existed for seventy years. Its aim is to ensure high standards in the education, training, and practice of homeopathy. A good example of the scientific rigor and frequency of homeopathic practice is the recently published articles from a survey done in France (Grimaldi-Bensouda 2014, 2016). The EPI3 project followed 8,559 patients attending GP practices. The homeopathic patients studied used half as many painkillers in the form of NSAIDS and fewer drugs for sleep, anxiety, and depression.

Homeopathy is based on several principles. The first of these is the materia medica, which is the physicians' desk reference of substances. The second principle is the matching of the patient's clinical picture with the medicine or remedy. This includes signs and symptoms as well as mental or emotional components. The third principle is the use of ultra-molecular homeopathic solutions. The fourth principle is that the homeopathic medicine facilitates the body's own physiological reaction to healing itself. This is quite different from regular pharmacology, which, in most cases, only suppresses symptoms.

The safety of homeopathic medicines is incredible. They have no pharmacologic action and, thus, no adverse side effects. There are no drug interactions, and toxic overdosing is impossible. They are easy to take for children and adults, with application under the tongue. The dissolvable sugar pellets or drop containing tiny amounts of sugar can even be used pre- and post-surgery. The simplicity and safety of this approach is part of what drew me to homeopathy. I hope you can appreciate this as a new tool in your journey toward health. You can contact CEDH for a listing of clinical homeopathy practitioners in your area. Alternatively, you can look for homeopaths locally or by referral from one of your health care practitioners. I have no hesitation in confirming the safety of this approach. It may be a very useful choice to add to your recovery process.

In addition to many clinical trials, several hundred basic science studies confirm the biologic activity of homeopathic medicines. Homeopathy can affect gene expression. This alone is enough to help me understand how something so dilute and safe can still have a measurable impact on well-being. Historical comparisons between homeopathy and allopathic medicine have been done many times. One example is that homeopathy is considerably more successful in reducing death rates from cholera, typhoid, and scarlet fever. The death rates from these diseases were 50-88 percent lower in homeopathic hospitals than conventional hospitals. One further example is the terrible flu epidemic of 1918. The hospital mortality rate using homeopathy was 1-5 percent, while the mortality with allopathic medicine was 30 percent. Most of the research conducted on homeopathic medicines has been published in peer-reviewed journals and has shown positive clinical results. This is particularly noted in treatment of respiratory allergies, influenza, fibromyalgia, rheumatoid arthritis, childhood diarrhea, post-surgical abdominal surgery recovery, attention-deficit disorder, and in the reduction of the side effects of conventional cancer treatments.

I particularly like a quote by Peter Fisher, MD, who was recently deceased. I heard him speak at the CEDH International meeting in Chicago in June 2016. He said,

> The reason why people find [homeopathy] so challenging is that we are used to thinking about pharmacology in molecular terms. If you take homeopathic medicine to be analysed, a pharmacologist would say its water and ethanol and sugar, and that's true. But if you take a floppy disk to a chemist he will say it is ferric oxide and vinyl. The information is stored in physical form: the alignment of the dipoles of ferric oxide. We shouldn't write off homeopathy simply because the dose-response relationship is reversed. We just don't know enough about ultra-dilute solutions.

Peter Fisher was qualified in homeopathy and rheumatology and was physician to Her Majesty Queen Elizabeth II. He was also the clinical and research director of the Royal London Hospital for Integrated Medicine in London, UK.

I would like to focus on some of the homeopathic treatments of vascular conditions. I hope you will also read the chapter on the new MS, which I call microvascular syndrome. This concept is a parallel to the neurovascular effects of many brain illnesses or injuries. Hence, any advantage we can achieve using the safe effects of homeopathy can be a great assist.

Homeopathic treatments for arterial/vascular insufficiency include the following:

- Arnica montana: a vascular protector for capillaries and veins
- Hamamelis virginiana: effects the venous system, including the manifestations of venous inflammation
- Phosphorus: used in conditions linked to arteriosclerosis, prevention of strokes, and arteriography of the lower limbs
- Secale cornutum: used for arterial insufficiency, ischemia, skin trophic disorders, ischemic stroke, and brain vascular disorders

To decide which of the above to use, at what strengths, and how frequently, you will need the assistance of an experienced homeopathic physician. You will find one in your vicinity, if you take the time to look.

Where do we go from here? To use homeopathy optimally in conjunction with regular Western medicine, Dr. Dumont suggests we develop a system to recommend/prescribe appropriate homeopathic medicines. He wisely suggests that we develop algorithms and engage health care professionals trained in clinical homeopathy to properly prescribe and monitor responses. Ideally, we should develop a system to track responses to each specific treatment and include these on an online database, perhaps in conjunction with the CEDH. I hope that a number of health care professionals, attuned to homeopathy, will embark on this venture together.

29: Oxygen and My Personal Journey With MS

As noted previously, I was diagnosed with MS in August 1996, just before my 43 birthday. At that time, I was practicing anesthesiology in a small city in British Columbia, Canada. I had grown up on a small mixed farm in the Canadian prairies. After medical school, I did four years of family practice in a small town. There, I diagnosed three patients with MS which, at that time, was the average number diagnosed by a family medicine practitioner during a lifetime of practice.

In 1983, I started a five-year program in anesthesiology in Calgary. This included two years of laboratory research to study the pharmacology of how anesthetics work on the brain. Hence, this meant two years of learning a lot about the neurobiology of the brain and neuroscience. Following this, I took an academic position on a tenure track at the University of Saskatchewan. During this time, I spent another four years on brain research, including helping establish a centre of excellence for stroke research.

After this period, my family and I moved to a small city on Vancouver Island. This move was an effort to reduce my stress markers, which included frequent migraine headaches, borderline high blood pressure, intermittent periods of fatigue of undetermined origin, and a history of recurring depression treated with a tricyclic antidepressant. Everything improved for one year, but then I returned to my workaholic ways, and everything started to recur.

My health began to deteriorate rapidly in the summer of 1996. By the end of that summer, I was diagnosed with MS by Dr. D. Paty at the University of British Columbia. Dr. Paty wrote the chapter on MS diagnosis in a major textbook on MS (Burks 2000). In my case, Dr. Paty recommended six months off work. I continued to worsen, whereupon he suggested a further six months off. If an MS attack or event is longer than three months, it removes the possibility of it being relapsing-remitting MS. It is typically called either secondary-progressive or primary-progressive MS. The last two diagnoses are particularly ominous in that it is thought that no recovery is possible and that it is a downhill slide at varying speeds.

I was able to sustain some recovery and improvement of quality of life through changes in my diet and lifestyle. I talk about these in two earlier books, *Who is in Control of your Multiple Sclerosis?* (2005) and *Winning the Pain Game* (2007). In both of these, I alluded to the autoimmune theory of MS. In late 2009, I learned of a potential conflicting theory that suggested a relative blockage of the veins draining the brain and spinal cord might be a factor in MS. This would shift the emphasis from damage to the blood-brain barrier (BBB) and brain via an autoimmune attack and subsequent inflammation to damage to neurons and the brain due to lack of oxygen.

As I recount earlier in this book, on November 29, 2010, I went to California to have a venous angioplasty of both of my jugular veins as well as my azygos vein. The short-term effect was profound. For a period of six to eight months, I had far fewer migraine headaches, almost normal bowel and bladder function, some reduced fatigue, and some improvement in my cognition. I was impressed and began a journey to learn as much as I could about this different approach and its role in promoting recovery. I already had significant exposure to stroke research, and this helped somewhat, but it lacked adequate answers. I had a second similar procedure in November 2017 in Brooklyn, New York, by Dr. S. Sclafani.

Finally, in the latter part of 2014, at the recommendation of two friends who are well versed in hyperbaric oxygen and diving technology, I read a new book called *Oxygen and the Brain—The Journey of our Lifetime* (James 2014) by Dr. Philip James from Dundee, Scotland. This was a seminal and life-changing event for me. It helped fit all the puzzle pieces together. The relative lack of oxygen in the brain following a stroke is similar to the relative lack of oxygen in the brain in MS. It was already known that many of the neurons survive in peripheral areas of the stroke, called the penumbra or watershed. However, these neurons do not have adequate oxygen to produce enough energy to function optimally, hence the term "idling neurons." However, once additional oxygen is added, the neurons often begin to function. I am sure this sounds like a miracle, but it is just the body achieving its needs, so it can function its best and heal on its own. Dr. James' book started me on my journey of enhanced recovery secondary to oxygen therapy.

I have always liked the dictum, "When the student is ready, the teacher will appear." I feel I was finally ready to hear the principles and concepts within Dr. James' book when I read it at the beginning of 2015. It had a profound influence on me. Soon after, I embarked on my oxygen therapy journey. I have had more than 350 treatments by doing 40 within the first 50 days and 1 or 2 per week since. Each oxygen therapy session lasts about an hour, at a pressure of 1.75-2 atm. Also, I like to do one treatment before a long-distance flight and as soon as possible after a flight. For the divers reading this, please note that hyperoxygenating before flying is not the same as diving on air before flying, which is strongly discouraged due to the risk of decompression sickness.

I have been fortunate in that twice in early 2016, I was able to spend time with Dr. James in Scotland. Prior to this, we had almost a year of interaction via email and telephone conference. In addition, he was one of the keynote speakers at the fifth annual Canadian Neurovascular Health Society Conference in Vancouver, BC in October 2015. We always have provocative, entertaining, and informative discussions. I have learned a great deal from Dr. James and look forward to a long association with him. I am especially grateful to have been included as one of the authors in a book about MS and oxygen. I certainly feel oxygen therapy is a key piece of the puzzle in MS recovery.

Today's best understanding of MS is that it is an injury to the BBB with subsequent triggering of inflammation. Both scenarios may persist, even to the degree of forming scar tissue, which can be seen on pathology examination as well as with imaging with MRI. If the unidentified bright object image (UBO) or white matter hyperintensity (WMH) on MRI is only edema (swelling), then it is reversible. At this time, imaging experts are unable to distinguish between edema or swelling bright spots and those of scar tissue. If the images indicate the formation of hard scar tissue, then it is relatively irreversible.

In 1983, in the *Lancet,* Dr. Philip James published the case report consistent with fat embolus being a trigger of MS (James 1983). He went on to talk about the similarities between decompression syndrome (the bends) and MS. In fact, these two clinical syndromes look identical on MRI. A growing amount of evidence supports Dr. James' concepts.

To begin, the pathology literature recognizes that almost all MS lesions are in the areas of tiny veins within the brain. Why might this be so? The concentration of oxygen in the plasma of the blood continues to get lower as the blood travels farther from the heart through the carotid arteries, through the small arterioles into the capillaries, and into the smallest veins or venules. The lowest concentration of oxygen is almost always at the site where the brain injury of MS occurs. It is at these same sites that the fat emboli do the most damage. Unprotected fat is a major trigger for free radical production, with secondary injury to the nearby tissues, especially the endothelium. This happens most dramatically where the oxygen concentration is lowest, hence, in the small or micro veins. If this fat or other emboli, such as LPS from a leaky gut, bump up against the side wall of the vein, called endothelium, then this can trigger local inflammation and injury to the BBB. This is most common when the veins are long and, therefore, farthest from the heart and lowest in oxygen. This local hypoxia makes the endothelium especially vulnerable to embolus of any type, including a tiny clot from slowed blood flow. Hypoxia alone can cause the death of neurons (Mander 2004) when present with inflammation.

The second question is why people with MS have more of these fat emboli than the regular population. One possibility is the presence of right-to-left shunt within the heart. The most common of these is called a patent foramen ovale (PFO), found in 20-25 percent of the population. Typically, the fat injury happens in bone or fatty tissue and then travels to the heart via the venous system. The fat injury leaves the heart, travels to the lungs, is filtered by the lungs, and then goes back to the heart to be pumped to the brain and other organs. The above pattern of blood flow is short-circuited in someone with a PFO. In this case, there is a shunt, the PFO, which permits the blood to bypass the lungs and go directly to the brain. Women have a higher frequency of PFO than men. A majority of migraine headaches are triggered by embolic phenomena. Many more people who suffer from migraines have a PFO, about 50 percent more than the regular population. We also know the incidence of migraine headaches is three times as common in women as in men. Curiously, this is the same incidence of MS. Perhaps this is more than a coincidence. Is there a higher frequency of PFO in the MS population? We do not know. However, this could be determined by a study using cardiac ultrasound with a bubble component, which is a safe and accepted method of diagnosing PFO. Alternatively, this can be done by screening with an ear pulse oximeter probe and a coordinated Valsalva maneuver (Billinger 2013).

The third question to consider comes from my frequent contact with MS patients over the last twenty years. I have noted that a large proportion of my patients, mostly women, describe an accident or injury that they feel triggered their MS. Many of them come up with this spontaneously, and the majority of others admit to this with careful questioning. In addition, many recall sustaining a concussion or traumatic brain injury before their diagnosis. Is it possible that a mild, moderate, or even significant soft-tissue injury triggers the first event, causing the injured BBB? Even a mild traumatic brain injury causes a pruning of the affected areas of blood vessels in the brain. This means a tearing and blood leak from some of these tiny vessels, especially veins, because they are thinner and more fragile. Might this aggravate the local area of hypoxia, helping to initiate the cascade of BBB injury and secondary inflammation?

The fourth question is why people with significant MS frequently have relatively obstructed jugular and azygos veins. I suggest this is because the area that is drained by these obstructed veins is relatively more hypoxic. The evidence by Dr. Petrov, a European cardiologist, suggests this is the case (Petrov 2016). Petrov sampled the blood around the obstruction of veins, typically above the valve of the jugular veins and tested it for oxygen saturation, oxygen content, and carbon dioxide content. He found that prior to relieving the obstruction in the neck vein, the oxygen saturation and oxygen content were lower, and the carbon dioxide content was higher. This difference was resolved once the obstruction was treated with venous balloon angioplasty. This is consistent with the oxygenated blood coming from the heart, relatively bypassing the area that had obstructed outflow. This makes a great deal of sense to me. Wherever the hypoxia is worse, the blood-brain injury and inflammation will also be worse.

The final question I would like to address is the association between leaky gut syndrome and a leaky BBB. Evidence has continued to mount that there is a direct association. This makes sense to me. One of the major triggers of inflammation in the brain is lipopolysaccharide (LPS). This compound is a part of the cellular wall of gram-negative bacteria in the gut. In a recent article in the *Annals of Neurology*, LPS was used as the trigger, in the presence of hypoxia, for BBB breakdown, inflammation, and demyelination (Desai 2016). LPS could be another source of emboli moving throughout the body and either initiating or aggravating injury to the BBB and secondary inflammation. I suggest the above reinforces how, where, and when these triggering events of MS occur. Since reading Dr. James' book, I have had 350 oxygen therapy sessions at 1.75 atm. When I cannot access one of these chambers, I travel with an oxygen concentrator. I could not have written this book without this intervention. It has helped my cognition dramatically.

30: Oxygen and Cognitive Function

My goal in this chapter is to give you a simple, safe, and readily available method to improve your cognitive function. It is not a drug; it is simply oxygen. We breathe oxygen every day, taking in the 21 percent of oxygen in the atmosphere around us. If the brain does not receive enough oxygen, hypoxia occurs, and cognitive function is reduced. Many call this brain fog. Supplemental oxygen is safe, yet anxiety exists in the medical field regarding the use of oxygen. Dr. John West, a world expert on breathing physiology, discusses the importance of oxygen and helps to dispel this anxiety in a recent *New England Journal of Medicine* article (West 2017). I will review his article and provide some recommendations that you can apply at home, safely and economically, because of the development of the oxygen concentrator. A great paper supports the connection between oxygen, homeostasis, and disease (Semenza 2011).

I congratulate Dr. West's elegant presentation on "Oxygen Conditioning" for people living at higher altitudes. He estimates 140 million people live at higher altitudes. This is in the range of one mile high (approximately 1,600 meters) and includes places like Mexico City, Denver, and Colorado Springs. He describes the benefit of oxygen conditioning in a straightforward and nonthreatening manner. Please, allow me to read between the lines as to what he may be trying to tell us for those of us who do not live at increased altitude. Oxygen enrichment of room air, called "oxygen conditioning," can relieve hypoxia caused by high altitudes (West 1995, 2015, 2016). Anyone who has a reduced ability to exchange and distribute oxygen to the tissues potentially suffers from cognitive dysfunction of the brain (West 1992). In addition, anyone with either blood flow problems or swelling within regions of the brain is also in this category. As discussed, inflammation in the brain is a key factor in Alzheimer's, MS, depression, stroke, and traumatic brain injury. One of the four components of inflammation is swelling or edema. This edema occurs outside the red blood cells and usually within the vessel wall and outside the vessel wall. As a consequence, when oxygen is released from the saturated hemoglobin of the red blood cell, it must travel an extra distance if swelling is present. If oxygen supply to the area is also compromised, this extra distance causes hypoxia, which impairs cognitive function. When this occurs, less energy will be produced in the mitochondria, the cell's energy factory, due to lack of oxygen.

Do you truly want better cognitive function? Most of us use our brains for work or creative pursuits and want optimal cognitive function. Hyperbaric oxygenation is one method to achieve this. Having been used for over fifty years, hyperbaric oxygenation has provided us with a great deal of information and research upon which to base oxygen use. In the chapter on hyperbaric oxygenation, you learned that this can increase the dissolved oxygen in the blood by twelve to fifteen times. Many people cannot access hyperbaric oxygen because of its cost and/or geographic availability. However, there is a way that you can achieve an increase in dissolved oxygen by three to five times in the comfort of your own home. This is through the use of an oxygen concentrator and an appropriate mask.

Oxygen concentrators have been available for at least thirty years. They work by taking in room air, which is composed of

21 percent oxygen, 78 percent nitrogen, and small amounts of carbon dioxide and argon. These machines extract the oxygen from the air and concentrate it to greater than 95 percent. Oxygen concentrators have virtually replaced home oxygen tanks, and many hospitals in Canada now use oxygen concentrators in place of huge liquid oxygen tanks. They eliminate the need for regular delivery of tanks of oxygen. Oxygen concentrators are compact, relatively quiet, and are simply plugged into a wall outlet. Purchase of one of these concentrators may require a physician's signature. This will be easiest if you are willing to pay for the oxygen concentrator rather than apply for coverage from your medical insurance. These units, supplying 5-12 litres of oxygen per minute, cost between $1500-$2000. They run for 40,000 hours and are quite economical for the amount of electricity required. The only other items you will need are a mask, nasal prongs, and possibly a tubing device, called pillow oxygen.

Who in the population would benefit from oxygen supplementation? People with end-stage or severe lung problems are treated with supplemental oxygen. Hospitals suggest an oxygen saturation point below 92 percent to medically indicate oxygen supplementation, and this is often funded by the insurance company. My question is, why not treat anyone below 97 percent oxygen saturation if they have symptoms suggestive of cognitive dysfunction? As stated previously, my goal is optimal health and performance, not just survival. This can be the difference between waking up fuzzy headed in the morning to being clearheaded and optimally functioning. If your goal for the day is simply to watch television and take it easy, then supplemental oxygen or oxygen conditioning is not for you. However, if your goal is optimal cognitive function, including executive decision-making, problem-solving, or creativity, then read on.

The first major group, other than those with lung problems (West 1995), that should consider oxygen supplementation are those with sleep apnea (Owens 2012). Evidence suggests that central sleep apnea is due to part of the brain functioning poorly, usually due to lack of energy and oxygen. Thus, I strongly recommend oxygen supplementation at night whether you have central sleep apnea, obstructive sleep apnea, or a combination of the two. If people are already on a CPAP (Continuous Positive Airway Pressure) machine, then they simply need to supply extra oxygen to the intake. I believe that central sleep apnea is due to regional hypoxia within the breathing centre of the brain, and this can be minimized with the addition of extra oxygen. The extra oxygen through the night will probably improve sleep quality, improve the brain healing through the night, and permit an awake, energized individual in the morning. You may ask, "Why hasn't my respiratory physician told me about this already?" They are likely practicing within the standard protocols that they have been taught, and they have not had the opportunity to learn about optimal brain function and oxygen conditioning. All respiratory physicians will be familiar with Dr. West's writing, if not his last review article in the *New England Journal of Medicine* (West 2017).

People who snore, are overweight, or both are the next large group that might benefit from oxygen conditioning at night. When we lie down, our abdominal contents push up on the diaphragm. This is aggravated by a fat belly, reducing the space required for the lungs to inflate. The immediate consequence is a dramatic ventilation perfusion mismatch. Ventilation is the small tubes of the lungs delivering fresh air to the alveoli, tiny air sacs that provide a huge surface for gas exchange. Your lungs equal the same surface area as a football field. The gas exchange is oxygen entering the blood and carbon dioxide leaving the blood. The perfusion is the tiny blood vessels adjacent to your alveoli. When you lie flat, the optimal contact between blood flow and air entry is more poorly matched. The consequence of this is reduced oxygenation of the blood as it travels through the lungs from the heart. The more fat around the belly, the worse this becomes.

In my more than twenty years of experience as an anaesthesiologist, I can confirm that almost everyone's oxygen saturation falls when they lie down because of the scenario described above. I learned this, because I always recorded the patient's supine pulse oximeter oxygen saturation reading on my anaesthetic chart before giving the individual any drugs. In addition, before starting any anaesthetic, I routinely gave 100 percent oxygen for either four minutes or four deep and complete breaths. Typically, this raises an individual's oxygen saturation and broadens the safety time in the initiation of anaesthesia and intubation (securing of the airway). I present this discussion, because you may not be aware of this long-practiced and well-researched use of supplemental oxygen by anesthesiologists.

The third group of people to consider oxygen supplementation includes those with a brain injury or illness, such as stroke, traumatic brain injury, ALS, brain cancer, or MS. Each of these conditions will have inflammation within the brain and, therefore, swelling or edema within parts of the brain. This swelling increases the distance required for the dissolved oxygen to travel once it leaves the hemoglobin of the red blood cell in the blood vessel. By supplementing the oxygen to the individual, we can potentially improve this borderline oxygen supply or hypoxia. Most of this improvement is from increasing the dissolved oxygen in the blood. You are changing the hemoglobin saturation of the pulse oximeter relatively little.

Unfortunately, my colleagues have been taught the oxygen hemoglobin saturation curve is all that matters. It is not. What matters is how much dissolved oxygen arrives at the cell, especially neurons and oligodendrocytes (these make myelin or nerve insulation). Dr. John Nunn, and more recently Slesserev (2006), confirmed in human subjects that by breathing 100 percent oxygen with a good "rebreathing" mask, dissolved oxygen increases four to five times.

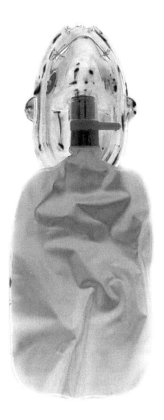

A more recent study revealed high-flow nasal oxygen saves lives (Matthay 2015). Remember, the brain uses 20 percent of the oxygen collected in the lungs but has only 2 percent of the body's blood supply. This fact illustrates the importance of these suggestions. If the neurons and other brain cells are hypoxic, their function is reduced.

In addition, the hypoxic cells produce an excess amount of reactive oxygen species or free radicals. These injure the cells further. This is important, because the naysayers of oxygen supplementation worry that extra oxygen produces extra-reactive oxygen species. This is not the case. The advantage of an increased oxygen supply is increased functioning of the mitochondria or energy-making part of the cell. (This is presented in chapter 7.) If the cell has adequate energy, it can control and minimize the injury from the reactive oxygen species. It will create more glutathione and other antioxidants, which suppress the reactive oxygen species. If the mitochondria have adequate oxygen, they can produce thirty-four molecules of ATP energy instead of just two molecules being produced by the glycolysis/lactate pathway. Thus, supplemental oxygen benefits cells rather than producing a negative impact via reactive oxygen species.

In recent years, we have learned another critical lesson: optimal deep sleep is vital for the brain cleaning itself and waste removal. When we are in stage III sleep, without medication, the brain is able to squeeze itself like a sponge with a tremendous removal of metabolic waste products and toxins. If our brain is unhealthy, hypoxic, or overmedicated, this doesn't happen. This "brain wash" is critical for optimal brain function. On a personal note, my sleep quality is improved on the days when I have hyperbaric oxygenation. In addition, for the last ten months, I have used supplemental oxygen at night, in the range of 28 percent oxygen. This has improved the quality of my sleep dramatically, and I suspect at least a portion of this is the improved brainwash. My wife's sleep quality has also improved, and we both feel more rested and refreshed in the morning.

I realize that, at age sixty-five, twenty-two years after being diagnosed with MS, I fit in the above category of brain illness. I live quite close to sea level, but as is typical with MS, I sleep poorly. My sleep was dramatically improved by my venous angioplasty, but this benefit diminished after some six months. It is now seven and a half years since I had my first procedure of venous angioplasty. I happily report that the ongoing use of supplemental oxygen is certainly one way to treat the regions of relative hypoxia that occur in individuals experiencing a brain illness. It is exceedingly safe, and there is virtually no downside. I have recommended supplemental home oxygen to more than one hundred patients in recent months, and many have found similar benefits.

Two methods are available for obtaining supplemental oxygen at night once you have an oxygen concentrator on-site in your home. The first is via nasal prongs, as seen in the emergency room, hospital ICU, or on medical TV shows. You simply set the flow on the oxygen concentrator at 5 L/min and wear the prongs at night. A second option that we have developed after the first prototype by Dr. Phillip James is "pillow oxygen." Multiple holes are made in a plastic oxygen tube, and then the tube is inserted between the pillow and the pillowcase. The tube is connected to the oxygen concentrator, which is set to a flow of 5 L/min per person. This latter option is equally safe and may be more comfortable than wearing nasal prongs, especially if you are up and down throughout the night to go to the washroom.

In conclusion, perhaps the story of a patient might help you understand how beneficial supplemental oxygen can be to the brain. L.B. had metastatic cancer, began having a lot of unpleasant nightmares, and was waking frequently at night. When reviewed, it was realized she had a lot of lung metastases, and her pulse oximetry saturation on lying flat was 89-90 percent. She was started on nasal prongs of oxygen at 5 L/min, and her nightmares disappeared. As a consequence, she had several more months of a much better quality of life simply by adding supplemental oxygen.

31: Neuroplasticity and the PoNS Device

Contributed by Dr. Teri Jaklin, ND

"Any man could, if he were so inclined, be the sculptor of his own brain." — Santiago Ramón y Cajal, *Advice for a Young Investigator*, 1879

While the concept of neuroplasticity has been familiar to me for some time, it was Norman Doidge's second book, *The Brain's Way of Healing*, that made it understandable on an everyday level (Doidge 2015). The idea of the brain being plastic (as in neuroplasticity) means the brain has the capacity to create new neural pathways to repair those lost to brain injury of any kind. While this concept has been around for nearly a century, like any good idea bound to change the face of how we see the brain, it is just now gaining widespread acceptance. Maybe part of the acceptance issue is that neuroplasticity has never been "owned" by one medical or professional specialty. It is as applicable in psychology as it is in neurology, physiotherapy, and education, to name a few. It also disproves the widely held belief that once the brain is injured, there is no coming back. Whenever we are training the brain anew, we are calling on its plasticity to get us there. When I was first wrapping my head around the idea, I thought of Plasticine, the putty-like modeling clay we had as kids, and being able to mush one bad creation up to build another.

Quality research on this phenomenon abounds in Doidge's book; however, it was the work of Dr. Paul Bachy-Rita MD, PhD, and the PoNS (portable neuromodulation stimulator) device that hooked me (Doidge 2015). By the time I finished chapter seven, I had picked up the phone and called the Tactile Communication and Neurorehabilitation Laboratory (TCNL) at the University of Wisconsin and asked if I could have one. Janet, the research assistant on the other end of the line, gently told me, "No, you can't have one of the devices, but you sound like a good candidate for our study in advanced multiple sclerosis."

At that time, data published on the use of PoNS in mild and moderate MS already showed an improvement in gait during the course of a 14-week study (Tyler 2014), and with my personal mission to get on my feet again, I jumped at the opportunity to participate.

I qualified as advanced MS due to impaired mobility. My mobility had been compromised a number of years earlier as result of a series of orthopedic knee, foot, and ankle injuries, along with thirty plus years of MS affecting my mobility. I had mild to moderate numbness in my hands and feet (but my dexterity was not greatly compromised), some bladder issues, and moderate fatigue, but my cognition and balance were fine.

Interestingly, in other TCNL trials over the years, versions of PoNS had also been used effectively to restore balance in a woman whose inner ear was destroyed by antibiotics, treat the effects of traumatic brain injury (TBI), restore voice in a singer with MS, in stroke recovery, Parkinson's disease, and even to help a blind man regain vision. It even helped Montel Williams overcome his MS-related balance issues enough to get back on his snowboard, and their research is now being actively supported by the US military, who see great promise for its use with veterans who suffer with PTSD.

What does PoNS do? Simply put, it expedites neuroplasticity. It enhances the body's natural ability to create neuropathways when used with mental and physical exercises specific to the functions that have been lost. Then the brain begins to create new neural networks under the old adage, "Neurons that fire together wire together." Researchers found that the device stimulates the entire brain so it doesn't matter where the damage is or even if it can be seen.

Although the research has been focused on more obvious brain injuries, researchers at the TCNL have found that by affecting the entire brain, it is also stimulating neurons that govern sleep, balance, mood, movement, and sensation, opening up endless possibilities.

The PoNS device I used looks like the one in the picture below. The new models, the ones that will soon be available commercially, are much fancier. It has 144 electrodes on one side that, when placed on the tongue, provide a wonderful conductive interface close to the brain. Once activated, it emits an electrical charge that directly stimulates the brain. This heightens the body's receptivity to new messages, such as those delivered through targeted exercise.

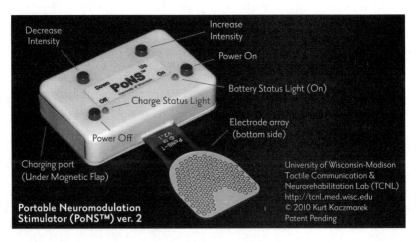

Solving the Brain Puzzle

Just to be clear, on its own, it probably has a limited positive effect. To make a noticeable difference, it requires an active process. Remember, this device *enhances* plasticity. It stimulates, but you do the work in the form of targeted daily exercise to retrain your brain.

I spent the first two weeks of the study at the lab in Wisconsin getting to know the team, doing baseline testing (both mental and physical), getting acquainted with the device, and learning my first exercise routines. The study protocol was to use the PoNS device three times daily for twenty minutes each time. Each session was different and was adjusted over time as my body responded. As you might expect, the training was heavily weighted on gait, balance, and coordination training, but to my bewilderment, the first stop on each of the monthly follow-up visits was with Dr. Yakov Verbny, a neurophysiologist, who ran a series of tests specific to my eyes. Now, you may be asking yourself the same questions I did. The eyes? What the heck? It turns out three key areas govern the restoration of good movement, and one of them is the eyes! I was intrigued to learn the role of eye strength and function in walking and that, like any other muscle, nerve innervations can be compromised here too—and improved through targeted eye exercises. At different points in the study, one of my PoNS sessions was specifically designed eye exercises. To my surprise, the strength in my eyes changed over time. By the end of the study's first phase, the nystagmus (repetitive uncontrolled movement of the eyes) I had experienced for decades was gone. I use these same eye exercises regularly as part of my own overall recovery program and integrate them clinically with some of my more compromised patients to initiate plasticity process in their healing process. You would be fascinated to experience how fatiguing twenty minutes of eye exercises can be!

When it came to the actual targeted exercises, the morning session included sustained core and balance, which was a series of exercises focused on restoring a strong core and training the body how the arms and legs function in relation to that core to enable walking. A midday session consisted of breathing awareness training (BAT) followed by an evening session dedicated to coordinated movement, which was mostly a stationary bike but was sometimes swimming. As a meditator, I was interested to learn that a relaxed state promotes neuroplastic healing. The BAT consisted of a guided meditation with theta brainwave music, and I always noted a positive difference in my abilities after I completed it.

The first phase of the trial was six months. Each month I spent time at the TCNL in Wisconsin, where I was re-assessed, and my exercise program was tweaked to push me forward.

I mentioned earlier that my goal was to walk again. What I began to notice even before the end of the two introductory weeks was a strength and confidence in standing that made all aspects of life a little easier. Even though I had never really suffered from any cognitive issues, such as the dreaded MS cog-fog, I did notice my mind was sharper, and by the four-month point, I was able to walk significantly farther with a walker than the few steps I was capable of when I began.

In the fifth month of the study, I was standing and moving more independently, as much as three to five unsupported steps at a time! That may not sound like much to you, but to someone who hadn't taken any real steps in a few years, it was a marathon. I was able to stand long enough to have a good smooch with my husband and hug my patients again.

Just as I was taking a few steps forward, there it was, the colossal step back. I began to experience pain and instability in my (already unstable) right knee. This was not a consequence of the PoNS but the ongoing deterioration initiated by a horseback riding accident at the age of eighteen, some thirty-five years prior. It wasn't the first time I'd had problems with that knee. In 2010, a meniscus tear was laparoscopically repaired with a warning that it would eventually need replacing. The significance of this setback was that I was actually up on the knee enough to reactivate the injury. It sounds odd, but it was a backhanded way of measuring progress. As fate would have it, an appointment that had been made months earlier came up with an orthopedic surgeon. She gave me two options. If I was comfortable on my scooter for the rest of my life, the first option was far less invasive. If my intention was to walk again, the second option was a total knee replacement. The team at the TCNL in Wisconsin considered this new development and endorsed the knee surgery and my continuation in the study.

Although I was in good physical shape as I went into what I knew would be a brutal surgery, I was completely unprepared for the physical and metabolic consequences of major surgery with power tools. Ugh. When I awoke, I was unable to move from the waist down. By the time I resumed the study two months later, it was like starting way beyond the beginning. In addition to learning how to wiggle my toes again, I dealt with unbelievable physiologic setbacks, including the profound constipation that accompanies IV antibiotic and narcotic use, severe blood sugar swings, and a thyroid crash, not to mention the side effects of the anesthesia, drugs administered to keep me from feeling the fact that an operating room team was working on me with saws and hammers!

Equally shocking and distressing to a naturopathic doctor was the quality of the food in the hospital and rehab facility. We quickly installed a plug-in cooler in my room with some seriously green soup and other yummies to promote healing.

The new knee was amazing and totally pain-free, but just when I thought I was truly on the road to recovery, at about the one-year point after surgery, I had a three-month period of unexplained severe nerve pain that literally drove me out of my mind, making me depressed, angry, homicidal, and, on two separate occasions, suicidal.

Most interesting to me, in an observational kind of way, was that the entire muscle chain on my right side had lost all strength and tone from my shoulder to my toes. The remaining "good" side, my left, had always been my weaker side, so I was left with my weak side and my right side, which was now reduced to wet-noodle status. For months, my incredible husband, Mike, helped me with every single move, including lifting me onto the treatment table, where I did my PoNS sessions. As a committed clinician (or a clinician who should be committed) my workplace was adapted, and I returned to work just fifteen days after the surgery. Later, I seriously pondered the sanity of that move.

In January 2017, I finished phase two of the PoNS study. While on a chart my progress had slipped back a bit, at the end of the day, I was amazed at how far I had come since the surgery. I am grateful for having had the PoNS as part of that surgical recovery.

Overall, the PoNS experience has been positive. Some key extra-curricular lessons include how important regular routine is, how, if we are serious about change we must be serious about changing the way we do things now, and how we can't try to fit something into an already crazy life and expect great results. The crazy must be tamed to make ample room for the new activity.

It is impossible to determine exactly how I benefited from the use of this device, especially with the complication of a total knee replacement. However, as I continue with my recovery and an exercise program, now unrestricted by my participation in the study, I am able to work out for more than twenty minutes at a time, and my strength and ability are improving exponentially. It is clear to me that anything is possible in my Plasticine brain!

Before I left the lab one final time last January, I spoke with the research team for some insight on when we might see the PoNS device in the hands of clinicians in the real world. There are still many hurdles to clear and much education to be done to overcome skepticism in the current therapeutic model before they can get it into marketplace. Continued clinical trials are required to gain FDA and Health Canada approval, development of therapeutic interventions for each indication, the training of therapists, and so on.

While neuroplasticity radically reverses ages of scientific dogma, and the PoNS device is poised to revolutionize the way we treat brain injury through the simple principle of how the brain is capable of controlling and changing the body, changing dogma in science happens at a glacial pace.

The good news is that rather than waiting for the PoNS device to hit the market as the next best thing, you can still activate neuroplasticity, harness and re-enable your body's own healing process, and begin your path of change right now.

Remember what I said about meditation setting the stage for neuroplastic healing? I begin each of my workouts with a twenty to fifty minute body scan meditation. I fall back on the lessons learned and experiences gained from my incredible PhD physiotherapist/TCNL research assistant, Georgia— and Janet and Kim too! Together, they had the deepest pool of knowledge, an eclectic combination of classical clinical physiotherapy, dance, yoga, and the uncanny ability to create precisely what my body needed to maintain forward momentum at all times. To these ladies, I am eternally grateful.

As I was cut loose from my PoNS team, I continued to draw on their wisdom. I also draw upon the wisdom of other movement therapists whom I have worked with over the years and who have incorporated the principles of neuroplasticity in their training. I would like to leave you with the three principles of neuroplasticity that stick with me the most and guide me in sitting, standing, walking, and even lying down.

1. Perfect practice makes perfect

I think of this as mindful movement—every move counts. This means in retraining the brain you don't want to confuse it with sloppy messages. Remember the old adage, "Neurons that fire together wire together"? To have neurons firing together, they need a consistent and clear message. This means it does not benefit you to take more steps just to get your count up. You are better to take two or three perfect steps and then do seated exercises that support your walking ability. Thanks to Georgia, I have a library of these insights that I will use forever. I recommend you find a movement therapist who uses the principles of neuroplasticity to assess your own needs and build on your strengths. Eventually, those neurons firing together will wire together in a new neural network, and those steps will be easier and easier.

2. Practice makes permanent

The only way to stay moving is to stay moving. It is not something that can happen by taking a bottle of supplements or a pharmaceutical. Our bodies are made to move, not sit all day. One of the great gifts of the PoNS device was the routine of doing something several times per day. The odds of me continuing three times per day are highly unlikely, but my new goal is twice per day five days per week, which is doable. In my world, it will include any combination of core and stability exercises, treadmill, meditation, yoga, stationary bike, and swimming. So many options, so little time! What is the best way to start a new habit? Break an old one. Get up and walk at lunch, set an alarm to stretch every hour, create a regular workout routine, and stick to it *whether you want to or not*. Those last words are italicized, because they were Georgia's words of encouragement when my jaw was on the floor as she first introduced the concept of "three times per day."

3. The body receives the stimulus, whether it is real or perceived

You can stimulate neural firing by visualizing the workout too. This can be helpful in a number of situations: 1) if your ability is severely compromised, and you need somewhere to start, 2) if you are unable to work out, for example, in a car travelling from Ontario to Wisconsin, or maybe on the commuter train or even sitting on a chair, you can go through your targeted routine in your mind. If you find your technique getting sloppy partway through an exercise routine, sit down and visualize the rest of the program in real time.

It is fantastic that the most recent scientific evidence shows that neuroplasticity can be harnessed and optimized to prevent and treat neurodegenerative diseases, brain injury, stroke, and mental disorders.

Beyond the TCNL, researchers are debunking old beliefs and have proved that progression of disability in MS has nothing to do with a failure of the brain's plasticity, despite what MS patients have been told for decades (Tomassini 2012). When I was diagnosed in the mid-1980s, the first thing I was told was to take it easy—don't exercise; it will only make things worse.

Through the new neuroscience, we can now be reassured that brain plasticity is preserved, and physical and mental ability can be improved with practice even with a high level of brain injury. No matter how old you are or how severe the injury, the brain has a unique way of doing a workaround—it's called neuroplasticity. This is promising not only for people with MS but also for those with all nature of brain injuries.

I'd like to close with a quote from Mitch Tyler, one of the lead researchers at the TCNL (Tactile Communication and Neurorehabilitation Laboratory) clinic: "The collective 'we' of research is just beginning to scratch the surface of engaging Neuroplasticity at its most fascinating levels."

It is my sincerest hope that this chapter brings you a greater understanding of how neuroplasticity can play a significant role in your recovery and your life, whether you have a PoNS device or not.

If you are interested in the PoNS device, go to Helius Medical Technologies.com online.

32: Exercise and Whole-body Vibration

We have all heard the recommendation that exercise is good for us. Is this true with regard to brain function? The answer is a resounding *yes*. In this chapter, I explain why exercise can make a huge difference in brain function and preservation. In addition, I talk about how you can minimize the length of time you exercise but still have reasonable benefits. Finally, I talk about whole-body vibration exercise, which can have specific attributes and may be a way to begin for those challenged with mobility issues.

To begin, I would like to talk about brain-derived neurotrophic factor (BDNF). This is a protein known to be increased in concentration in the blood and in the brain secondary to exercise. BDNF plays a critical role in activity-dependent processes within the brain. This includes synapse development and nerve plasticity. BDNF is involved in memory formation, including learning and behavioural synaptic plasticity. It increases the effectiveness and number of neuron connections. It also promotes the development of immature neurons and enhances the survival of adult neurons.

Exercise is most effective if done daily and maintained for up to ninety days. The benefits persist for at least seven days thereafter. In short, ongoing exercise is key and should be done at least three times a week (Zoladz 2010).

Physical exercise can prevent or delay several different metabolic disorders, including diabetes. It can also enhance mood and cognitive function. The review cited above helps us understand how BDNF can make a difference. Exercise regulates BDNF in the hippocampus. BDNF benefits our cerebral cortex, hippocampus, and midbrain (substantia nigra, pons, medulla oblongata, thalamus, and hypothalamus). This important substance is found primarily in circulating platelets within the blood. BDNF may be produced by endothelial cells and is known to cross the blood-brain barrier in both directions. Hence, if it is increased in the blood, then it is also increased in the brain tissue.

BDNF is known to be decreased in major depression. There is also some suggestion that it is reduced in schizophrenia. Blood concentrations of BDNF are also significantly lower in established type 2 diabetes mellitus.

The magnitude of the increase in BDNF from exercise is dependent on the intensity of the exercise. Physical activity has been described as "the best buy in medicine." (Loprinzi 2013, 2015). Hopefully, that will get your attention, because it certainly got mine.

Executive function is described as a coordinated operation of various processes to accomplish a particular goal in a flexible manner. As you might guess, this is a very important skill for leaders and executives. Executive function encompasses three main factors.

1. Mental flexibility/set shifting.
2. Monitoring and updating working memory.
3. Inhibition of prepotent response. This means suppressing inappropriate dominant or habitual responses, when necessary (Allan 2016).

Executive function typically declines in old age and in degenerative brain illnesses. This is important, because executive function plays a key role in carrying out tasks, including chronic illness management. Executive function becomes less efficient due to inactivity, in the presence of obesity, and in the presence of systemic inflammation. Physical activity improves executive function (Allan 2016). In older adults, regular aerobic exercise can improve task switching and selective attention and can reduce one's susceptibility to being distracted. It can also increase memory span.

Resistance training can benefit in measures of reasoning, while Tai Chi improves measures of attention and processing speed. These are felt to help brain function in three ways. First, they increase BDNF. Second, the growth of new blood vessels in the brain is felt to be stimulated by the increase of blood flow to the brain during exercise. Third, exercise reduces pro-inflammatory markers, which improves executive function.

Any exercise can increase BDNF, but some types are more effective. Suggestions are as follows:

- Find something you enjoy.
- Incorporate choices with a high reward/failure ratio. This means doing something that is a bit risky.
- Do something daily.
- Add some sprints for short intervals.
- Increase your exercise intensity for 30 seconds every two minutes seven to eight times.
- Practice complex motor skills, such as martial arts or tennis, or add agility and balance skills to your workout.
- Exercise with others, because this stimulates the brain and is one of the best motivators of active lifestyle.
- Get outside (vitamin D and sunshine may help BDNF production).

- Try new things outside the gym, such as learning a new language or learning to play a musical instrument, or even memorize poetry.
- Volunteer.
- Let the brain work. Read, do puzzles, such as crosswords or Sudoku, or play Scrabble.

Depression reduces optimal function of the brain at almost any age. Similarly, exercising often can be as effective as psychological counselling, such as cognitive behavioral therapy or antidepressant medication (Sjosten 2006). This is particularly true in mild or moderate depression. However, no evidence supports a combination of cognitive behavioural therapy, antidepressants, and exercise producing greater effectiveness than one used individually. This is humbling to me, as I spent nearly twenty years on an antidepressant called imipramine (one of the early tricyclic antidepressants). I realize now that regular exercise may have been enough for most of that time. Recent research suggests that aerobic exercise may be comparable to established antidepressant drug regimens (Carson in Greenblatt 2016).

Changing Brain Structure and Function: Nerve Regeneration and Neuroplasticity

Looking at the brain through an MRI and other neuroimaging techniques has shown that brain injury or depression causes the loss (atrophy) of nerve cells and reduced rewiring of circuits throughout the brain. Changes in the hippocampus and frontal cortex are especially critical to mood stability, learning, and memory. Each of these are at risk in any brain illness. In addition, chronic stress exposes our brains to stress hormones, reduces the forming of new nerve cells, and prunes the branches at the end of neurons (dendrites). Consequently, the overall signalling ability of our brain's neurons is compromised, which reduces our ability to cope with stress. Does this sound familiar? It does to me, so listen up!

BDNF is a key component in optimizing neuron growth, replacement, and interaction (synapse selectivity). Exercise regulates this nerve growth factor.

Exercise also activates the endocannabinoid system. New data suggests this comes much before the beta endorphin system in the "runner's high." The endocannabinoid called anandamide and BDNF are highly correlated during exercise and fifteen minutes afterwards. In addition, exercise and endocannabinoids independently regulate hippocampal plasticity. An increase in cannabinoid signalling in the hippocampus is required for exercise-induced nerve cell growth in number and size. In short, exercise is good for all of us!

The Inflammation Component in Exercise

Exercise is a near-universal assist in almost all brain problems, because it helps alleviate stress, obesity, and diabetes. Each of these are a challenge, because they all aggravate inflammation. Activity also reduces the production of inflammatory products (cytokines) and reduces C-reactive protein. C-reactive protein is my favourite marker of inflammation, because it is readily available in almost all laboratories.

Sleep and Exercise

Slow-wave sleep, stage 3, is the key component of sleep that allows our body and brain to repair itself the best. This stage of sleep is increased with regular exercise (Passos 2011). During slow-wave sleep, the body releases more growth hormone, so the body and brain heal better. These are good things. Once sleep improves, the body rests better, and we feel more awake and energized the following morning.

In one study, Giselle Passos found that moderate aerobic exercise helped sleep onset by 40–54 percent. It also reduced wait time by 36 percent, increased total sleep time by 21–37 percent, improved sleep efficiency by 18 percent (Passos 2011). Personally, I need and like all the above.

Whole-body Vibration Plate and Exercise

I first saw one of these in operation almost ten years ago in South Africa. A woman with MS would go to see her kinesiologist three times a week. Part of her treatment was to stand on the plate for twenty minutes each visit. It was impressive, because she was very challenged walking into the facility but would walk almost normally on the way out. Her kinesiologist was following a key paper on vibration and MS (Schuhfried 2005). I realize this stimulus does not last more than several minutes; however, it dramatically improves people's balance, enhances their fitness, and can dramatically increase their confidence to do forms of exercise, such as walking. This is a particularly good way to help people with mobility issues secondary to a brain challenge, whether MS, a stroke, or a traumatic brain injury.

In learning how these units work, I discovered humans have three kinds of muscle-twitch fibres: slow, fast, and super-fast twitch. Slow-twitch fibres are primarily for endurance and are used in walking. They use fat as a fuel source. Fast twitch fibres are for quick bursts of energy, such as sprinting. Super-fast twitch fibres are sudden moves from a life-threatening situation. An example is touching your hand on a hot stove element and rapidly jerking it away. This super-fast twitch also turns on slow- and fast-twitch fibres. A vibration plate causes involuntary muscle contractions. It is these contractions that provide neuromuscular, cardiovascular, and flexibility benefits. Whole-body vibration is safe, and countless hours have been performed with no adverse effects. This is well-documented in more than one hundred research articles in peer-reviewed journals, such as *Spine, Journal of Bone and Mineral Research*, and *Medicine and Science in Sports and Exercise.*

Whole-body vibration is different than traditional exercise and has a few competitive advantages. It can provide a more effective and efficient exercise without the constraints associated with regular training. These include reduced joint stress due to lengthy repetitions and time commitments. The research confirms it provides similar strength gains to conventional resistance training but within a fraction of the time. Fifteen minutes of vibration exercise produces results similar to thirty to forty-five minutes of conventional training. In this way, whole-body vibration provides an effective solution to those who may benefit from weight training but are unable to engage in such activities. I think particularly of people with neurological challenges, such as stroke, traumatic brain injury, or MS.

What is the science behind vibration? The movement of the vibration plate with an attitude of about 1 cm simulates the body's natural stretch reflex. This is similar to the knee-jerk reaction that occurs when your physician taps your knee ligament with a reflex hammer. Without thinking about it, your body responds with a strong involuntary muscle contraction, causing your leg to kick forward. Whole-body vibration allows these strong muscle contractions to be repeated at a rapid rate. The other advantage is that it involves nearly 100 percent muscle recruitment, whereas in conventional training, there is only an average of 40 percent muscle recruitment.

This is particularly important for rehabilitation patients trying to add stability and strength to all muscles around the joints and to athletes looking to maximize strength gains. The gentle, rapid contractions of up to 3,000 times per minute allow the muscle to work optimally introducing blood to even the smallest blood vessels. Therefore, peripheral circulation is improved. This also allows the body to carry off any waste products at a much faster rate. The increased flow also provides increased oxygen, which is why some people use an oxygen mask, such as EWOT (exercise while oxygen training) while on the vibration machine.

Can whole-body vibration replace traditional exercise? While this is not the intent, published clinical research shows that whole-body vibration training is a safe and acceptable alternative to cardiovascular exercise. This is particularly important for those who cannot participate in regular exercise because of functional limitations, drugs, or heart disease limitations, such as heart failure. If the individual combines resistance, strength training, and whole-body vibration, they can get rapid results while minimizing the stress on the body and joints. In whole-body vibration, the body is loaded naturally with vibration rather than with weights, and this reduces the incidence of injury and joint degradation. Vibration amplifies any motion performed on a vibration plate by a factor of eight to ten. Ten minutes of whole-body vibration training can provide better results than forty-five minutes of traditional strength training.

The neuromuscular benefits are partly due to the fact that vibration can trigger an involuntary contraction in 100 percent of the muscles by firing slow and fast-twitch fibres. Typically, 40 percent of our fibres are slow twitch, and 60 percent are fast twitch. In addition, whole-body vibration can cause up to three times more circulation than running on a treadmill. This increased circulation can improve the dilation of the blood vessel wall. The consequence of this is a more rapid transport of much healthier blood throughout the body. In some instances, this can increase healing and reduce recovery time by up to 60 percent. It provides flexibility benefits as well. Vibration causes an increase in muscle flexibility and pliability and can improve circulation and warm up the muscles prior to exercise. Finally, it provides significant bone density benefits. When vibration is applied to the soft tissues and bone, it causes quite an improvement in the density and strength of both. The muscle contractions generated through vibration can play a major role on the G forces exerted on bone. Consequently, there is more bone build up and less bone breakdown. Studies have confirmed an acceleration of the regeneration of bone within defects. Bone density improvements of up to 12 percent in one year have been documented in clinical studies with no side effects of note.

Body vibration training can be beneficial to cardiovascular health. Ongoing training can reduce arterial stiffness and blood pressure. In fact, the benefits of circulation from the rapid contraction of muscle fibres can provide almost the same benefits as that seen from regular cardiovascular exercise. Every clinical study involving whole-body vibration reports an increase in the volume of oxygen uptake by the body and improved heart-lung efficiency. Blood pressure tends to be lowered to a more normal range. Overall, whole-body vibration provides a low-risk, effective, and comfortable alternative to traditional cardiovascular exercise. This is particularly important to someone who has limited range of mobility, strength, or balance secondary to their neurological challenge. This is a key reason why I've included it in this book.

Stroke treatment and prevention can both be impacted by vibration. Stroke patients typically have problems with posture control and balance. Whole-body vibration training can improve the proprioceptive control posture.

Proprioception is the sense of knowing where your body is in space and time. When this is lost, we become extremely eye dependent. However, this can be retrained, and whole-body vibration can greatly assist this. Clinical studies provide evidence that stroke patients benefit from combined whole-body vibration and balance training more than from a comprehensive inpatient rehabilitation program. This improvement is in terms of trunk stability, postural control, and muscle tone. Therefore, it is a safe and effective means of neuromuscular stimulation and improved quality of life for stroke patients. For many of the same reasons, I like to use it in MS patients as well. In summary, whole-body vibration improves strength, proprioception, gait, and balance in patients who are suffering from neurological diseases as well as people who are not.

Much of the early work with vibration plates was done for people in the space program. In the early 1960s, Russian space program scientists were the first to apply vibration to the entire body. They found that vibrating their cosmonauts prior to sending them into space put their bodies in peak physical condition and allowed them to stay in a zero-gravity environment up to three times longer than without vibration. It had been recognized that when people were in the much-reduced gravity situation, they suffered major muscle wasting and even bone wasting, which is osteopenia and even osteoporosis. The vibration plate is able to effectively increase gravity. Another way to think of this is if you were on the moon, you would have one-sixth of Earth's gravity. Similarly, if you were on Jupiter, you would have two-and-a-half times the gravity of Earth.

What are some of the general benefits of vibration of the entire body?

1. Lower back and disk degeneration improvements
2. Promotes energy and endurance

3. Can do specific strengthening exercises once a patient has shown improved function
4. Stronger more effective core muscles
5. Increases bone mineral density, which can help reverse bone loss and combat osteoporosis
6. Enhances blood circulation and lymphatic drainage
7. Improves flexibility and agility
8. Increases range of motion, balance, and mobility
9. Increases metabolic rate, which is critical to weight loss and maintenance
10. Reduces joint/ligament stress
11. Neuromuscular stimulation and enhancement, which can improve joint proprioception, muscle rehabilitation, and retraining muscle-holding patterns
12. Reduces back pain and stiffness and can improve spinal curvature and vertebral spacing
13. Can elevate human growth hormone, testosterone, collagen, and serotonin production while supressing cortisol, the hormone triggered by stress

When you purchase one of these machines, you need to consider if you will purchase it for 2 G or even up to 10 G. I suggest most people start in a more modest range of 4-6 G. The second component to consider is the frequency of movement. This is measured in hertz and typically means the number of movements per second. The next consideration is what direction these movements are in. Level 1 units are typically only in one direction, alternating sides. Level 2 units operate in three directions, usually with a low amplitude and a high frequency. These are called tri-planar, because they move in three directions. These are particularly good at increasing muscle strength and increasing bone density. The level 3 machines are effectively a combination of levels 1 and 2. Correspondingly, they have two motors to permit this combination. As a consequence, they are more expensive and perhaps more complicated than most of us would use at home. I suggest you ask a qualified physiotherapist or kinesiologist regarding the purchase and operation of one of these units. The human tolerant safety factor is in the range of 15-50 Hz. The amount of G forces you select must also be done with care. Start small, and work your way up. In addition, you should have your joints, particularly your knees, in a flexed position, because you need to increase the resilience as you work on this unit.

Common sense still applies to exercise. Hence, do something you enjoy, or do it with someone you enjoy being with. Today, I walk with my wife and golf with friends. When I'm on an elliptical with oxygen, I listen to music that I enjoy and look out on our organic farm/garden. I enjoy both of these. In the future, I plan to add tennis. It's been years since I played, but why not?

Regular exercise permits increasing strength, flexibility, mobility, and stamina. Similarly, it protects blood vessels, strengthens the heart, and improves blood flow to the brain. Cognitive skills are enhanced. Therefore, you can stave off declining memory, think better, and learn. Remember, sitting is the new smoking. By spending a little more time on your feet, you lengthen your chromosomal telomeres, and this can increase your lifespan. Exercise reduces tension, stress, fatigue, and anger and promotes more sleep and enjoyment. The result is an improved quality of life. What more could we ask for?

33: Microbiome, Brain Issues, and Gut Flora Transplant (GFT) or Fecal Microbiota Transplant (FMT)

Everyone who has worked as a nurse or physician in a hospital or been a patient will know how each patient is very bowel focused. In some ways, knowing what we know now, they are more correct than anyone accepted or realized. Almost any chronic illness, immune or "autoimmune," can be helped considerably by a healthier gut microbiome (Mullin 2011, 2017).

Our gut (from the mouth to the anus) hosts ten trillion microbes, which is ten times our human cells! The number and type of microbes varies for each region—mouth, stomach, small intestine and the colon, which has the greatest number. Our host-bacteria associations must be seen as of mutual benefit. In short, like it or not, we are a team. Like any team, we must work together and support each other, or every player will suffer. As the host body, without this team approach, we will become sick in a multitude of ways. Perhaps now you can see why our food diversity, fermented foods, prebiotics, and probiotics can support our team. Damage to the team comes from many sources: antibiotics, glyphosate (Shehata 2012), vaccination, major antacids (PPIs), and processed foods, to name a few. We can help our microbe team by what we put in our mouth.

A final rescue, if needed, is possible with gut flora transplant (GFT) or fecal microbiota transplant (FMT). I will now use the new term, Gut Flora Transplant (GFT) as this term is more correct because if properly prepared there are no feces in the implant . I had this myself in 2016 and will outline the procedure later in the chapter. Case reports of GFT (FMT) have shown good outcomes in Parkinson's, MS (Borody 2011), and chronic fatigue syndrome. The literature to date has used FMT but the Taymount Clinics have adopted GFT as the preferred term. Taymount has now performed 30,000 implants worldwide. I suspect that this is more than everyone else combined. I will use FMT if quoting the term from a published article but will put GFT in brackets behind it to help you help us with more correct, safer and more palatable term Gut Flora Transplant (GFT).

According to Meng-Que Xu et al., "FMT (GFT) achieved a successful cure rate in recurrent C. difficile infection. Although there is a deficiency of randomized controlled trials for FMT (GFT), the present review reveals that FMT (GFT) could be a promising rescue therapy in extra-intestinal disorders associated with the gut microbiome, including metabolic diseases, neuropsychiatric disorders, autoimmune disease, allergic disorders, and tumors" (Xu 2015).

Our intestinal microbiome is key in nutrition defense against nasty microbes (bacteria, fungi, and viruses), immune system development, and performance of the gut wall function (i.e., degree of leaky gut syndrome). In addition, our cells interact and cross talk. This is one of our greatest epigenetic controls. Epigenetics suggests turning genes on and off for a favourable and healthier outcome.

Our individual gut microbiome is influenced by our sanitation, social behaviours, and genetics. Sanitation can be positive or negative. For example, chlorinated water can have negative effects on our microbiota, but it makes our water safer from some things, such as nasty strains of E. Coli. Social behaviour can be as simple as a child eating and playing in soil, which is beneficial but often discouraged. Similarly, the quaternary "hand wash" units at the entry to public buildings do more harm than good. Soap and water works better against the dreaded C. difficile bacteria. The compounds in some hand cleansers are very harmful to us. In fact, the FDA has recently warned against their use (Commissioner FDA 2018).

The four predominant bacteria phyla (groups) in the human gut are Bacteroidetes, Firmicutes, Actinobacteria and Proteobacteria. If the first two, Bacteroidetes and Firmicutes, are reduced, then chances increase for the development of IBD (inflammatory bowel disease), and CDI (clostridia difficile infection). Similarly, an increase in Proteobacteria (including a subgroup called Enterobacteriaceae) is found in IBD and MS patients. Meanwhile, the increased presence of Bacteroides fragilis, a commensal or innocent bystander, can prevent and cure inflammatory disease via the effect of its symbiosis factor, Polysaccharide A.

It is beyond the scope of this book to address all possible health issues potentially impacted by improved microbiota. Suffice it to say that strong evidence suggests that FMT(GFT) solves C. difficile. In addition, increasing evidence in Nature indicates that FMT (GFT)may be impactful in MS (Branton 2016). There is also a strong association between MS and irritable bowel syndrome. An excellent article by Aric Lodgson describes how the BBB (Blood Brain Barrier) connects the microbiome and the brain (Lodgson 2018). Finally, brain microbiota disruption is implicated in demyelinating lesions in MS (Branton 2016).

When my personal journey with MS began twenty-two years ago, I did not envision a link to my gut flora, now known as the microbiome. Nor did I envisage having a gut flora transplant. However, in March 2016, I had my GFT at the Taymount Clinic in the United Kingdom. I have continued with a top-up from Taymount once a month since. We now know diet changes can modulate the gut microbiome in MS patients (Saresella 2017). More on my personal experience later. For the moment, how did we get here? One of the fastest-growing topics in the literature today is the awareness, investigation, and increasing understanding of the importance of the gut in virtually all animals, including humans. The question could arise: who is supporting whom? In reality, it is an incredible synergy that changes our epigenetics, our sense of well-being, and even our longevity. I can think of nothing that treats us so simply but impacts us so greatly. The blood-brain barrier connects the microbiome and the brain (Clapp 2017).

Over the last few years, under the leadership of Dr. Enid Taylor, naturopath, and Glenn Taylor, microbiologist, the Taymount Clinic has conducted more than 30,000 fecal microbial implants. The initial interview, when one is still at home, determines if dysbiosis is present. Anyone with a significant health challenge can apply for consideration of treatment of GFT. Patients should become gluten-free prior to GFT (FMT). The treatment begins with a one-month period of a very good stool softener. Clients are encouraged to have at least one colonic irrigation one to two weeks prior to arriving at the Taymount Clinic. This colonic irrigation is repeated on the first day at the Taymount Clinic. Then, immediately after the colonic, patients receive their first rectal instillation of the donor implant. Following the implant, patients are placed in several positions to facilitate movement of the 50–60 cc of fluid throughout the colon. The instillation, but not the colonic, is repeated daily. If a patient is only being treated to control C. difficile, then only four more treatments are required. All other dysbiosis issues are treated by five installations the following week and two further implants are sent home with the client to be self-administered.

Donor implants are collected under major safety protocols. They are all evaluated with DNA typing for the numbers and diversity of microbes, thus ensuring quality of transplantable microorganisms. In addition, all donors have been comprehensively tested for critical viruses and have no chronic viral illness, such as hepatitis B or C or HIV/AIDS. Each donor unit is stored at -80°C for three months, and the original donor is tested again for all the same viruses, as some of these may be lingering and declare themselves within that three-month time frame. I believe this is the safest, most diverse, and healthiest GFT (FMT) available in the world. The Taymount Clinic also provides this same quality donor material to Taymount Bahamas, a clinic in Germany, one in Slovakia. Other affiliates are in process, and I am hopeful Canada can join the International Taymount Clinic group in 2018 as Taymount Canada.

In March 2016, I had a series of ten microbiota implants in the UK. The process was done carefully and completely. I was pleased by how professional the procedure was completed. I complied with the daily Bimuno, which is a prebiotic that enhances growth of Bifido bacteria. This is superior to Bifidus probiotics, because this enhances the growth of your own "wild" type bacteria. These function and maintain much better than ordinary probiotic Bifidus. The probiotic Bifidus are typically many generations away from wild and tend to not persist within our microbiota. Kefir is a fermented food highly recommended by Dr. Enid Taylor (Taylor 2013).

The newest probiotic now taken by all the Taymount donors is Symprove. This product has been tested extensively by a quality third-party investigator in London, UK, with excellent results. Symprove is able to succeed where almost all other probiotics do not. It will soon be readily available in North

America. Currently, it must come from the UK. On a personal note, I recommend the Symprove passion fruit flavour. I found the natural flavour quite a challenge to swallow. www.symprove.com has a wealth of research results from university-led studies comparing it with other forms of probiotics. Synprove out-performs all other types of probiotics as it survives the stomach acid, arrives in sufficient numbers immediately to have a beneficial effect and thrives in the large intestine, to the benefit of the host. Its actions are facultative, not being part of the microbiome, but supporting and enhancing it.

By the eighth day from beginning my GFT, I noted increased energy and brain clarity. This pleased me immensely. In addition, my IBS symptoms have virtually disappeared. Studies have confirmed that quality microbiota implants like these are good at persisting within our bodies. However, we must look after them by staying gluten-reduced, better gluten-free and possibly dairy-free and by avoiding antibiotics and glyphosate-containing foods.

The Taymount Clinic routinely sends two implants home with patients, and more are available to purchase. I use a further GFT approximately monthly. Overall, I have been quite pleased with the results, hence this lengthy chapter discussing GFT.

It seems that everything happens for a reason. Little did I know that when my best friend from medical school suggested that hospitals have become plague centres, he was right. By being admitted to hospital, you dramatically increase your risk of developing methicillin resistant staph aureus (MRSA) or Clostridium difficile (C. difficile). These are the two most common killing bacterial infections today despite a plethora of antibiotics. At present, your chance of a speedy death once admitted to hospital is ten times as likely as that of dying in a motor vehicle accident. C. difficile is now found throughout our communities. In fact, only a couple of strains of this

Solving the Brain Puzzle

organism are particularly lethal. Almost all other strains are normal inhabitants with helpful benefits within our gastro-intestinal tract. Meanwhile, these two key strains of C. diffi-cile are difficult to treat, with the standard antibiotic therapy working about 15 percent of the time. However, four to five installations of a quality GFT have a better than 95 percent recovery rate.

When did C. difficile become recognized as such a danger? This occurred in the intensive care units in the hospitals in the 1980s. When a patient had a severe infection or even a fever of unknown cause, without a specific organism cultured, that person was typically put on three different broad-spec-trum antibiotics. This triple therapy was often lifesaving but sometimes caused the patient to develop pseudomembranous colitis. This latter condition occurs because of extreme over-growth of C. difficile, which produces a severe toxin. In fact, during my oral exams in anaesthesiology in 1988, one of my questions was about severe sepsis in a patient on the ward. This was an appropriate question, because, in Canada, anaes-thesiology residents spend six months in intensive-care train-ing during their five-year residency. Fortunately, I answered appropriately, the patient survived, and I passed my exam. Since that time, we have come to understand and treat the microbiome as a "virtual organ" that is equal in importance to our liver or our kidneys. So, a gut flora transplant is not unlike a liver or kidney transplant in importance. In addi-tion, a typical microbial transplant is a lot easier, safer, rela-tively painless and, as yet, quite unavailable in many medical centres today. In reality, GFT is not a medical procedure and if its donors are carefully selected, and samples are tested for critical viruses at least twice and prepared appropriately, then GFT has essentially no human epithelial cells. Therefore, vir-tually no immune reaction should occur, as might be expected with an organ transplant.

We now know that the brain's function is influenced by the bacteria within the intestinal tract. This is frequently called the gut-brain axis, and it is pivotal in understanding brain well-being. To help you understand this symbiosis, I want to give excerpts from a talk by Dr. William Shaw of Great Plains Laboratories, called "Microorganisms and their effect on mental health." This includes all brain health, so it is very pertinent to this book.

In 1957, a test showed that virtually all people with mental health illness had an abnormal protein in their urine. This finding in the literature noted by Dr. Shaw, and he went on to develop his organic acid testing on urine samples. In 2010, he published it in *Nutritional Neuroscience* (Shaw 2010). This publication was the culmination of fifteen years of work and showed that there was an abnormal phenylalanine metabolite created by some bacteria. This metabolite is formed in the gastrointestinal tract relative to which particular strains of Clostridium are present. He found these proteins especially common in the urine samples from patients with autism and schizophrenia (Shaw 2010). These researchers noted that these substances were present in all mental and neurological illnesses, including MS and Parkinson's disease. The two proteins that Dr. Shaw especially concentrates on are HPHPA and 4-Cresol. These are not produced by Clostridium difficile but rather by some of the other strains of Clostridium. This means that by using a sophisticated urine test, we are able to confirm that an overabundance of certain Clostridium species may be dramatically affecting our mental health or neurological brain health.

The evaluation of the organic acid test is, in many ways, like the testing we do in newborns to check for inborn errors of metabolism. Dr. Shaw's initial interest was in a young child who had developed psychosis during hospitalization. He confirmed that the patient's urine demonstrated an excess of these abnormal proteins. These are from six different strains of Clostridium, with the dominant ones being Clostridium sporogenes and Clostridium botulinum. This is the same botulism that is significant in food poisoning. People can be carriers of this particular organism, and it may not cause problems in them. Alternatively, these individuals have a low-grade infection, and it may be noted simply as a "bad cold." This means they do not get severely ill, and rarely would they be diagnosed as severe food poisoning or botulism. You may know much more about Clostridium difficile or it's more popular name, C. diff. However, there are six critical strains of Clostridia that are actually much more common than C. diff. I will now outline how these can make such a difference to one's health.

The structure of the protein HPHPA is similar to the catecholamine neurotransmitter dopamine. You may remember hearing the importance of dopamine in Parkinson's. If the proteins HPHPA or 4-Cresol are in excess, then they dramatically block the conversion of dopamine to norepinephrine (noradrenaline). The secondary effects of this are an excess amount dopamine and a reduced or inadequate amount of norepinephrine. It is the excess of dopamine that psychiatrists are trying to block when they prescribe antipsychotics to control hallucinations. These drugs block some of the effect of excess dopamine. Dopamine is a very reactive molecule compared to other neurotransmitters. In addition, dopamine degradation or breakdown naturally produces a large number of oxidative species, otherwise known as free radicals. Ordinarily, over 90 percent of dopamine is stored in the little vesicles or sacs at the end of nerve terminals. When there is an excess of dopamine, some of it leaks into the cell space, where it creates toxic issues. The breakdown products of dopamine injure neuron structure and function. This excess amount of dopamine especially injures the cells that ordinarily produce dopamine, such as the Substantia Nigra. These cells are critically destroyed prior to Parkinson's symptoms developing.

Once one uses an organic acid urine test to confirm that these patients have a dramatic excess of these particular strains of Clostridium bacteria, treatment is possible. The first published treatment of these organisms was reported in the *Journal of Child Neurology* (Sandler 2000). Eight of these ten patients got better with the use of oral vancomycin, an antibiotic. The treatment of these Clostridia organisms is particularly challenging, because many of them live as spores as well. These are tiny pieces of protein that are very resistant to treatment and can linger on surfaces. According to Dr. Shaw, today's preferred mode of treatment is more of a pulse treatment of either vancomycin or metronidazole. In this instance, one takes the regular amount for two to three weeks and then for one day and then stops for two days and then uses it every third day up to a month. The amount of antibiotic is no different than treating it daily for ten days, but it has a much better response by eliminating more of the spores because of the longer duration of pulse therapy.

I may sound ridiculous with my above comments when compared to the microbiota heath concepts in the previous chapter. However, please allow me to explain. First, antibiotics can still be lifesaving and life altering, if used judiciously. Second, if we can help resolve a mental or neurological illness with a course of pulse antibiotics, then we should use them. Then we can focus on helping the microbiota recover to a more optimal one, as this is a large part of how the illness began in the first place. All the suggestions in the previous chapter still apply. In many cases, these should be enough. However, if the above-recommended choices are not enough, the newest option is GFT.

Before closing I want to emphasize that I believe improved microbiome diversity is critical to the recovery of any neurodegenerative disease including MS, Parkinson's and Alzheimer's. Furthermore, it is being shown to have an impact on our mental health challenges, TBI, diabetes mellitus and even cardiovascular disease. The recent article by Menni "Gut microbial diversity is associated with lower arterial stiffness in women" and hence reduced atherosclerosis helps highlight why so many health problems improve as the blood vessels and therefore blood flow improve (Menni 2018). Better blood flow means better oxygenation and less hypoxia and less inflammation. The latter two are cornerstones to illness recovery. Taymount UK has established clinics in the Bahamas (Taymount Bahamas), Slovakia, Germany and is anticipating Taymount Canada.

34: Mindfulness, Meditation, Gratitude, and Rotary

The practices listed in the title of this chapter can perhaps be best understood as a practice of being present. A common misconception about meditation is that it offers an escape from the world. Instead, I suggest it is a matter of being present to the degree that you ignore all past experiences that are frustrating you, annoying you, and stressing you out. Traditionally, much of mindfulness and meditation practices, including yoga, come from Eastern contemplative practices in philosophy. Even when these are applied to our contemporary western scientific models, they are still incredibly successful and useful. The concept of mind-body-spirit is to focus at calming the mind, so the spirit within can heal the body and the mind. In the last seventy-five years, over two thousand articles on mindfulness have been published in the English language. Most of this is based on mindfulness-based stress reduction or mindfulness-based cognitive therapy and transcendental meditation (TM). I would like to credit much of the information in this chapter to Dr. Healy Smith and Dr. Gregory Thorkelson. They did an excellent job on this topic in the book edited by Drs. James Greenblatt and Kelly Brogan called *Integrative Therapies for Depression* (Greenblatt 2016).

In addition, I would like to credit Dr. Lucinda Sykes, whom I met initially at a retreat in Mexico but who has been teaching mindfulness to people in Canada for more than twenty years.

It is best to define meditation as a technique and as a state of mind being attained through the technique. Our initial impression is always that it is something practiced by monks, nuns, mystics, and ascetics. Frequently, meditations are broken down into two main categories depending on the direction in which our awareness is focused. The first of these, as was initially suggested by transcendental meditation, is that of focused attention or concentrated meditation. In this technique, the mind is focused on a particular object, such as the breath or a mantra. The second category is more of an open monitoring invitation, where one cultivates an open, nonreactive, nonjudgmental, moment-to-moment awareness of the sensations and events that enter one's mind.

Mindfulness is a state of awareness as a way of paying attention. Mindfulness has been defined as bringing one's full attention to the present moment in an accepting, compassionate, nonjudgmental, nonreactive, non-striving way. Jon Kabat-Zinn, a leader in bringing meditation into clinical use, defines mindfulness as "paying attention in a particular way: on purpose, in the present moment, and nonjudgmentally. With this in mind, mindfulness can be cultivated through formal meditation practice and through application. This can occur during one's daily life, for example, noticing moment to moment one's experience while walking, eating, or washing one's hands."

Historical consensus suggests meditation has been practised for most of human history. Our earliest records of meditation are found in the teachings of Hindu Vedas of ancient India as far back as 1,500 BC. Almost all global cultures and religions have their own traditions of meditative practice that cultivate elevated mind states. Examples include yogic and

Buddhist traditions or the plainsong chat of a Trappist Catholic monk or to the spontaneous personal prayers in a field or forest of the Jewish Chassid. Similarly, it can be compared to the intentional silence of the Quaker meeting or to the visionary stillness of an indigenous shaman.

In the 1970s, Herbert Benson, a cardiologist and professor of Harvard Medical School, directed his research toward meditation. He focused on a version of transcendental meditation that he separated from its religious roots. In his text, called *The Relaxation Response* (2000), he identified meditation as an antidote to the stress response, thereby balancing a chronically activated sympathetic nervous system. Most of us in Western society are forced to be continuously busy, and we live in an adrenaline mode most of the time. This is not healthy. Sure, we may get a lot done, but it comes at a tremendous cost. I was at least a year off work with my MS diagnosis before I started to figure part of this out.

I have included the following article by Lucinda Sykes as an effort to emphasize how each of must improve our yin-yang or sympathetic-parasympathetic life balance if we are to achieve optimal health. I will introduce two methods to assist you on your path. Perhaps most important is that recognition of the importance of this will empower you to work on it sooner rather than later. Look in your community for resources that work for you. Yoga is an excellent beginning. Another modality increasingly available where I live is mindfulness training.

Breathing: A Simple Way to Help Yourself Relax

By Lucinda Sykes, MD

The practice of breath awareness is a simple way to help yourself relax. Here's an explanation of two reliable methods that have been adapted from ancient traditions of meditation and yoga.

Breath awareness is especially useful for times when you know you don't have to think about or accomplish anything. For example, you might practice breath awareness as you're resting at home, riding a bus, sitting in a waiting room, or even while you're lying in an MRI scanner—any time there's no need to do or think about things, at least for the moment.

You can practice breath awareness briefly, maybe for a minute or two during a busy day, or for longer periods, such as during a long sleepless night. Whenever you choose to turn to it, breath awareness is available.

Method One: Feeling Your Breath

Breath awareness means body awareness—you feel your body breathing.

Right now, how do you actually know that you're breathing? What sensations are you experiencing? Maybe you're feeling the air entering and leaving your nose. Or you feel your chest moving, expanding, relaxing. Or you feel your abdomen breathing somehow, or your back. You could be feeling the clothing touching your skin as you breathe, or maybe you're experiencing deeper inner sensations of breathing. In any case, there's no correct or better way to feel yourself breathing. You just feel what you feel. Your body is breathing, and you experience sensations happening, moment by moment.

You'll probably notice a pause or stillness between the out-breath and the in-breath: the out-breath ending in stillness, and the in-breath arising from stillness. This too is part of breath awareness: you experience your body moving and resting as you breathe.

Thinking about breathing differs from actually feeling it. Do you recognize this difference?

For example, right now, as you read these words, you're probably having ideas, you're thinking about breathing, thinking about breath awareness. You're reading, focused on your thoughts.

But now, turn your attention away from reading this text, and feel instead how your body is actually breathing right now. Notice the various sensations that are happening as you breathe—the involvement of your nose or your chest or your abdomen. Now your attention is focused to body experience. No words are necessary.

This is a practice of awareness. You don't need to need to change or improve how you're breathing. Your body knows how to breathe. Just be aware of the experience, breathing now.

You'll probably notice that some breaths are longer, others are shorter, some breaths are deeper, others shallower. And many times the breath seems irregular. The breath is faster and then slower. This is all natural; nothing you need to change.

You might pay attention to only one or two breaths or follow along with a series of breaths, experiencing each breath happening just as it is.

Your eyes may be open or closed as you feel your breath. (See below, "Common Questions about Breath Awareness.")

If you're lying down or reclining in a chair, you might like to rest your hands on your abdomen or chest as you breathe.

> ### The Feeling of Breathing
>
> Bring attention to the feeling of your body breathing right now.
>
> Notice how sensations are developing and changing, moment by moment.
>
> You might follow sensations of a particular region—nose? Chest? Back? Abdomen? Or maybe feel your entire body, your overall experience of breathing.
>
> You're following a cycle of sensations: experiencing the in-breath and the out-breath and the pause or stillness between breaths.
>
> Notice you don't need to think about this experience. Each moment offers new sensations you can experience.

Method Two: Guiding Your Breath

With this second method of breath awareness, you continue to feel your breath, but you guide your breath too—you let each out-breath last a little longer than the preceding in- breath. This is how the body typically breathes during states of relaxation: the out-breath tends to continue a little longer than the in-breath. So, to help yourself relax, guide your breath in this way.

Here's how: as you're feeling your in-breath begin, start counting slowly and regularly, beginning with the number one. This is silent counting, within yourself.

When the in-breath ends, notice the number you've reached. Then, as the out-breath begins, start counting again in the same slow, measured way, starting at one. As your out-breath releases, prolong it, letting it continue a little longer than the in-breath.

For example, if you reached three during the in-breath, release the out-breath more slowly, so the out-breath continues for a count of four, five, six, or even seven.

Then start a new count with the next in-breath, breathing naturally. There's no need to slow or otherwise influence the in-breath. You'll likely notice that some in-breaths are faster than others. Such irregularity is natural. But again, during the out-breath, prolong the release of breath just a little, so the out-breath is longer than the preceding in-breath.

Continue in this way for as long as it feels comfortable. At any point, you can return to simple breath awareness, as described in method one.

Tips

Don't be too ambitious; you don't have to slow your breath more and more. Trying too hard to manipulate the breath eventually becomes stressful, not relaxing. This gentle practice encourages your body to settle into its natural pattern of relaxed breathing. You don't need to force change.

Some people prefer to alternate between methods one and two. For example, you might choose to follow mainly with Method one, and then, occasionally, slow the outbreath with method two.

Common Questions

How can I practice breath awareness with open eyes?

Even with open eyes, you can let your eyes rest by looking toward a neutral spot, an object or area that's unmoving and visually uninteresting. For example, this could mean looking toward an empty chair or a blank spot on the wall or the floor. If you're lying on your back, you can look up to a neutral spot on the ceiling.

As your eyes relax, they may partially close or become a little unfocused. From time to time, blink naturally, as often as you want. Even though light is entering your eyes, you're paying attention to the inner feeling of your body breathing.

I forget to feel my breath because I'm thinking. How can I stop thinking?

This is a common misunderstanding: people mistakenly expect that the thinking mind should be quiet during breath awareness. This isn't necessary.

You don't need to silence your mind as you feel your breath. Thoughts happen often during breath awareness. Thinking may even seem to continue in the background while you're feeling your breath.

Recognize that you're not trying to stop thinking; you're simply preferring to feel your breath.

Each time you're distracted, notice that you've been thinking, and then come back to the feeling of your body breathing.

Even when your mind is busy, your body is breathing. At any time, you can choose to feel the breath happening.

And you don't need to criticize yourself when you forget to feel your breath. Forgetting and remembering are normal in this practice. Each time you forget, come back to the feeling of breathing. Stay with it until you forget again. Yes, it's that simple!

This completes the contribution by Lucinda Sykes.

A Pattern of Breathing for Relaxation

By Bill Code, MD

I learned a breath technique directly from Dr. A. Weil while completing my two-year fellowship training in integrative medicine from 2006 to 2008. Dr. Weil describes it as one of the most helpful interventions as described by the patients themselves in all his years of practicing medicine. The benefit can be as dramatic as controlling the onset of some rapid heart rates and simple arrhythmias. I believe it does this by increasing our calming or vagal tone and, therefore, parasympathetic tone. This helps counterbalance the sympathetic or adrenalin-like state some of us develop or even get from too much caffeine.

I suggest you practice this technique at least twice a day and up to twice more when you need it. It consists of four breath cycles of four, seven, and eight. To begin, place your tongue on your hard palate, above your upper teeth. Blow out all of your breath. Then breath in through your nose for a count of four. Then hold this breath for a count of seven. Then breathe out through pursed lips for a count of eight. Repeat all this for three more times.

I find this helpful anytime I am anxious, such as before a stressful interview or before giving a talk. I even use it while driving to calm my irritation with traffic. I cannot change others, but I can change myself. I hope the above suggestions help you achieve more balance in your life. If you do, your personal health journey will likely be better overall.

Gratitude and Rotary

Gratitude, as explained by University of California psychology professor Robert Emmons on Mercola.com (Emmons 2016), involves two key components. The first is "an affirmation of goodness." When you feel gratitude, you affirm that you live in a benevolent world. Second, "gratitude is a recognition that this source of goodness comes from outside yourself; that other people (or higher powers) have provided you with 'gifts' that improve your life in some way."

Gratitude has been studied and shown to have benefits for every major organ system in your body. This can be as simple as the ritual of saying grace at every meal. It creates a deeper connection to your food while stimulating digestion.

I expect you can readily connect gratitude to generosity. This might seem counterintuitive, since "giving" means giving of some of your own physical or emotional resources. Science has confirmed generosity and happiness are actually wired together in the brain.

"Service above Self," which is the motto of Rotary International, exemplifies generosity. Rotary has 1.2 million men and women worldwide who regularly support this concept in their lives. I have been a Rotarian for more than twenty years. The like-minded friends and contacts I have through this organization have rebuilt my confidence that my MS diagnosis stole from me in 1996.

Denise and I just completed a Rotary-coordinated trip to Asia with Sustainable Cambodia (see www.sustainable-cambodia.org). We were excited to see more than ten years of cooperation with local villages enhancing the quality of life through clean water, sanitation, and education for many Cambodians—some of the poorest people on the planet. We travelled with Americans, Australians, Canadians, and others, both Rotarians and non-Rotarians. It was a memorable and eye-opening journey.

Almost everyone lives in a community where Rotary and other community organizations exist and where one can experience gratitude, generosity, and a purpose in life. Please, use the resources around you, as it is a useful and key component of healing.

35: Laser, PBMT (Photobiomodulation Therapy)

I first learned about photobiomodulation therapy from Norman Doidge's second book, *The Brain's Way of Healing* (2015). He devotes forty-five pages to a chapter called "Rewiring of Brain with Light: Using Light to Awaken Dormant Neural Circuits." This began my quest to learn more about this safe and relatively inexpensive modality for brain recovery. The journey has been exciting and has culminated with asking Thor Laser engineer and owner, James Carroll, to speak at two of our successive Canadian Neurovascular Health meetings in Ottawa in October 2016 and Vancouver 2017. He stated there are now more than 550 clinical trials involving lasers in the scientific literature. New information is appearing in the literature almost daily.

I needed some new choices for people stalled in their recovery path that would require minimal effort or work on their part. As I stated earlier, I have learned that many of us need a jump start toward becoming well. Once we get that burst of energy and or enthusiasm, we are ready to take the next step. A series of PBMT treatments may be the first piece of the puzzle to trigger our recovery journey. In some ways, this can be likened to a heart patient having a coronary artery bypass.

Anyone who heeds this wakeup call and changes their diet and lifestyle tends to do well.

This concept and the newly available "pod" lasers by Thor in our small city allowed me to do a pilot study on twenty MS patients for twelve treatments, fifteen minutes each. One of the pods looked like a tanning bed. The study was supported by my long-time friend, Josh Crawford. He was particularly interested after many years as a caregiver of patients with traumatic brain injuries.

We had an interesting set of responses in our small pilot study. Almost everyone had a relative increase in energy. This is not surprising, because 85 percent of MS patients have fatigue. One of the twenty clients eliminated her vertigo (balance issues) after just two pod treatments. She was ecstatic. Another client found it reduced her muscle spasticity, so she could walk ten blocks instead of just two. Some clients noticed improved bladder function with reduced frequency and urgency. I was one of these and was delighted with this improvement. Some of us noted reduced headache and some reduction in associated neck tension. Suffice it to say that the outcome was successful, and more studies are indicated.

What do you know about light therapy? The Egyptians and Romans understood the significance of sunlight and well-being. The Romans had laws about houses and sufficient sunlight. Florence Nightingale understood this early with her treatment of patients from the Crimean War. You may have experienced phototherapy for jaundice as a newborn, as did one of our children. Our second child was full term but had neonatal (newborn) jaundice.

My background as a family physician had exposed me to treatment using a "bili-light" for jaundiced newborns, especially premature infants. This is simply a light in the blue spectrum that can penetrate the skin and convert the fat-soluble bilirubin to a water-soluble form. This has two major benefits. First, the water-soluble bilirubin is much less able to cross the blood-brain barrier and injure the brain, so-called kernicterus. In addition, the water-soluble bilirubin is better removed from the body via the kidneys.

In modern medicine, this light therapy practice was implemented in Essex, UK, by a nurse, Sister J. Ward, after World War II. This was especially a concern, because it made physicians better at saving the lives of premature infants. Their immature brains are especially susceptible to newborn jaundice injury. Sister Ward was already known for her skill in rearing puppies, so she was put in charge of newborn babies. She took the most delicate of her charges and put them in fresh air in a sunlit courtyard. Other staff were anxious, but Sister Ward's infants improved. One day, she demonstrated to a physician in charge that a baby's tummy was no longer yellow in places that were exposed to the sun. Then, serendipity intervened. A blood sample from a jaundiced baby was accidentally left on a sunlight windowsill for several hours. Lab measurement revealed that the blood bilirubin was normal. These amazing results were repeated, and the same occurred. Doctors R.H. Dobbs and R.J. Cremer followed up on this brilliant observation by Sister Ward. They began using light to treat jaundice in newborns, and this became mainstream.

In his book, Dr. Doidge states, "we are not as opaque as we imagine ourselves to be. In fact, we have more spaces between our visible components than we can begin to appreciate. This is why some wavelengths of light, especially infrared and near infrared can penetrate several centimeters of tissue, including through bone" (Doidge 2015). Included within this is the realization that the skull does not block light, X-rays, or MRI, but it does block ultrasound. Hence, we can use light for therapy for the brain just as Sister Ward did. This response is not limited to bilirubin alone. In fact, all cells respond to certain frequencies of light, as all cells use mitochondria for their energy source. Similarly, all mitochondria have cytochromes in their makeup, and light affects these. Could it become any more obvious to us? Yes, all cells need energy to do their regular functions and to heal. Because light increases their energy, the cells can proceed to heal. In addition, the inflammatory processes in the cells are controlled, so healing is further enhanced. Finally, the major upside is there is virtually no risk or toxicity to light therapy. A startling example is low-level light treatment ameliorates immune thrombocytopenia (low platelets) (Yang 2016). Now I hope you can understand why I am so excited about PBMT as a valuable addition to your toolbox in your healing journey.

Initially, PBMT was called "cool laser" and then called Low Level Laser Therapy (LLLT). It has been used for more than thirty years to promote cell growth and recovery from injury. Research shows PBMT can enhance stem cell function (Arany 2016). Light in particular wavelengths is able to affect the activity in one or more of the body's inner (endogenous) photoreceptors. This can signal and trigger cell pathways and alter cell and tissue metabolism and cell proliferation. The most effective wavelengths are visible near red up to near infrared (NIR), which are in the range of 590–850 nanometers per second. Light in this range of the spectrum can penetrate tissue. However, this does not cause cancer the way that ultraviolet light potentially can. Studies confirm that PBMT facilitates wound and retinal healing. This latter retinal component means it also works on brain cells. Retinal cells at the back of the eye are specialized brain cells. In addition, PBMT improves recovery rates from ischemia, hypoxia, and re-oxygenation. In addition, NIR (near infrared) light promotes cell proliferation in fibroblasts and endothelial cells. This feature is exquisitely important in blood-brain barrier and circulation recovery. PBMT also reduces oxidative stress and has neuroprotective effects against the injury of neurons of the eye. These injuries are secondary to mitochondrial dysfunction. Better mitochondrial function means better energy, so everything in the cell and beyond can function better.

Mitochondrial Cytochrome C Oxidase as a Photoreceptor for PBMT

The word "chrome" means this part of the cell's mitochondria is light sensitive. Hence, every cell in the body is light sensitive, because every single cell in the body needs mitochondria to provide its energy.

PBMT can enhance cell function in several ways. First, it can increase the speed of ATP (energy production) by affecting the cytochrome chain in the mitochondria. Second, PBMT can improve energy production when there is hypoxia, because it helps release nitric oxide, so the oxygen available can more easily bind to the cytochrome, and more energy can be produced.

One of the fortunate consequences of PBMT has revealed that shining this particular wavelength of light on the bones can increase the release of new stem cells by six to eight times. The literature reveals that these stem cells can work elsewhere in the body. One example is improved recovery from heart attack even without shining the laser onto the heart itself.

A recent excellent article by Michael R. Hamblin, of Harvard, was published in December 2016 (Hamblin 2016). Its title was "Shining light on the head: photobiomodulation for brain disorders." In this review article, Hamblin divides brain problems into three broad groups.

1. Traumatic (stroke, traumatic brain injury, global ischemia)

2. Degenerative diseases (dementia, Alzheimer's, Parkinson's)
3. Psychiatric disorders (depression, anxiety, PTSD)

There is some evidence that PBMT can help all the above. In fact, it can be suggested for cognitive enhancement in normal healthy people.

Photobiomodulation was accidentally discovered in 1967. Endre Mester, a Hungarian, asked for a ruby laser but, unknown to him, he received one of much less power. However, he observed his new laser stimulated hair growth and improved wound healing in his experimental rats. LLLT was born and is now called photobiomodulation (PBMT), because there are uncertainties as to the exact meaning of the words "low-level laser."

Three clinical trials for stroke have been done to date. The best results have been in mild and moderately severe stroke. The better results tend to be in those when used in early intervention. In addition, these trials used a single event of PBMT. A series would likely be even more successful. Dr. Doidge has described chronic stroke rehabilitation treatment as a component of enhancing neuroplasticity (Doidge 2015).

PBMT for TBI

Studies to date are only in animal models. These studies have been reasonably successful when used with metabolic combinations to reverse memory and learning deficits in TBI mice.

Margaret Naeser and collaborators have tested PBMT in human subjects with a prior TBI (Naeser 2011). Symptoms of moderate and severe TBI include lasting and major symptoms, such as headaches, cognitive impairment, and difficulty sleeping. These problems often prevent them from working or living any kind of normal life. Initial case studies were positive. Later in a series of eleven patients, Naeser found improved executive function (often reduced by TBI), improved learning ability, better sleep, and fewer PTSD symptoms (Naeser 2011). Family members noted better social function and better ability to perform interpersonal and occupational activities (Naeser 2014, 2015). A later case report by Henderson and Morries of a patient showed reduced depression, anxiety, headache, and insomnia (Henderson 2015). Overall, there was better cognitive abilities and quality of life with accompanying changes confirmed on SPECT imaging.

PBMT for Alzheimer's Disease

A convincing study reported in 2011 in the *Journal of Alzheimer's Diagnosis* was done on a mouse model (De Taboada 2011). De Taboada et al. demonstrated that PBMT attenuated the amyloid beta peptide neuropathology. In humans, a small pilot study on nineteen patients investigated PBMT on people with dementia and mild cognitive impairment. Participants with moderate to severe impairment showed significant improvement after twelve weeks. They also reported better sleep, fewer angry outbursts, and reduced anxiety and wandering. Most benefits declined over the next four weeks.

A Russian study reported by I.V. Maksimovich using an inside-the-brain blood vessel probe for PBMT showed great results (Maksimovich 2015). The PBMT group had improved cerebral microcirculation leading to a permanent (one- to seven-year) reduction in dementia and better cognitive recovery.

Parkinson's Disease and PBMT

The majority of animal model studies were done in John Mitro-fanis' lab in Australia and reported in *Frontiers in Neuroscience* (Johnson 2015). In two different animal models, the results have been promising. The only clinical report in humans is in abstract form, where they studied eight patients with late-stage Parkinson's in a non-controlled, non-randomized study. They used external PBMT on the surface of the skull to study the benefits on severity of their symptoms of balance, gait, freezing, cognitive function, rolling in bed, and difficulties with speech. All patients improved some. There was a statistically significant reduction in problems with gait, cognitive function, freezing, and difficulty with speech ratings.

PBMT for Psychiatric Disorders

The first clinical study in depression and anxiety was reported by Schiffer, in a pilot study of ten patients (Schiffer 2009). A single treatment improved their depression at two weeks. A second study on major depression with six PBMT sessions significantly reduced depression scores.

Cognitive Enhancement

Several reports have been done on lab animals and humans. A positive effect was noted in each of these subjects. A study by N. J. Blanco in the *Journal of Neuropsychology* showed participants receiving topical laser had enhanced Wisconsin Card Sorting Task (WSCT) (Blanco 2015). This is considered the gold standard in executive function, which is compromised in normal aging and several neuropsychological disorders. They also showed that this topical treatment to the right forehead, but not the left, improved the attention-bias modification in humans with depression.

Finally, a study by Salgado revealed that twenty-five elderly women were able to enhance their brain blood flow (Salgado 2014). This positive effect was shown in the middle cerebral artery and the basilar artery. This is exciting, because brain blood flow is key in major dementias (Alzheimer's and vascular dementia).

Conclusion

Hamblin went on to suggest to many investigators that PBMT for brain disorders will become one of the most important applications of light therapy in coming years. As all populations age, and together with ever-lengthening lifespans, then dementia, Alzheimer's, and Parkinson's diseases will become global health problems. No drug has been effective and, in fact, pharmaceutical companies have closed neuro drug research programs. It is a similar state of affairs with regard to stroke, except for clot-busting drugs, and TBI is the same problem. New indications for PBMT, such as brain damage after heart attack (global ischemia), post-operative cognitive dysfunction (POCD), and autism spectrum disorders may well emerge.

36: Hyperbaric Oxygen Therapy (HBOT) and Brain Recovery

"There is no more scientific and critical action than to correct lack of oxygen" — *Prof. Philip B. James*

Hyperbaric oxygen therapy is a decades-old procedure, but it is still poorly understood by most people and, therefore, instills fear in some. There is no good reason for this. HBOT is misunderstood by most medical doctors in North America and Europe. Consequently, they have missed out on a valuable tool. The world expert on HBOT and the brain is undoubtedly Dr. Philip James. His book, *Oxygen and the Brain*, has been life-changing for me (James 2014). It elegantly outlines the brain and the illnesses/injuries that can be greatly helped with extra oxygen (HBOT). Similarly, I am delighted to be working with Dr. James and Dr. Duncan Black, vascular surgeon, on an oxygen approach to MS book.

In this chapter, I briefly outline some key points. When you are ready for more, please go directly to Dr. James' book. It's all there (James 2014).

The three tenets of optimal health or health recovery are: 1) circulation, 2) oxygen delivery to all regular body cells, and 3) delivery of nutrients (simple sugars or free fatty acids) for energy and subsequent removal of metabolic by-products (carbon dioxide and other waste products) via the lungs and kidneys. This is an over-simplification, but this chapter is focused on oxygen delivery to our cells (as opposed to our microbiome).

Oxygen enters the airway and lungs, then either attaches to the haemoglobin molecule of red blood cells or is dissolved directly into the liquid blood component (plasma). Final delivery of all oxygen to the cells is from oxygen dissolved in the liquid around the cells. Yes, that's right, all oxygen that finally arrives at the cells is dissolved. Medical doctors and laypeople alike have become confused by the importance of haemoglobin in this process. Yes, it's important, but we have become "slaves" or misguided interpreters of oxygen saturation as determined by pulse oximetry. Physicians often misinterpret oxygen saturation via a pulse oximeter as being an indication for no oxygen therapy. This is in error. It is a great assist but only that. It is not the "be all and end all" clinicians make it out to be. Remember, my background is anesthesiology, and I trained when pulse oximeters became available. This device greatly helped the safety of patients in the operating room.

However, the pulse oximeter at the fingertip is only a relative indicator of dissolved oxygen in the tissue, especially the brain, which is the most oxygen-requiring tissue in the body. For example, if at sea level or 760 mm mercury of pressure, 21 percent oxygen from air results in a dissolved oxygen of about 120 mm mercury when the pulse oximeter reads 99 percent. Yet, when a pulse oximeter reads 92 percent, the dissolved oxygen is about 60 mm mercury or half the other reading. Similarly, the oxygen in the brain cell is less than 20 mm mercury. If the brain is swollen or inflamed, the oxygen level is even lower. If you have had a stroke or embolus (from fat or a nitrogen bubble), the oxygen level is even lower still. Now the brain neuron may not have enough oxygen to function or control free radicals or inflammation. This explains regions of probable hypoxia, especially in the brain. The same occurs in peripheral wounds, for example, leg ulcers. Just because the fingertip reads 92% or above on the pulse oximeter, the swelling and inflammation in the wound makes oxygen concentration considerably less and thereby extra oxygen will benefit the healing process.

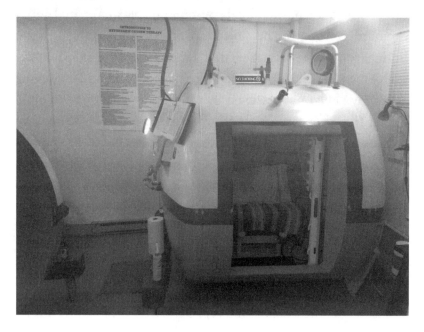

If one is in a chamber pressurized to 2.0 atmospheres absolute and breathing pure oxygen, then the circulating dissolved oxygen is increased 12–14 times. Furthermore, we know this hyperbaric oxygenation promotes neural stem cell proliferation and protects the learning and memory ability in neonatal hypoxic-ischemic brain damage (Wei 2015). In addition, a course of twenty or more of these treatments over six weeks mobilizes our stem cells and these increase by six to eight times (Thom 2006).

I realize these partial pressure/atmospheres discussions are daunting for some. Therefore, I will give an example that may help. Your mother or grandmother has a leg ulcer on her swollen leg and is now in hospital. The nurse looks at the patient's pulse oximeter, and it reads 92 percent on room air. Unfortunately, you mother/grandmother is being short-changed, and the ulcer will heal very slowly, if at all. Amputation becomes the likely outcome, as the ulcer is now infected and becomes gangrenous. In Canada, the surgeon explains this to the patient and family, then books the surgery. This can be avoided! Twenty to forty treatments in a hyperbaric chamber (HBOT) will raise dissolved oxygen enough in the leg to heal the ulcer. Forty years or more of research, published in the literature, confirms this is true (Fosen 2014).

Let me describe this very scenario in a ninety-four year-old woman whom I know. She had a leg ulcer for nearly two years and did not want to end her days with a leg amputation. She began a series of HBOT treatments. Not only did the ulcer heal, she and her family noted how it improved her mental clarity. Happily, she was able to cancel her amputation, and now, two years later, she continues HBOT twice a week, because it helps her brain function better too.

By being in HBOT, her dissolved oxygen concentration increased ten to twelve times above normal compared to normal room air at sea level. This increased level of oxygen permitted the inflammation to decrease, treated the infection, and allowed the mitochondria in the cells to produce energy more effectively. The outcome is dramatic in that healing occurs (Fife 2016).

Before leaving this discussion of healing of leg ulcers, I want to restate that brain cells need more oxygen to function optimally than any other body cell type. As a result, the need for increased oxygen is nowhere as dominant as in healing brain tissue. Therefore, if you are in need of a rapid or urgent reversal of your reduced brain function, I suggest you seek out HBOT. In much of the world, you will have to pay privately for this treatment. This is unfortunate, but this does allow you access to this treatment without a specialist's referral. This latter is difficult to achieve, so we are better off on our own recognizance.

In Dr. James' book, he describes in detail and with examples many of the brain problems that can benefit from oxygen therapy (James 2014). (I have mentioned protocols in many chapters, namely Traumatic Brain Injury and Stroke.) Perhaps oxygen therapy for MS has the best data so far. Much of this began with the 1983 *New England Journal of Medicine* article by Drs. Fischer, Marks, and Reich in a controlled study of MS patients (Fischer 1983). Based on this, Dr. James and his team initiated a national charity for MS to permit MS patients to have HBOT in their community safely and for minimal costs through the use of volunteers. There are more than sixty centres are around the United Kingdom, Ireland, Jersey, and Gibraltar.

To date, the national charity centres have done more than 3.5 million treatments over thirty-six years without a single significant mishap. In 2018 I spoke at the annual meeting of this group held at Warwick University. Many people attending have stabilized or improved their MS with weekly HBOT treatments safely run by trained volunteers. Some have done this for over thirty years as Professor James initiated this program thirty-six years ago. I have visited three of these centres and have had oxygen therapy numerous times. I am convinced this has slowed my MS disease progression. To date, I have done more than 350 such treatments. I also use HBOT for treating my migraine/cluster headaches, which usually resolve quickly in the chamber. If HBOT is unavailable, I use a rebreathing mask and 12 L/min of oxygen flow from an oxygen concentrator for an hour a day preferably with exercise.

The general protocol listed at the end of chapter 21 (Stroke) is an excellent one to follow for almost all brain issues. It does not go above two atmospheres, so it is exceedingly safe. If mechanisms of HBOT on the brain is your passion, read the following article "Effect of hyperbaric oxygenation on brain hemodynamics, hemoglobin oxygenation and mitochondrial NADH" (Meirovithz 2007). One of my favourite articles is on how HBOT induces antioxidant gene expression (Godman 2010). We now know additional oxygen can enhance over 8000 of our genes. I appreciate this positive effect every time I do another of my weekly sessions.The short story is that a modest increase of 50 to 100% over normal pressure, with oxygen delivered by mask or hood, can make a great difference. If you are unable to access oxygen under pressure, then purchase an oxygen concentrator as discussed in the oxygen therapy chapter.

I use 28% oxygen overnight most nights and this improves my rest and mental clarity in the morning. I do this with nasal prongs. In addition, I do at least one session of oxygen under pressure at 1.5 to 2.0 atmospheres absolute. People at sea level live at 1.0 atmospheres of pressure, so this is a modest increase in pressure. You have likely experienced the same pressure difference if you have travelled on a commercial airliner.

Perhaps Edward Teller, the world-famous physicist, said it best in his letter to the *Journal of American Physicians and Surgeons in 2003* :

On Hyperbaric Oxygenation

Dr. Richard Neubauer of Lauderdale-by-the-Sea, Florida, has explained to me that the time has come to make hyperbaric oxygenation [see pp. 117–120] more available and to obtain scientific approval and third-party reimbursement. Reviewing the literature that he has sent me, I find that this modality is unequivocally of potential value in acute anoxic states. Certainly, carbon monoxide and cyanide poisoning have been accepted indications for a number of years, but the value of hyperbaric oxygenation in other anoxic situations has been shown in animal studies. In acute ischemic stroke, treatment with hyperbaric oxygenation within the first four hours reduces morbidity and mortality significantly. Benefits have also been shown in traumatic brain injury. There is a scarcity of chambers to handle these situations and a serious lack of knowledge among professionals concerning indications and dosage.

Functional brain imaging after hyper- baric oxygenation clearly demonstrates varying degrees of recoverable brain function in many patients suffering the chronic sequelae of stroke, traumatic brain injury, or anoxic encephalopathy. Cost savings even from late utilization of hyperbaric oxygenation could be substantial.

I would like to comment on two issues from personal experience.

I had a stroke a number of years ago, and Dr. Neubauer made a chamber available to me. Although I may have recovered from the stroke spontaneously, I feel that the pressurized oxygen gave me every advantage. I have had this chamber for more than 6 years. I take six treatments per week at 1.35 atmospheres absolute (ATA) for one hour each and have had more than 3,000 exposures. I am 95 years old and work five days a week doing research, lecturing, and writing papers. Oxygen toxicity has never been a problem. I suggest investigation of the effectiveness of this procedure in permitting scientists or executives to maintain whatever mental acuity they have, using neuropsychologic and intelligence testing as well as functional brain imaging. I understand that Dr. Neubauer and Clark Kirk, Sr., began a project with this hypothesis in 1972. Psychological studies have shown a transient rise in the intelligence quotient (IQ), which seems to fall off after a period of time. I have not given it the opportunity to wear off. Whether I would be as mentally alert without this treatment I am not sure, but I would be hesitant to stop my daily sessions.

A totally unexplored area with which I have personal experience requires extensive investigation. This is the application of hyperbaric oxygenation in chronic obstructive pulmonary disease. My wife of many years suffered from this, and when the chamber was installed in my home, she was bedridden and severely emaciated. Her pulmonologist expected her to die within two months. Drs. Richard Neubauer and William Maxfield suggested supplemental oxygenation at very low pressures of 1.1-1.25 ATA for 20 minutes twice a day. This was indeed helpful. Mici became more alert, began to gain weight, and no longer needed constant supplemental oxygen, although she did use oxygen at night. The pressure was gradually increased to 1.35 ATA for 40 minutes twice a day. Mici gained 35 pounds and became bright, alert, and ambulatory. If the technician missed a single treatment, she would deteriorate. She had five wonderful unexpected years. One hopes that home chambers may become readily available.

I also wish to comment on the overwhelming evidence of the effectiveness of hyperbaric oxygenation in cerebral palsy and the brain-injured child. Reproducibility of results from around the world is compelling. Although double-blind cross-over controlled studies are the standard of the scientific community, effectiveness has been demonstrated by Dr. Neubauer and a number of others, using each patient as his own control, and documented by sequential functional brain imaging. Experience is such that a double-blind study may be immoral.

In the long-term history of hyperbaric oxygenation, many of the problems have resulted from inappropriate pressures and treatment protocols. The proper dose in many conditions has not been fully ascertained and may vary as does insulin dose in a diabetic. I feel that the lower-pressure protocol and use of functional brain imaging will eventually make hyperbaric oxygenation a standard treatment.

Edward Teller, Ph.D. (1908-2003)
July 9, 2003 *Journal of American Physicians and Surgeons*

Epilogue

In this book, I have attempted to empower you to improve your health, especially your brain health. I have concentrated on brain recovery for two reasons:

- I have my own brain challenges, with MS, migraines, and depression.
- The brain is missed, left out, or stated to have no recovery options. This is not true.

The brain has a few key issues to solve to maintain or recover brain health. These are oxygen, circulation (venous and arterial), and associated gut-brain interactions. Because the gut bacteria influence brain health and the health of the entire body, it is important to choose options that promote the health of the gut microbiota.

The secrets to gut health and, therefore, brain health are primarily in what you eat, breathe, and drink. The first secret is to minimize toxic inputs by eating mainly organic foods, breathing clean air, drinking pure water, and minimizing electronic smog (EMF). The second secret is to eat the best quality and variety of whole, fresh foods that you can. Aim for 50 different foods per week. This will improve the variety and number of microbes in your gut. Furthermore, if you have a significant health challenge, then add supplements appropriately.

This book contains many tips and suggestions based on in-depth research, evidence in the literature, and experience working with clients. Select those that you feel may be useful. It may take two to three months of consistent effort with any therapy before you feel the benefits. Remember, your body strives to heal itself, so provide the therapeutic elements, be proactive, be consistent, and be patient, and you will be on your way to winning the brain game.

In my personal journey, many of the pieces of the puzzle have helped me—certainly some more than others—but this is where an individual's genetic makeup and environmental circumstances are unique. If I had to choose a single piece of the puzzle beyond the obvious nutrition piece, I would choose oxygen therapy. I don't believe I could have written this book without the over 350 hyperbaric oxygenation sessions I have gone through over the last three years.

Bibliography

A Better Route to High Dosage Without Psychoactivity ... Accessed May 12, 2018. http://www.bing.com/cr?IG=65BACF554D74483AA1F66A6368D01E96& CID=0B27C562DC786E6514EFCE8CDDD76F74&rd=1&h=uiJi5DPGOs_hWW- fhYvFT5BlD8d_sjMzgjsZwWkpHHOc&v=1&r=http://www.beyondthc.com/ wp-content/uploads/2013/03/Juicing-33.pdf&p=DevEx.LB.1,5555.1.

Abel, Ernest L. *Marihuana: The First Twelve Thousand Years*. Springer Science Business Media, 2014.

Abrams, D. I., H. P. Vizoso, S. B. Shade, C. Jay, M. E. Kelly, and N. L. Benowitz. "Vaporization as a Smokeless Cannabis Delivery System: A Pilot Study." *Clinical Pharmacology & Therapeutics*82, no. 5 (2007): 572-78. doi:10.1038/sj.clpt.6100200.

Abrams, D. I., P. Couey, S. B. Shade, M. E. Kelly, and N. L. Benowitz. "Cannabinoid-Opioid Interaction in Chronic Pain." *Clinical Pharmacology & Therapeutics*90, no. 6 (2011): 844-51. doi:10.1038/clpt.2011.188.

Abrams, Donald I., and Andrew Weil. *Integrative Oncology*. Oxford: Oxford University Press, 2014.

Aggarwal, Sunil K. "Cannabinergic Pain Medicine." *The Clinical Journal of Pain*29, no. 2 (2013): 162-71. doi:10.1097/ajp.0b013e31824c5e4c.

Ahern, Shauna James. *Gluten-free Girl: How I Found the Food That Loves Me Back - & How You Can Too*. Wiley, 2009.

Alexander, Dominik D., Paige E. Miller, Mary E. Van Elswyk, Connye N. Kuratko, and Lauren C. Bylsma. "A Meta-Analysis of Randomized Controlled Trials and Prospective Cohort Studies of

Eicosapentaenoic and Docosahexaenoic Long-Chain Omega-3 Fatty Acids and Coronary Heart Disease Risk." *Mayo Clinic Proceedings*92, no. 1 (2017): 15-29. doi:10.1016/j.mayocp.2016.10.018.

Alexander, J. S., R. Chervenak, B. Weinstock-Guttman, I. Tsunoda, M. Ramanathan, N. Martinez, S. Omura, F. Sato, G. V. Chaitanya, A. Minagar, J. Mcgee, M.h. Jennings, C. Monceaux, F. Becker, U. Cvek, M. Trutschl, and R. Zivadinov. "Blood Circulating Microparticle Species in Relapsing–remitting and Secondary Progressive Multiple Sclerosis. A Case–control, Cross Sectional Study with Conventional MRI and Advanced Iron Content Imaging Outcomes." *Journal of the Neurological Sciences*355, no. 1-2 (2015): 84-89. doi:10.1016/j.jns.2015.05.027.

Allan, Julia L., David Mcminn, and Michael Daly. "A Bidirectional Relationship between Executive Function and Health Behavior: Evidence, Implications, and Future Directions." *Frontiers in Neuroscience*10 (2016). doi:10.3389/fnins.2016.00386.

Alpini, D. C., P. M. Bavera, A. Hahn, and V. Mattei. "Chronic Cerebrospinal Venous Insufficiency (CCSVI) IN Meniere Disease. Case or Cause?" *ScienceMED*4, no. 1 (2013): 9-15.

Amar, Mohamed Ben, and Stéphane Potvin. "Cannabis and Psychosis: What Is the Link?" *Journal of Psychoactive Drugs*39, no. 2 (2007): 131-42. doi:10.1080/02791072.2007.10399871.

Amminger, G. Paul, Miriam R. Schäfer, Konstantinos Papageorgiou, Claudia M. Klier, Sue M. Cotton, Susan M. Harrigan, Andrew Mackinnon, Patrick D. Mcgorry, and Gregor E. Berger. "Long-Chain ω-3 Fatty Acids for Indicated Prevention of Psychotic Disorders." *Archives of General Psychiatry*67, no. 2 (2010): 146. doi:10.1001/archgenpsychiatry.2009.192.

Anand, Praveen, Garth Whiteside, Christopher J. Fowler, and Andrea G. Hohmann. "Targeting CB2 Receptors and the Endocannabinoid System for the Treatment of Pain." *Brain Research Reviews*60, no. 1 (2009): 255-66. doi:10.1016/j.brainresrev.2008.12.003.

Andreae, Michael H., George M. Carter, Naum Shaparin, Kathryn Suslov, Ronald J. Ellis, Mark A. Ware, Donald I. Abrams, Hannah Prasad, Barth Wilsey, Debbie Indyk, Matthew Johnson, and Henry S. Sacks. "Inhaled Cannabis for Chronic Neuropathic Pain: A Meta-analysis of Individual Patient Data." *The Journal of Pain*16, no. 12 (2015): 1221-232. doi:10.1016/j.jpain.2015.07.009.

Arany, Praveen R. "Special Issue on Stem Cells and Photobiomodulation Therapy." *Photomedicine and Laser Surgery*34, no. 11 (2016): 495-96. doi:10.1089/pho.2016.4216.

Arata, M., and Z. Sternberg. "Neuroendocrine Responses to Transvascular Autonomic Modulation: A Modified Balloon Angioplasty in Multiple Sclerosis Patients." *Hormone and Metabolic Research*48, no. 02 (2015): 123-29. doi:10.1055/s-0035-1547235.

Artuch, Rafael, Gloria Brea-Calvo, Paz Briones, Asunción Aracil, Marta Galván, Carmen Espinós, Jordi Corral, Victor Volpini, Antonia Ribes, Antoni L. Andreu, Francesc Palau, José A. Sánchez-Alcázar, Plácido Navas, and Mercè Pineda. "Cerebellar Ataxia with Coenzyme Q10 Deficiency: Diagnosis and Follow-up after Coenzyme Q10 Supplementation." *Journal of the Neurological Sciences*246, no. 1-2 (2006): 153-58. doi:10.1016/j.jns.2006.01.021.

Atamna, Hani, Justin Newberry, Ronit Erlitzki, Carla S. Schultz, and Bruce N. Ames. "Biotin Deficiency Inhibits Heme Synthesis and Impairs Mitochondria in Human Lung Fibroblasts." *The Journal of Nutrition*137, no. 1 (2007): 25-30. doi:10.1093/jn/137.1.25.

Bab, I., O. Ofek, J. Tam, J. Rehnelt, and A. Zimmer. "Endocannabinoids and the Regulation of Bone Metabolism." *Journal of Neuroendocrinology*20, no. S1 (2008): 69-74. doi:10.1111/j.1365-2826.2008.01675.x.

Bachhuber, Marcus A., Brendan Saloner, Chinazo O. Cunningham, and Colleen L. Barry. "Medical Cannabis Laws and Opioid Analgesic Overdose Mortality in the United States, 1999-2010." *JAMA Internal Medicine*174, no. 10 (2014): 1668. doi:10.1001/jamainternmed.2014.4005.

Bahi, Amine, Shamma Al Mansouri, Elyazia Al Memari, Mouza Al Ameri, Syed M. Nurulain, and Shreesh Ojha. "β-Caryophyllene, a CB2 Receptor Agonist Produces Multiple Behavioral Changes Relevant to Anxiety and Depression in Mice." *Physiology & Behavior*135 (2014): 119-24. doi:10.1016/j.physbeh.2014.06.003.

Baker, David, Gareth Pryce, Gavin Giovannoni, and Alan J. Thompson. "The Therapeutic Potential of Cannabis." *The Lancet Neurology*2, no. 5 (2003): 291-98. doi:10.1016/s1474-4422(03)00381-8.

Bambico, F. R., N. Katz, G. Debonnel, and G. Gobbi. "Cannabinoids Elicit Antidepressant-Like Behavior and Activate Serotonergic Neurons through the Medial Prefrontal Cortex." *Journal of Neuroscience*27, no. 43 (2007): 11700-1711. doi:10.1523/jneurosci.1636-07.2007.

Barody, T. "Fecal Microbiota Transplantation (FMT) in Multiple Sclerosis (MS)." *Am J Gastroenterol*106:S352.

Bartholomew, Mel. *Square Foot Gardening*. Emmaus, PA: Rodale Press, 1981.

Bartzokis, George, Po H. Lu, Kathleen Tingus, Douglas G. Peters, Chetan P. Amar, Todd A. Tishler, J. Paul Finn, Pablo Villablanca, Lori L. Altshuler, Jim Mintz, Elizabeth Neely, and James R. Connor. "Gender and Iron Genes May Modify Associations Between Brain Iron and Memory in Healthy Aging." *Neuropsychopharmacology*36, no. 7 (2011): 1375-384. doi:10.1038/npp.2011.22.

Beaulieu, Pierre. "Cannabinoids for Postoperative Pain." *Anesthesiology*106, no. 2 (2007): 397. doi:10.1097/00000542-200702000-00028.

Beggs, Clive B., Alessia Giaquinta, Massimiliano Veroux, Ester De Marco, Dovile Mociskyte, and Pierfrancesco Veroux. "Mid-term Sustained Relief from Headaches after Balloon Angioplasty of the Internal Jugular Veins in Patients with Multiple Sclerosis." *Plos One*13, no. 1 (2018). doi:10.1371/journal.pone.0191534.

Bendsen, N. T., R. Christensen, E. M. Bartels, and A. Astrup. "Consumption of industrial and ruminant trans fatty acids and risk of coronary heart disease: a systematic review and meta-analysis of cohort studies." *European Journal of Clinical Nutrition*65, no. 7 (2011): 773-83. doi:10.1038/ejcn.2011.34.

Bennett, Michael H., Christopher French, Alexander Schnabel, Jason Wasiak, Peter Kranke, and Stephanie Weibel. "Normobaric and Hyperbaric Oxygen Therapy for the Treatment and Prevention of Migraine and Cluster Headache." *Cochrane Database of Systematic Reviews*, 2015. doi:10.1002/14651858.cd005219.pub3.

Bennett, Michael H., Jan P. Lehm, and Nigel Jepson. "Hyperbaric Oxygen Therapy for Acute Coronary Syndrome." *Cochrane Database of Systematic Reviews*, 2015. doi:10.1002/14651858.cd004818.pub4.

Berer, Kerstin, Lisa Ann Gerdes, Egle Cekanaviciute, Xiaoming Jia, Liang Xiao, Zhongkui Xia, Chuan Liu, Luisa Klotz, Uta Stauffer, Sergio E. Baranzini, Tania Kümpfel, Reinhard Hohlfeld, Gurumoorthy Krishnamoorthy, and Hartmut Wekerle. "Gut Microbiota from Multiple Sclerosis Patients Enables Spontaneous Autoimmune Encephalomyelitis in Mice."

Proceedings of the National Academy of Sciences114, no. 40 (2017): 10719-0724. doi:10.1073/pnas.1711233114.

Bergamaschi, Mateus M., Regina Helena Costa Queiroz, Marcos Hortes Nisihara Chagas, Danielle Chaves Gomes De Oliveira, Bruno Spinosa De Martinis, Flávio Kapczinski, João Quevedo, Rafael Roesler, Nadja Schröder, Antonio E. Nardi, Rocio Martín-Santos, Jaime Eduardo Cecílio Hallak, Antonio Waldo Zuardi, and José Alexandre S Crippa. "Cannabidiol Reduces the Anxiety Induced by Simulated Public Speaking in Treatment-Naïve Social Phobia Patients." Neuropsychopharmacology36, no. 6 (2011): 1219-226. doi:10.1038/npp.2011.6.

Biesiekierski, Jessica R., Simone L. Peters, Evan D. Newnham, Ourania Rosella, Jane G. Muir, and Peter R. Gibson. "No Effects of Gluten in Patients with Self-Reported Non-Celiac Gluten Sensitivity After Dietary Reduction of Fermentable, Poorly Absorbed, Short-Chain Carbohydrates." Gastroenterology145, no. 2 (2013). doi:10.1053/j.gastro.2013.04.051.

Billinger, Michael, Markus Schwerzmann, Wilhelm Rutishauser, Andreas Wahl, Stephan Windecker, Bernhard Meier, and Christian Seiler. "Patent Foramen Ovale Screening by Ear Oximetry in Divers." The American Journal of Cardiology111, no. 2 (2013): 286-90. doi:10.1016/j.amjcard.2012.09.030.

Blanco, Nathaniel J., W. Todd Maddox, and Francisco Gonzalez-Lima. "Improving Executive Function Using Transcranial Infrared Laser Stimulation." Journal of Neuropsychology11, no. 1 (2015): 14-25. doi:10.1111/jnp.12074.

Bolay, Hayrunnisa, Uwe Reuter, Andrew K. Dunn, Zhihong Huang, David A. Boas, and Michael A. Moskowitz. "Intrinsic brain activity triggers trigeminal meningeal afferents in a migraine model." Nature Medicine8, no. 2 (2002): 136-42. doi:10.1038/nm0202-136.

Boldt, Ethan. "Liver Cleanse: Detox Your Liver in 6 Easy Steps." Dr. Axe. December 06, 2017. Accessed December 24, 2017. https://draxe.com/liver-cleanse/.

Booven, Derek Van, Sharon Marsh, Howard Mcleod, Michelle Whirl Carrillo, Katrin Sangkuhl, Teri E. Klein, and Russ B. Altman. "Cytochrome P450 2C9-CYP2C9." Pharmacogenetics and Genomics, 2010, 1. doi:10.1097/fpc.0b013e3283349e84.

Borgelt, Laura M., Kari L. Franson, Abraham M. Nussbaum, and George S. Wang. "The Pharmacologic and Clinical Effects of Medical Cannabis."

*Pharmacotherapy: The Journal of Human Pharmacology and Drug Therapy*33, no. 2 (2013): 195-209. doi:10.1002/phar.1187.

Borody, Thomas J., and Alexander Khoruts. "Fecal Microbiota Transplantation and Emerging Applications." *Nature Reviews Gastroenterology & Hepatology*9, no. 2 (2011): 88-96. doi:10.1038/nrgastro.2011.244.

Bounous, G., P. A. Kongshavn, and P. Gold. "The Immunoenhancing Property of Dietary Whey Protein Concentrate." *Clin Invest Med*11, no. 4 (August 1988): 271-78.

Brady, C. M., R. Dasgupta, C. Dalton, O. J. Wiseman, K. J. Berkley, and C. J. Fowler. "An Open-label Pilot Study of Cannabis-based Extracts for Bladder Dysfunction in Advanced Multiple Sclerosis." *Multiple Sclerosis Journal*10, no. 4 (2004): 425-33. doi:10.1191/1352458504ms1063oa.

Brandt, Eric J., Rebecca Myerson, Marcelo Coca Perraillon, and Tamar S. Polonsky. "Hospital Admissions for Myocardial Infarction and Stroke Before and After the Trans-Fatty Acid Restrictions in New York." *JAMA Cardiology*2, no. 6 (2017): 627. doi:10.1001/jamacardio.2017.0491.

Branton, W. G., J. Q. Lu, M. G. Surette, R. A. Holt, J. Lind, J. D. Laman, and C. Power. "Brain microbiota disruption within inflammatory demyelinating lesions in multiple sclerosis." *Scientific Reports*6, no. 1 (2016). doi:10.1038/srep37344.

Bredesen, Dale E. "Reversal of Cognitive Decline: A Novel Therapeutic Program." *Aging*6, no. 9 (2014): 707-17. doi:10.18632/aging.100690.

Bredesen, Dale E., and Joe LeMonnier. *The End of Alzheimer's: The First Program to Prevent and Reverse Cognitive Decline*. Waterville, ME: Thorndike Press, A Part of Gale, a Cengage Company, 2017.

Brewster, Kerry. "Sydney Doctor Claims Poo Transplants Curing Diseases." ABC News. March 19, 2014. Accessed December 1, 2017. http://www.abc.net.au/news/2014-03-18/sydney-doctor-claims-poo-transplants-curing-diseases/5329836.

Brogan, Kelly, MD. *A Mind of Your Own: The Truth About Depression and How Women Can Heal Their Bodies to Reclaim Their Lives*. Harperwave, 2017.

Brown, Kirsty, Daniella Decoffe, Erin Molcan, and Deanna L. Gibson. "Diet-Induced Dysbiosis of the Intestinal Microbiota and the Effects on Immunity and Disease." *Nutrients*4, no. 12 (2012): 1095-119. doi:10.3390/nu4081095.

Brownstein, David. *Overcoming Thyroid Disorders*. West Bloomfield, MI.: Medical Alternatives Press, 2008.

Brundin, Lena, Maria Björkqvist, Åsa Petersén, and Lil Träskman-Bendz. "Reduced orexin levels in the cerebrospinal fluid of suicidal patients with major depressive disorder." *European Neuropsychopharmacology*17, no. 9 (2007): 573-79. doi:10.1016/j.euroneuro.2007.01.005.

Bruno, Aldo, Luigi Califano, Diego Mastrangelo, Marcella De Vizia, Benedetto Bernardo, and Francesca Salafia. "Chronic Cerebrospinal Venous Insufficiency in Ménière's Disease: Diagnosis and Treatment." *Veins and Lymphatics*3, no. 3 (2014). doi:10.4081/vl.2014.3854.

Burks, Jack S., and Kenneth P. Johnson. *Multiple Sclerosis: Diagnosis, Medical Management, and Rehabilitation*. New York: Demos, 2000.

Burstein, Sumner H. "The Cannabinoid Acids." *Pharmacology & Therapeutics*82, no. 1 (1999): 87-96. doi:10.1016/s0163-7258(98)00069-2.

Campbell, V. A., and A. Gowran. "Alzheimer's Disease; Taking the Edge off with Cannabinoids?" *British Journal of Pharmacology*152, no. 5 (2009): 655-62. doi:10.1038/sj.bjp.0707446.

Capkun, Gorana, Frank Dahlke, Raquel Lahoz, Beth Nordstrom, Hugh H. Tilson, Gary Cutter, Dorina Bischof, Alan Moore, Jason Simeone, Kathy Fraeman, Fabrice Bancken, Yvonne Geissbühler, Michael Wagner, and Stanley Cohan. "Mortality and Comorbidities in Patients with Multiple Sclerosis Compared with a Population without Multiple Sclerosis: An Observational Study Using the US Department of Defense Administrative Claims Database." *Multiple Sclerosis and Related Disorders*4, no. 6 (2015): 546-54. doi:10.1016/j.msard.2015.08.005.

Carlini, Elisaldo A., and Jomar M. Cunha. "Hypnotic and Antiepileptic Effects of Cannabidiol." *The Journal of Clinical Pharmacology*21, no. S1 (1981). doi:10.1002/j.1552-4604.1981.tb02622.x.

Carlsson, Cynthia M. "Lowering homocysteine for stroke prevention." *The Lancet*369, no. 9576 (2007): 1841-842. doi:10.1016/s0140-6736(07)60830-7.

Carpenter, D., and C. Sage. "BioInitiative Report: A Rationale for a Biologically-based Public Exposure Standard for Electromagnetic Fields (ELF and RF)." The BioInitiative Report. 2012. http://www.bioinitiative.org/.

Carroccio, Antonio, Giovambattista Rini, and Pasquale Mansueto. "Non-Celiac Wheat Sensitivity Is a More Appropriate Label Than

Non-Celiac Gluten Sensitivity." *Gastroenterology*146, no. 1 (2014): 320-21. doi:10.1053/j.gastro.2013.08.061.

Carroll, C. B., P. G. Bain, L. Teare, X. Liu, C. Joint, C. Wroath, S. G. Parkin, P. Fox, D. Wright, J. Hobart, and J. P. Zajicek. "Cannabis for Dyskinesia in Parkinson Disease: A Randomized Double-blind Crossover Study." *Neurology*63, no. 7 (2004): 1245-250. doi:10.1212/01.wnl.0000140288.48796.8e.

Carter, G. T., P. Weydt, M. Kyashna-Tocha, and D. I. Abrams. "Medicinal Cannabis: Rational Guidelines for Dosing." IDrugs: The Investigational Drugs Journal. May 2004. Accessed April 25, 2018. https://www.ncbi.nlm.nih.gov/pubmed/15154108.

Carter, Gregory T., Mary E. Abood, Sunil K. Aggarwal, and Michael D. Weiss. "Cannabis and Amyotrophic Lateral Sclerosis: Hypothetical and Practical Applications, and a Call for Clinical Trials." *American Journal of Hospice and Palliative Medicine*®27, no. 5 (2010): 347-56. doi:10.1177/1049909110369531.

Centonze, D., M. Bari, B. Di Michele, S. Rossi, V. Gasperi, A. Pasini, N. Battista, G. Bernardi, P. Curatolo, and M. Maccarrone. "Altered Anandamide Degradation in Attention-Deficit/hyperactivity Disorder." *Neurology*72, no. 17 (2009): 1526-527. doi:10.1212/wnl.0b013e3181a2e8f6.

Cersosimo, Maria G., and Eduardo E. Benarroch. "Neural Control of the Gastrointestinal Tract: Implications for Parkinson Disease." *Movement Disorders*23, no. 8 (2008): 1065-075. doi:10.1002/mds.22051.

Chow, Roberta T., Gillian Z. Heller, and Les Barnsley. "The Effect of 300 MW, 830 Nm Laser on Chronic Neck Pain: A Double-blind, Randomized, Placebo-controlled Study." *Pain*124, no. 1 (2006): 201-10. doi:10.1016/j.pain.2006.05.018.

Christiansen, Christian Fynbo, Steffen Christensen, Dóra Körmendiné Farkas, Montserrat Miret, Henrik Toft Sørensen, and Lars Pedersen. "Risk of Arterial Cardiovascular Diseases in Patients with Multiple Sclerosis: A Population-Based Cohort Study." *Neuroepidemiology*35, no. 4 (2010): 267-74. doi:10.1159/000320245.

Cichewicz, Diana L. "Synergistic Interactions between Cannabinoid and Opioid Analgesics." *Life Sciences*74, no. 11 (2004): 1317-324. doi:10.1016/j.lfs.2003.09.038.

Cichewicz, Diana L., Victoria L. Haller, and Sandra P. Welch. "Changes in Opioid and Cannabinoid Receptor Protein following Short-Term Combination Treatment with Δ9-Tetrahydrocannabinol and Morphine." Journal of Pharmacology and Experimental Therapeutics. April 01, 2001. Accessed April 25, 2018. http://jpet.aspetjournals.org/content/297/1/121.

Claire Hodges' Account - Marihuana and Multiple Sclerosis. Accessed May 01, 2018. http://rxmarijuana.com/Hodges.htm.

Clapp, Megan, Nadia Aurora, Lindsey Herrera, Manisha Bhatia, Emily Wilen, and Sarah Wakefield. "Gut Microbiota's Effect on Mental Health: The Gut-brain Axis." *Clinics and Practice*7, no. 4 (2017). doi:10.4081/cp.2017.987.

Cline, John C. "Nutritional Aspects of Detoxification in Clinical Practice." *Alternative Therapies*, May 2015, 54-62.

Cline, John, and Patrick Grant. *Detoxify for Life: How Toxins Are Robbing You of Your Health and What You Can Do about It*. Stockton, CA: More Heart than Talent Pub., 2008.

Code, Bill, and Claudia Tiefisher. *Youth Renewed: A Common Sense Approach to Vibrant Health . . . at Any Age*. Calgary: Chameleon Publishing & Graphics, 2000.

Code, Bill, and Denise Code. *Winning the Pain Game: The Surprising Discoveries of a Pain Relief Doctor in His Research to Relieve His Chronic Pain*. Malibu, CA: Words of Wisdom Press, 2007.

Code, W. "NSAIDs and Balanced Analgesia." *Canadian Journal of Anaesthesia*40, no. 5 (1993): 401-05. doi:10.1007/bf03009506.

Code, William E. *Non-opiate Centrally Acting Analgesics: Scientific programme: 11th World Congress of Anaesthesiologists, 14-20 April 1996, Sydney, Australia*. London: World Federation of Societies of Anaesthesiologists, 1996.

Code, William E., and Denise Code. *Who's in Control of Your Multiple Sclerosis?* Montréal: Songlines Health Products, 2005.

Code, William E., Raymond W. Yip, Michael E. Rooney, Philip M. Browne, and Tomas Hertz. "Preoperative naproxen sodium reduces postoperative pain following arthroscopic knee surgery." *Canadian Journal of Anaesthesia*41, no. 2 (1994): 98-101. doi:10.1007/bf03009799.

Cohen, Anna S., Brian Burns, and Peter J. Goadsby. "High-Flow Oxygen for Treatment of Cluster Headache." *Jama*302, no. 22 (2009): 2451. doi:10.1001/jama.2009.1855.

Colasanti, Brenda K. "A Comparison of the Ocular and Central Effects of Δ9-Tetrahydrocannabinol and Cannabigerol." *Journal of Ocular Pharmacology and Therapeutics*6, no. 4 (1990): 259-69. doi:10.1089/jop.1990.6.259.

Coleman, Eliot. *Four-season Harvest: Organic Vegetables from Your Home Garden All Year Long*. White River Junction, VT: Chelsea Green Publishing, 1999.

Collin, C., P. Davies, I. K. Mutiboko, and S. Ratcliffe. "Randomized Controlled Trial of Cannabis-based Medicine in Spasticity Caused by Multiple Sclerosis." *European Journal of Neurology*14, no. 3 (2007): 290-96. doi:10.1111/j.1468-1331.2006.01639.x.

Commissioner, Office Of the. "Press Announcements - FDA Issues Final Rule on Safety and Effectiveness of Antibacterial Soaps." U S Food and Drug Administration Home Page. Accessed May 13, 2018. https://www.fda.gov/NewsEvents/Newsroom/PressAnnouncements/ucm517478.htm.

Consroe, Paul, Reuven Sandyk, and Stuart R. Snider. "Open Label Evaluation of Cannabidiol in Dystonic Movement Disorders." *International Journal of Neuroscience*30, no. 4 (1986): 277-82. doi:10.3109/00207458608985678.

Cook, Marc D., Jacob M. Allen, Brandt D. Pence, Matthew A. Wallig, H. Rex Gaskins, Bryan A. White, and Jeffrey A. Woods. "Exercise and Gut Immune Function: Evidence of Alterations in Colon Immune Cell Homeostasis and Microbiome Characteristics with Exercise Training." *Immunology and Cell Biology*94, no. 2 (2015): 158-63. doi:10.1038/icb.2015.108.

Cook, Michelle Schoffro. *The brain wash: a powerful, all-natural program to protect your brain against Alzheimer's, chronic fatigue syndrome, depression, Parkinson's, and other diseases*. Mississauga, Ont.: J. Wiley & Sons Canada, 2007.

Corey-Bloom, J., T. Wolfson, A. Gamst, S. Jin, T. D. Marcotte, H. Bentley, and B. Gouaux. "Smoked Cannabis for Spasticity in Multiple Sclerosis: A Randomized, Placebo-controlled Trial." *Canadian Medical Association Journal*184, no. 10 (2012): 1143-150. doi:10.1503/cmaj.110837.

Corrigan, F. M., C. L. Wienburg, S. E. Daniel, and D. Mann. "Organochlorine Insecticides In Substantia Nigra In Parkinsons Disease."

*Journal of Toxicology and Environmental Health, Part A*59, no. 4 (2000): 229-34. doi:10.1080/009841000156907.

Crane, Paul K., Rod Walker, Rebecca A. Hubbard, Ge Li, David M. Nathan, Hui Zheng, Sebastien Haneuse, Suzanne Craft, Thomas J. Montine, Steven E. Kahn, Wayne Mccormick, Susan M. Mccurry, James D. Bowen, and Eric B. Larson. "Glucose Levels and Risk of Dementia." *New England Journal of Medicine*369, no. 6 (2013): 540-48. doi:10.1056/nejmoa1215740.

Crippa, José Alexandre S, Guilherme Nogueira Derenusson, Thiago Borduqui Ferrari, Lauro Wichert-Ana, Fábio Ls Duran, Rocio Martin-Santos, Marcus Vinícius Simões, Sagnik Bhattacharyya, Paolo Fusar-Poli, Zerrin Atakan, Alaor Santos Filho, Maria Cecília Freitas-Ferrari, Philip K. Mcguire, Antonio Waldo Zuardi, Geraldo F. Busatto, and Jaime Eduardo Cecílio Hallak. "Neural Basis of Anxiolytic Effects of Cannabidiol (CBD) in Generalized Social Anxiety Disorder: A Preliminary Report." *Journal of Psychopharmacology*25, no. 1 (2010): 121-30. doi:10.1177/0269881110379283.

Cruz, Rogério Santos De Oliveira, Rafael Alves De Aguiar, Tiago Turnes, Rafael Penteado Dos Santos, Mariana Fernandes Mendes De Oliveira, and Fabrizio Caputo. "Intracellular Shuttle: The Lactate Aerobic Metabolism." *The Scientific World Journal*2012 (2012): 1-8. doi:10.1100/2012/420984.

Currais, Antonio, Oswald Quehenberger, Aaron M. Armando, Daniel Daugherty, Pam Maher, and David Schubert. "Amyloid Proteotoxicity Initiates an Inflammatory Response Blocked by Cannabinoids." *Npj Aging and Mechanisms of Disease*2, no. 1 (2016). doi:10.1038/npjamd.2016.12.

Czapp, Katherine. "Magnificent Magnesium." The Weston A. Price Foundation. September 23, 2010. Accessed May 15, 2017. https://www.westonaprice.org/health-topics/abcs-of-nutrition/magnificent-magnesium/.

Dal-Bianco, Assunta, Simon Hametner, Günther Grabner, Melanie Schernthaner, Claudia Kronnerwetter, Andreas Reitner, Clemens Vass, Karl Kircher, Eduard Auff, Fritz Leutmezer, Karl Vass, and Siegfried Trattnig. "Veins in Plaques of Multiple Sclerosis Patients – a Longitudinal Magnetic Resonance Imaging Study at 7 Tesla." *European Radiology*25, no. 10 (2015): 2913-920. doi:10.1007/s00330-015-3719-y.

Daniel, E., and E. P. Ryan. *The Molecular Basis of Plant Genetic Diversity.* InTech, 2012.

Das, Ravi K., Sunjeev K. Kamboj, Mayurun Ramadas, Kishoj Yogan, Vivek Gupta, Emily Redman, H. Valerie Curran, and Celia J. A. Morgan.

"Cannabidiol Enhances Consolidation of Explicit Fear Extinction in Humans." *Psychopharmacology*226, no. 4 (2013): 781-92. doi:10.1007/s00213-012-2955-y.

Dashti, Hussein M., Thazhumpal C. Mathew, Mousa Khadada, Mahdi Al-Mousawi, Husain Talib, Sami K. Asfar, Abdulla I. Behbahani, and Naji S. Al-Zaid. "Beneficial effects of ketogenic diet in obese diabetic subjects." *Molecular and Cellular Biochemistry*302, no. 1-2 (2007): 249-56. doi:10.1007/s11010-007-9448-z.

Daulatzai, Mak Adam. "Obesity and Gut's Dysbiosis Promote Neuroinflammation, Cognitive Impairment, and Vulnerability to Alzheimer's Disease: New Directions and Therapeutic Implications." *Journal of Molecular and Genetic Medicine*S1, no. 01 (2014). doi:10.4172/1747-0862.s1-005.

Davies, Andrew L., Roshni A. Desai, Peter S. Bloomfield, Peter R. Mcintosh, Katie J. Chapple, Christopher Linington, Richard Fairless, Ricarda Diem, Marianne Kasti, Michael P. Murphy, and Kenneth J. Smith. "Neurological deficits caused by tissue hypoxia in neuroinflammatory disease." *Annals of Neurology*74, no. 6 (2013): 815-25. doi:10.1002/ana.24006.

Davis, William. *Wheat Belly*. Harper-Collins, 2012.

Dawodu, Segun T., and Denise I. Campagnolo. "Traumatic Brain Injury (TBI) - Definition, Epidemiology, Pathophysiology." Overview, Epidemiology, Primary Injury. August 18, 2017. Accessed March 16, 2017. https://emedicine.medscape.com/article/326510-overview.

Dawson, Ted M., and Valina L. Dawson. "Neuroprotective and Neurorestorative Strategies for Parkinsons Disease." *Nature Neuroscience*5, no. Supp (2002): 1058-061. doi:10.1038/nn941.

Dean, Carolyn. *The Magnesium Miracle*. Ballantine Books, 2017.

Degenhardt, Louisa, Wai Tat Chiu, Nancy Sampson, Ronald C. Kessler, and James C. Anthony. "Epidemiological Patterns of Extra-medical Drug Use in the United States: Evidence from the National Comorbidity Survey Replication, 2001-2003." *Drug and Alcohol Dependence*90, no. 2-3 (2007): 210-23. doi:10.1016/j.drugalcdep.2007.03.007.

Denson, Thomas F., and Mitchell Earleywine. "Decreased Depression in Marijuana Users." *Addictive Behaviors*31, no. 4 (2006): 738-42. doi:10.1016/j.addbeh.2005.05.052.

Desai, Roshni A., Andrew L. Davies, Mohamed Tachrount, Marianne Kasti, Frida Laulund, Xavier Golay, and Kenneth J. Smith. "Cause and prevention of demyelination in a model multiple sclerosis lesion." *Annals of Neurology*79, no. 4 (2016): 591-604. doi:10.1002/ana.24607.

Devinsky, Orrin, Maria Roberta Cilio, Helen Cross, Javier Fernandez-Ruiz, Jacqueline French, Charlotte Hill, Russell Katz, Vincenzo Di Marzo, Didier Jutras-Aswad, William George Notcutt, Jose Martinez-Orgado, Philip J. Robson, Brian G. Rohrback, Elizabeth Thiele, Benjamin Whalley, and Daniel Friedman. "Cannabidiol: Pharmacology and Potential Therapeutic Role in Epilepsy and Other Neuropsychiatric Disorders." *Epilepsia*55, no. 6 (2014): 791-802. doi:10.1111/epi.12631.

Diamond, David M., and Uffe Ravnskov. "How statistical deception created the appearance that statins are safe and effective in primary and secondary prevention of cardiovascular disease." *Expert Review of Clinical Pharmacology*8, no. 2 (2015): 201-10. doi:10.1586/17512433.2015.1012494.

Ding, Zheng, Wesley C. Tong, Xiao-Xin Lu, and Hui-Ping Peng. "Hyperbaric Oxygen Therapy in Acute Ischemic Stroke: A Review." *Interventional Neurology*2, no. 4 (2013): 201-11. doi:10.1159/000362677.

Dirikoc, S., S. A. Priola, M. Marella, N. Zsurger, and J. Chabry. "Nonpsychoactive Cannabidiol Prevents Prion Accumulation and Protects Neurons against Prion Toxicity." *Journal of Neuroscience*27, no. 36 (2007): 9537-544. doi:10.1523/jneurosci.1942-07.2007.

Disanto, Giulio, Ute Meier, Gavin Giovannoni, and Sreeram V. Ramagopalan. "Vitamin D: A Link between Epstein–Barr Virus and Multiple Sclerosis Development?" *Expert Review of Neurotherapeutics*11, no. 9 (2011): 1221-224. doi:10.1586/ern.11.97.

Doidge, Norman. *Brains Way of Healing*. Penguin Group US, 2015.

Doidge, Norman. *The Brain That Changes Itself: Stories of Personal Triumph from the Frontiers of Brain Science*. London: Penguin Books, 2007.

Dolhun, R. "Blog of The Michael J. Fox Foundation for Parkinson's Research." The Michael J. Fox Foundation for Parkinson's Research | Parkinson's Disease.

Accessed May 16, 2018. https://www.michaeljfox.org/foundation/news.
html?navid=blog-home.

Dsouza, Deepak Cyril, Edward Perry, Lisa Macdougall, Yola Ammerman,
Thomas Cooper, Yu-Te Wu, Gabriel Braley, Ralitza Gueorguieva, and John
Harrison Krystal. "The Psychotomimetic Effects of Intravenous Delta-9-Tet-
rahydrocannabinol in Healthy Individuals: Implications for Psychosis." *Neuropsychopharmacology*29, no. 8 (2004): 1558-572. doi:10.1038/sj.npp.1300496.

Dunnett, Alenka J., Dianne Roy, Andrew Stewart, and John M. McPartland.
"The Diagnosis of Fibromyalgia in Women May Be Influenced by Menstrual
Cycle Phase." *Journal of Bodywork and Movement Therapies*11, no. 2 (2007):
99-105. doi:10.1016/j.jbmt.2006.12.004.

Edwards, L. L., E. M. M. Quigley, and R. F. Pfeiffer. "Gastrointestinal Dysfunction in Parkinson's Disease: Frequency and Pathophysiology." *Neurology*42, no. 4 (1992): 726. doi:10.1212/wnl.42.4.726.

Efrati, Shai, Haim Golan, Yair Bechor, Yifat Faran, Shir Daphna-Tekoah, Gal
Sekler, Gregori Fishlev, Jacob N. Ablin, Jacob Bergan, Olga Volkov, Mony
Friedman, Eshel Ben-Jacob, and Dan Buskila. "Hyperbaric Oxygen Therapy
Can Diminish Fibromyalgia Syndrome - Prospective Clinical Trial." *Plos
One*10, no. 5 (2015). doi:10.1371/journal.pone.0127012.

Eggenhofer, Elke, Franka Luk, Marc H. Dahlke, and Martin J. Hoogduijn.
"The Life and Fate of Mesenchymal Stem Cells." *Frontiers in Immunology*5
(2014). doi:10.3389/fimmu.2014.00148.

Eltzschig, Holger K., and Peter Carmeliet. "Hypoxia and Inflammation." *New England Journal of Medicine*364, no. 7 (2011):
656-65. doi:10.1056/nejmra0910283.

Emanuele, Enzo, Paolo Orsi, Marianna Boso, Davide Broglia, Natascia Bron-
dino, Francesco Barale, Stefania Ucelli Di Nemi, and Pierluigi Politi. "Low-
grade Endotoxemia in Patients with Severe Autism." *Neuroscience Letters*471,
no. 3 (2010): 162-65. doi:10.1016/j.neulet.2010.01.033.

Embry, Ashton. Direct MS. www.direct-ms.org/.

Embry, Matt. "MS Hope." www.mshope.com.

Emmons, R. "How Gratitude Can Improve Your Health and Wellbeing." Mercola.com. August 4, 2016. Accessed March 16, 2018. https://articles. mercola.com/sites/articles/archive/2016/08/04/ways-to-cultivate-gratitude. aspx.

Escolar, E., G. A. Lamas, D. B. Mark, R. Boineau, C. Goertz, Y. Rosenberg, R. L. Nahin, P. Ouyang, T. Rozema, A. Magaziner, R. Nahas, E. F. Lewis, L. Lindblad, and K. L. Lee. "The Effect of an EDTA-based Chelation Regimen on Patients with Diabetes Mellitus and Prior Myocardial Infarction in the Trial to Assess Chelation Therapy (TACT)." *Circulation: Cardiovascular Quality and Outcomes*7, no. 1 (2013): 15-24. doi:10.1161/circoutcomes.113.000663.

Escribano, Begona, Ana Colin-Gonzalez, Abel Santamaria, and Isaac Tunez. "The Role of Melatonin in Multiple Sclerosis, Huntingtons Disease and Cerebral Ischemia." *CNS & Neurological Disorders - Drug Targets*13, no. 6 (2014): 1096-119. doi:10.2174/1871527313666140806160400.

Estaki, Mehrbod, Jason Pither, Peter Baumeister, Jonathan P. Little, Sandeep K. Gill, Sanjoy Ghosh, Zahra Ahmadi-Vand, Katelyn R. Marsden, and Deanna L. Gibson. "Cardiorespiratory Fitness as a Predictor of Intestinal Microbial Diversity and Distinct Metagenomic Functions." *Microbiome*4, no. 1 (2016). doi:10.1186/s40168-016-0189-7.

Eubanks, Lisa M., Claude J. Rogers, Beuscher, George F. Koob, Arthur J. Olson, Tobin J. Dickerson, and Kim D. Janda. "A Molecular Link between the Active Component of Marijuana and Alzheimers Disease Pathology." *Molecular Pharmaceutics*3, no. 6 (2006): 773-77. doi:10.1021/mp060066m.

Feinman, Richard D. "Saturated Fat and Health: Recent Advances in Research." *Lipids*45, no. 10 (2010): 891-92. doi:10.1007/s11745-010-3446-8.

Feinman, Richard D., Wendy K. Pogozelski, Arne Astrup, Richard K. Bernstein, Eugene J. Fine, Eric C. Westman, Anthony Accurso, Lynda Frassetto, Barbara A. Gower, Samy I. Mcfarlane, Jörgen Vesti Nielsen, Thure Krarup, Laura Saslow, Karl S. Roth, Mary C. Vernon, Jeff S. Volek, Gilbert B. Wilshire, Annika Dahlqvist, Ralf Sundberg, Ann Childers, Katharine Morrison, Anssi H. Manninen, Hussain M. Dashti, Richard J. Wood, Jay Wortman, and Nicolai Worm. "Dietary carbohydrate restriction as the first approach in diabetes management: Critical review and evidence base." *Nutrition*31, no. 1 (2015): 1-13. doi:10.1016/j.nut.2014.06.011.

Fernández-López, David, Ignacio Lizasoain, Maria Moro, and José Martínez-Orgado. "Cannabinoids: Well-Suited Candidates for the

Treatment of Perinatal Brain Injury." *Brain Sciences*3, no. 4 (2013): 1043-059. doi:10.3390/brainsci3031043.

Fife, Caroline E., Kristen A. Eckert, and Marissa J. Carter. "An Update on the Appropriate Role for Hyperbaric Oxygen." *Plastic and Reconstructive Surgery*138 (2016). doi:10.1097/prs.0000000000002714.

Finsterer, Josef, and Sinda Zarrouk-Mahjoub. "Mitochondrial vasculopathy." *World Journal of Cardiology*8, no. 5 (2016): 333. doi:10.4330/wjc.v8.i5.333.

Fischer, Boguslav H., Morton Marks, and Theobald Reich. "Hyperbaric-Oxygen Treatment of Multiple Sclerosis." *New England Journal of Medicine*308, no. 4 (1983): 181-86. doi:10.1056/nejm198301273080402.

Fisher, Marc, and Joseph A. Hill. "Ischemic Stroke Mandates Cross-Disciplinary Collaboration." *Stroke*49, no. 2 (2018): 273-74. doi:10.1161/strokeaha.117.020014.

Flockhart Table ™ Indiana University, School of Medicine, Department of Medicine. Accessed May 01, 2018. http://medicine.iupui.edu/clinpharm/ddis/main-table/.

Fodale, V., L. B. Santamaria, D. Schifilliti, and P. K. Mandal. "Anaesthetics and postoperative cognitive dysfunction: a pathological mechanism mimicking Alzheimer's disease." *Anaesthesia*65, no. 4 (2010): 388-95. doi:10.1111/j.1365-2044.2010.06244.x.

Fosen, Katina M., and Stephen R. Thom. "Hyperbaric Oxygen, Vasculogenic Stem Cells, and Wound Healing." *Antioxidants & Redox Signaling*21, no. 11 (2014): 1634-647. doi:10.1089/ars.2014.5940.

Foti, Daniel J., Roman Kotov, Lin T. Guey, and Evelyn J. Bromet. "Cannabis Use and the Course of Schizophrenia: 10-Year Follow-Up After First Hospitalization." *American Journal of Psychiatry*167, no. 8 (2010): 987-93. doi:10.1176/appi.ajp.2010.09020189.

Fox, Molly, Leslie A. Knapp, Paul W. Andrews, and Corey L. Fincher. "Hygiene and the World Distribution of Alzheimer's Disease." *Evolution, Medicine, and Public Health*2013, no. 1 (2013): 173-86. doi:10.1093/emph/eot015.

Frat, Jean-Pierre, Arnaud W. Thille, Alain Mercat, Christophe Girault, Stéphanie Ragot, Sébastien Perbet, Gwénael Prat, Thierry Boulain, Elise Morawiec, Alice Cottereau, Jérôme Devaquet, Saad Nseir, Keyvan Razazi, Jean-Paul Mira, Laurent Argaud, Jean-Charles Chakarian, Jean-Damien Ricard, Xavier Wittebole, Stéphanie Chevalier, Alexandre Herbland, Muriel Fartoukh,

Jean-Michel Constantin, Jean-Marie Tonnelier, Marc Pierrot, Armelle Mathonnet, Gaëtan Béduneau, Céline Delétage-Métreau, Jean-Christophe M. Richard, Laurent Brochard, and René Robert. "High-Flow Oxygen through Nasal Cannula in Acute Hypoxemic Respiratory Failure." *New England Journal of Medicine*372, no. 23 (2015): 2185-196. doi:10.1056/nejmoa1503326.

Friedman, Michael. "Treatment of Hypoxemia in Obstructive Sleep Apnea." *American Journal of Rhinology*15, no. 5 (2001): 311-13.

Funkhouser, Lisa J., and Seth R. Bordenstein. "Mom Knows Best: The Universality of Maternal Microbial Transmission." *PLoS Biology*11, no. 8 (2013). doi:10.1371/journal.pbio.1001631.

Galli, Jonathan A., Ronald Andari Sawaya, and Frank K. Friedenberg. "Cannabinoid Hyperemesis Syndrome." *Current Drug Abuse Reviews*4, no. 4 (2011): 241-49. doi:10.2174/1874473711104040241.

Gaoni, Y., and R. Mechoulam. "Isolation, Structure, and Partial Synthesis of an Active Constituent of Hashish." *Journal of the American Chemical Society*86, no. 8 (1964): 1646-647. doi:10.1021/ja01062a046.

Glass, Michelle, and John K. Northup. "Agonist Selective Regulation of G Proteins by Cannabinoid CB1and CB2Receptors." *Molecular Pharmacology*56, no. 6 (1999): 1362-369. doi:10.1124/mol.56.6.1362.

Godman, Cassandra A., Rashmi Joshi, Charles Giardina, George Perdrizet, and Lawrence E. Hightower. "Hyperbaric Oxygen Treatment Induces Antioxidant Gene Expression." *Annals of the New York Academy of Sciences*1197, no. 1 (2010): 178-83. doi:10.1111/j.1749-6632.2009.05393.x.

Gómez-Pinilla, Fernando, Zhe Ying, Roland R. Roy, Raffaella Molteni, and V. Reggie Edgerton. "Voluntary Exercise Induces a BDNF-Mediated Mechanism That Promotes Neuroplasticity." *Journal of Neurophysiology*88, no. 5 (2002): 2187-195. doi:10.1152/jn.00152.2002.

Gooriah, Rubesh, Alina Buture, and Fayyaz Ahmed. "Evidence-based Treatments for Cluster Headache." *Therapeutics and Clinical Risk Management*, 2015, 1687. doi:10.2147/tcrm.s94193.

Gottlieb, Joshua D., Alan Schwartz, Samer S. Najjar, and Stephen S. Gottlieb. "Hypoxia, Not the Frequency of Sleep Apnea, Causes Acute Hemodynamic Stress in Patients with Congestive Heart Failure." *Journal of Cardiac Failure*15, no. 6 (2009). doi:10.1016/j.cardfail.2009.06.351.

Greenblatt, James, and Kelly Brogan. *Integrative therapies for depression: redefining models for assessment, treatment, and prevention*. Boca Raton: CRC Press, Taylor & Francis Group, 2016.

Greer, George R., Charles S. Grob, and Adam L. Halberstadt. "PTSD Symptom Reports of Patients Evaluated for the New Mexico Medical Cannabis Program." *Journal of Psychoactive Drugs*46, no. 1 (2014): 73-77. doi:10.1080/02791072.2013.873843.

Greif, Robert, Ozan Akça, Ernst-Peter Horn, Andrea Kurz, and Daniel I. Sessler. "Supplemental Perioperative Oxygen to Reduce the Incidence of Surgical-Wound Infection." *New England Journal of Medicine*342, no. 3 (2000): 161-67. doi:10.1056/nejm200001203420303.

Grimaldi-Bensouda, Lamiae, Bernard Bégaud, Michel Rossignol, Bernard Avouac, France Lert, Frederic Rouillon, Jacques Bénichou, Jacques Massol, Gerard Duru, Anne-Marie Magnier, Lucien Abenhaim, and Didier Guillemot. "Management of Upper Respiratory Tract Infections by Different Medical Practices, Including Homeopathy, and Consumption of Antibiotics in Primary Care: The EPI3 Cohort Study in France 2007-2008." *PLoS ONE*9, no. 3 (2014). doi:10.1371/journal.pone.0089990.

Grimaldi-Bensouda, Lamiae, Lucien Abenhaim, Jacques Massol, Didier Guillemot, Bernard Avouac, Gerard Duru, France Lert, Anne-Marie Magnier, Michel Rossignol, Frederic Rouillon, and Bernard Begaud. "Homeopathic Medical Practice for Anxiety and Depression in Primary Care: The EPI3 Cohort Study." *BMC Complementary and Alternative Medicine*16, no. 1 (2016). doi:10.1186/s12906-016-1104-2.

Guindon, Josee, and Andrea Hohmann. "The Endocannabinoid System and Pain." *CNS & Neurological Disorders - Drug Targets*8, no. 6 (2009): 403-21. doi:10.2174/187152709789824660.

Haacke, E. Mark, Wei Feng, David Utriainen, Gabriela Trifan, Zhen Wu, Zahid Latif, Yashwanth Katkuri, Joseph Hewett, and David Hubbard. "Patients with Multiple Sclerosis with Structural Venous Abnormalities on MR Imaging Exhibit an Abnormal Flow Distribution of the Internal Jugular Veins." *Journal of Vascular and Interventional Radiology*23, no. 1 (2012). doi:10.1016/j.jvir.2011.09.027.

Hagenbach, U., S. Luz, N. Ghafoor, J. M. Berger, F. Grotenhermen, R. Brenneisen, and M. Mäder. "The Treatment of Spasticity with Δ9-tetrahydrocannabinol in Persons with Spinal Cord Injury." *Spinal Cord*45, no. 8 (2006): 551-62. doi:10.1038/sj.sc.3101982.

Hahn, Ales. "Chronic Cerebrospinal Venous Insufficiency (CCSVI) IN Meniere Disease. Case or Cause?" *ScienceMED*4 (2103): 9-15.

Hamblin, Michael R. "Shining light on the head: Photo-biomodulation for brain disorders." *BBA Clinical*6 (2016): 113-24. doi:10.1016/j.bbacli.2016.09.002.

Hampson, A. J., M. Grimaldi, J. Axelrod, and D. Wink. "Cannabidiol and (-) 9-tetrahydrocannabinol Are Neuroprotective Antioxidants." *Proceedings of the National Academy of Sciences*95, no. 14 (1998): 8268-273. doi:10.1073/pnas.95.14.8268.

Hanning, C. D. "Postoperative cognitive dysfunction." *British Journal of Anaes-thesia*95, no. 1 (2005): 82-87. doi:10.1093/bja/aei062.

Hanuš, Lumír Ondřej. "Pharmacological and Therapeutic Secrets of Plant and Brain (endo)cannabinoids." *Medicinal Research Reviews*29, no. 2 (2009): 213-71. doi:10.1002/med.20135.

Harach, T., N. Marungruang, N. Duthilleul, V. Cheatham, K. D. Mc Coy, G. Frisoni, J. J. Neher, F. Fåk, M. Jucker, T. Lasser, and T. Bolmont. "Reduction of Abeta amyloid pathology in APPPS1 transgenic mice in the absence of gut microbiota." *Scientific Reports*7 (2017): 41802. doi:10.1038/srep41802.

Harch, Paul G., Edward F. Fogarty, Paul K. Staab, and Keith Van Meter. "Low Pressure Hyperbaric Oxygen Therapy and SPECT Brain Imaging in the Treat-ment of Blast-induced Chronic Traumatic Brain Injury (post-concussion Syn-drome) and Post Traumatic Stress Disorder: A Case Report." *Cases Journal*2, no. 1 (2009): 6538. doi:10.1186/1757-1626-0002-0000006538.

Harch, Paul G., Susan R. Andrews, Edward F. Fogarty, Daniel Amen, John C. Pezzullo, Juliette Lucarini, Claire Aubrey, Derek V. Taylor, Paul K. Staab, and Keith W. Van Meter. "A Phase I Study of Low-Pressure Hyper-baric Oxygen Therapy for Blast-Induced Post-Concussion Syndrome and Post-Traumatic Stress Disorder." *Journal of Neurotrauma*29, no. 1 (2012): 168-85. doi:10.1089/neu.2011.1895.

Hardell, Lennart, Michael Carlberg, Fredrik Söderqvist, and Kjell Hansson Mild. "Meta-analysis of Long-term Mobile Phone Use and the Association with Brain Tumours." *International Journal of Oncology*, 2008. doi:10.3892/ijo.32.5.1097.

Hart, Gillian. Methylation and Homocysteine. Accessed February 04, 2017. http://www.foodforthebrain.org/alzheimers-prevention/methylation-and-homocysteine.aspx.

Harten, A. E. Van, T. W. L. Scheeren, and A. R. Absalom. "A review of postoperative cognitive dysfunction and neuroinflammation associated with cardiac surgery and anaesthesia." *Anaesthesia*67, no. 3 (2012): 280-93. doi:10.1111/j.1365-2044.2011.07008.x.

Havas, Magda. "Electromagnetic Hypersensitivity: Biological Effects of Dirty Electricity with Emphasis on Diabetes and Multiple Sclerosis." *Electromagnetic Biology and Medicine*25, no. 4 (2006): 259-68. doi:10.1080/15368370601044192.

Havas, Magda. "Magda Havas Talks at NIEHS May 9, 2016 on Electrosmog and Electrohypersensitivity." YouTube. May 28, 2016. https://www.youtube.com/watch?v=fqMCjEs9oxE.

Henderson, Theodore A., Larry Morries, and Paolo Cassano. "Treatments for Traumatic Brain Injury with Emphasis on Transcranial Near-infrared Laser Phototherapy." *Neuropsychiatric Disease and Treatment*, 2015, 2159. doi:10.2147/ndt.s65809.

Hickey, Steve, and Hilary Roberts. *Tarnished Gold: The Sickness of Evidence-based Medicine*. Lexington, KY: Publisher Not Identified, 2011.

Hill, Kevin P. "Medical Marijuana for Treatment of Chronic Pain and Other Medical and Psychiatric Problems." *Jama*313, no. 24 (2015): 2474. doi:10.1001/jama.2015.6199.

Hoggard, M. L., K. E. Johnson, and D. Y. Shirachi. "Hyperbaric Oxygen Treatment on a Parkinson's Disease Patient: A Case Study." Hyperbaric Research & Studies. August 24, 2015. http://hyperbaricstudies.com/research-studies/hyperbaric-oxygen-treatment-on-a-parkinsons-disease-patient-a-case-study/.

Holdcroft, Anita, Mervyn Maze, Caroline Doré, Susan Tebbs, and Simon Thompson. "A Multicenter Dose-escalation Study of the Analgesic and Adverse Effects of an Oral Cannabis Extract (Cannador) for Postoperative Pain Management." *Anesthesiology*104, no. 5 (2006): 1040-046. doi:10.1097/00000542-200605000-00021.

Holmqvist, Staffan, Oldriska Chutna, Luc Bousset, Patrick Aldrin-Kirk, Wen Li, Tomas Björklund, Zhan-You Wang, Laurent Roybon, Ronald Melki, and

Jia-Yi Li. "Direct Evidence of Parkinson Pathology Spread from the Gastro-intestinal Tract to the Brain in Rats." *Acta Neuropathologica*128, no. 6 (2014): 805-20. doi:10.1007/s00401-014-1343-6.

Houston, Mark C. "New Concepts in Cardiovascular Disease." *Journal of Restorative Medicine*2, no. 1 (2013): 30-44. doi:10.14200/jrm.2013.2.0105.

Houston, Mark C. "Role of Mercury Toxicity in Hypertension, Cardiovascular Disease, and Stroke." *The Journal of Clinical Hypertension*13, no. 8 (2011): 621-27. doi:10.1111/j.1751-7176.2011.00489.x.

Huang, Xuemei, Alvaro Alonso, Xuguang Guo, David M. Umbach, Maya L. Lichtenstein, Christie M. Ballantyne, Richard B. Mailman, Thomas H. Mosley, and Honglei Chen. "Statins, Plasma Cholesterol, and Risk of Parkinsons Disease: A Prospective Study." *Movement Disorders*30, no. 4 (2015): 552-59. doi:10.1002/mds.26152.

Huestis, Marilyn A. "Human Cannabinoid Pharmacokinetics." *Chemistry & Biodiversity*4, no. 8 (2007): 1770-804. doi:10.1002/cbdv.200790152.

Hughes, G. R., R. A. Asherson, and M. A. Khamashta. "Antiphospholipid syndrome: linking many specialties." *Annals of the Rheumatic Diseases*48, no. 5 (1989): 355-56. doi:10.1136/ard.48.5.355.

Iadecola, Costantino. "From CSD to headache: A long and winding road." *Nature Medicine*8, no. 2 (2002): 110-12. doi:10.1038/nm0202-110.

ISBN: 978-1-930536-50-0

Izzo, A. A., and M. Camilleri. "Emerging Role of Cannabinoids in Gastrointestinal and Liver Diseases: Basic and Clinical Aspects." *Gut*57, no. 8 (2008): 1140-155. doi:10.1136/gut.2008.148791.

Izzo, Angelo A., Francesca Borrelli, Raffaele Capasso, Vincenzo Di Marzo, and Raphael Mechoulam. "Non-psychotropic Plant Cannabinoids: New Therapeutic Opportunities from an Ancient Herb." *Trends in Pharmacological Sciences*30, no. 10 (2009): 515-27. doi:10.1016/j.tips.2009.07.006.

Jadidi, Elham, Mohammad Mohammadi, and Tahereh Moradi. "High Risk of Cardiovascular Diseases after Diagnosis of Multiple Sclerosis." *Multiple Sclerosis Journal*19, no. 10 (2013): 1336-340. doi:10.1177/1352458513475833.

Jager, Gerry, and Renger F. Witkamp. "The Endocannabinoid System and Appetite: Relevance for Food Reward." *Nutrition Research Reviews*27, no. 01 (2014): 172-85. doi:10.1017/s0954422414000080.

James, P.B. "Fat Embolism In Multiple Sclerosis." *The Lancet* 319, no. 8285 (1982): 1356. doi:10.1016/s0140-6736(82)92418-7.

James, P. B. "Oxygen For Multiple Sclerosis." *The Lancet* 322, no. 8346 (1983): 396-97. doi:10.1016/s0140-6736(83)90362-8.

James, P. B. "Hyperbaric oxygen in multiple sclerosis." *Bmj* 292, no. 6521 (1986): 692. doi:10.1136/bmj.292.6521.692.

James, P.B. "Immunological treatment for multiple sclerosis." *The Lancet* 333, no. 8649 (June 3, 1989): 1272-273. doi:10.1016/S0140-6736(89)92372-6.

James, P.B. "Multiple sclerosis as a diagnosis." *The Lancet* 350, no. 9085 (1997): 1178-179. doi:10.1016/s0140-6736(05)63826-3.

James, P.B., D.J.D. Perrins, D.l.W. Davidson, and G.S. Plaut. "Hyperbaric Oxygen and Multiple Sclerosis." *The Lancet*325, no. 8428 (1985): 572-73. doi:10.1016/s0140-6736(85)91223-1.

James, Philip B. "Evidence for Subacute Fat Embolism as the Cause of Multiple Sclerosis." *The Lancet*319, no. 8268 (1982): 380-86. doi:10.1016/s0140-6736(82)91402-7.

James, Philip B. *Oxygen and the Brain: The Journey of Our Lifetime*. 1st ed. Best Publishing, 2014.

Jersey, Sean L., Robert T. Baril, Richmond D. Mccarty, and Christina M. Millhouse. "Severe Neurological Decompression Sickness in a U-2 Pilot." *Aviation, Space, and Environmental Medicine*81, no. 1 (2010): 64-68. doi:10.3357/asem.2303.2010.

Jessen, Nadia Aalling, Anne Sofie Finmann Munk, Iben Lundgaard, and Maiken Nedergaard. "The Glymphatic System: A Beginner's Guide." *Neurochemical Research*40, no. 12 (2015): 2583-599. doi:10.1007/s11064-015-1581-6.

Johnson, S. "The Multifaceted and Widespread Pathology of Magnesium Deficiency." *Medical Hypotheses*56, no. 2 (2001): 163-70. doi:10.1054/mehy.2000.1133.

Johnstone, Daniel M., Cécile Moro, Jonathan Stone, Alim-Louis Benabid, and John Mitrofanis. "Turning On Lights to Stop Neurodegeneration: The Potential of Near Infrared Light Therapy in Alzheimers and Parkinsons Disease." *Frontiers in Neuroscience*9 (2016). doi:10.3389/fnins.2015.00500.

Jones, N. A., A. J. Hill, I. Smith, S. A. Bevan, C. M. Williams, B. J. Whalley, and G. J. Stephens. "Cannabidiol Displays Antiepileptiform and Antiseizure

Properties In Vitro and In Vivo." *Journal of Pharmacology and Experimental Therapeutics*332, no. 2 (2009): 569-77. doi:10.1124/jpet.109.159145.

Jopling, Michael W., John A. Kurowski, and Suzanne M. Williams. "Patent Foramen Ovale—Its Correlation with Other Maladies and a Review of Detection Screening." *US Neurology*11, no. 02 (2015): 89. doi:10.17925/usn.2015.11.02.89.

Joutsa, Juho, Juha O. Rinne, Bruce Hermann, Mira Karrasch, Anu Anttinen, Shlomo Shinnar, and Matti Sillanpää. "Association Between Childhood-Onset Epilepsy and Amyloid Burden 5 Decades Later." *JAMA Neurology*74, no. 5 (2017): 583. doi:10.1001/jamaneurol.2016.6091.

Jovanovic, Tanja, Seth D. Norrholm, Nineequa Q. Blanding, Michael Davis, Erica Duncan, Bekh Bradley, and Kerry J. Ressler. "Impaired Fear Inhibition Is a Biomarker of PTSD but Not Depression." *Depression and Anxiety*27, no. 3 (2010): 244-51. doi:10.1002/da.20663.

Joy, Janet E., Stanley J. Watson, and John A. Benson. *Marijuana and Medicine Assessing the Science Base*. National Academy Press, 1999.

Ju, Yo-El S., Sharon J. Ooms, Courtney Sutphen, Shannon L. Macauley, Margaret A. Zangrilli, Gina Jerome, Anne M. Fagan, Emmanuel Mignot, John M. Zempel, Jurgen A.h.r. Claassen, and David M. Holtzman. "Slow Wave Sleep Disruption Increases Cerebrospinal Fluid Amyloid-β Levels." *Brain*140, no. 8 (2017): 2104-111. doi:10.1093/brain/awx148.

Julien, Boris, Pascale Grenard, Fatima Teixeira-Clerc, Jeanne Tran Van Nhieu, Liying Li, Meliha Karsak, Andreas Zimmer, Ariane Mallat, and Sophie Lotersztajn. "Antifibrogenic Role of the Cannabinoid Receptor CB2 in the Liver." *Gastroenterology*128, no. 3 (2005): 742-55. doi:10.1053/j.gastro.2004.12.050.

Juurlink, Bernhard HJ. "Lifestyle approaches to ameliorate diseases associated with oxidative stress and inflammation." In *Third European Conference on Scientific Publishing in Biomedicine and Medicine*, 1-20. Proceedings. Leiden, 2010.

Kang, Silvia S., Patricio R. Jeraldo, Aishe Kurti, Margret E. Miller, Marc D. Cook, Keith Whitlock, Nigel Goldenfeld, Jeffrey A. Woods, Bryan A. White, Nicholas Chia, and John D. Fryer. "Diet and Exercise Orthogonally Alter the Gut Microbiome and Reveal Independent Associations with Anxiety and Cognition." *Molecular Neurodegeneration*9, no. 1 (2014): 36. doi:10.1186/1750-1326-9-36.

Kaplan, Bonnie J., Julia J. Rucklidge, Amy Romijn, and Kevin Mcleod. "The Emerging Field of Nutritional Mental Health." *Clinical Psychological Science*3, no. 6 (2015): 964-80. doi:10.1177/2167702614555413.

Karler, Ralph, William Cely, and Stuart A. Turkanis. "The Anticonvulsant Activity of Cannabidiol and Cannabinol." *Life Sciences*13, no. 11 (1973): 1527-531. doi:10.1016/0024-3205(73)90141-0.

Karltunen, V., M. Ventilä, M. Hillbom, O. Salonen, H. Haapaniemi, and M. Kaste. "Dye Dilution and Oximetry for Detection of Patent Foramen Ovale." *Acta Neurologica Scandinavica*97, no. 4 (2009): 231-36. doi:10.1111/j.1600-0404.1998.tb00643.x.

Karltunen, V., M. Ventila, M. Ikaheimo, M. Niemela, and M. Hillbom. "Ear Oximetry: A Noninvasive Method for Detection of Patent Foramen Ovale: A Study Comparing Dye Dilution Method and Oximetry With Contrast Transesophageal Echocardiography." *Stroke*32, no. 2 (2001): 448-53. doi:10.1161/01.str.32.2.448.

Kathmann, Markus, Karsten Flau, Agnes Redmer, Christian Tränkle, and Eberhard Schlicker. "Cannabidiol Is an Allosteric Modulator at Mu- and Delta-opioid Receptors." *Naunyn-Schmiedebergs Archives of Pharmacology*372, no. 5 (2006): 354-61. doi:10.1007/s00210-006-0033-x.

Kaup, Allison R., and Kristine Yaffe. "Reassuring News About Football and Cognitive Decline?" *JAMA Neurology*74, no. 8 (2017): 898. doi:10.1001/jamaneurol.2017.1324.

Kidd, P. M. "Neurodegeneration from Mitochondrial Insufficiency: Nutrients, Stem Cells, Growth Factors, and Prospects for Brain Rebuilding Using Integrative Management." *Alter Med Rev*10, no. 4 (2005): 268-93.

Kilsdonk, I. D., M. D. Steenwijk, P. J. Pouwels, J. J. Zwanenburg, F. Visser, P. R. Luijten, J. Geurts, F. Barkhof, and M. P. Wattjes. "Perivascular Spaces in MS Patients at 7 Tesla MRI: A Marker of Neurodegeneration?" *Multiple Sclerosis Journal*21, no. 2 (2014): 155-62. doi:10.1177/1352458514540358.

Kim, H-J, H-K Park, D-W Lim, H-J Kim, I-H Lee, H-S Kim, J-S Choi, G-R Tack, and S-C Chung. "Effects of Oxygen Concentration and Flow Rate on Cognitive Ability and Physiological Responses in the Elderly." *Neural Regen Res*8, no. 3 (2013): 264-69.

Kim, Hyun, Chang-Ho Yun, Robert Joseph Thomas, Seung Hoon Lee, Hyung Suk Seo, Eo Rin Cho, Seung Ku Lee, Dae Wui Yoon, Sooyeon Suh, and Chol Shin. "Obstructive Sleep Apnea as a Risk Factor for Cerebral White Matter Change in a Middle-Aged and Older General Population." *Sleep*, 2013. doi:10.5665/sleep.2632.

Koppel, B. S., J. C. M. Brust, T. Fife, J. Bronstein, S. Youssof, G. Gronseth, and D. Gloss. "Systematic Review: Efficacy and Safety of Medical Marijuana in Selected Neurologic Disorders: Report of the Guideline Development Subcommittee of the American Academy of Neurology." *Neurology*82, no. 17 (2014): 1556-563. doi:10.1212/wnl.0000000000000363.

Kortekaas, Rudie, Klaus L. Leenders, Joost C. H. Van Oostrom, Willem Vaalburg, Joost Bart, Antoon T. M. Willemsen, and N. Harry Hendrikse. "Blood-brain barrier dysfunction in parkinsonian midbrain in vivo." *Annals of Neurology*57, no. 2 (2005): 176-79. doi:10.1002/ana.20369.

Kranich, Jan, Kendle M. Maslowski, and Charles R. Mackay. "Commensal Flora and the Regulation of Inflammatory and Autoimmune Responses." *Seminars in Immunology*23, no. 2 (2011): 139-45. doi:10.1016/j.smim.2011.01.011.

Kummerow, Fred A. "The negative effects of hydrogenated trans fats and what to do about them." *Atherosclerosis*205, no. 2 (2009): 458-65. doi:10.1016/j.atherosclerosis.2009.03.009.

Laat, Bas De, Koen Mertens, and Philip G De Groot. "Mechanisms of Disease: antiphospholipid antibodies—from clinical association to pathologic mechanism." *Nature Clinical Practice Rheumatology*4, no. 4 (2008): 192-99. doi:10.1038/ncprheum0740.

Labus, Jennifer S., Emily B. Hollister, Jonathan Jacobs, Kyleigh Kirbach, Numan Oezguen, Arpana Gupta, Jonathan Acosta, Ruth Ann Luna, Kjersti Aagaard, James Versalovic, Tor Savidge, Elaine Hsiao, Kirsten Tillisch, and Emeran A. Mayer. "Differences in Gut Microbial Composition Correlate with Regional Brain Volumes in Irritable Bowel Syndrome." *Microbiome*5, no. 1 (2017). doi:10.1186/s40168-017-0260-z.

Lahat, Adi, Alon Lang, and Shomron Ben-Horin. "Impact of Cannabis Treatment on the Quality of Life, Weight and Clinical Disease Activity in Inflammatory Bowel Disease Patients: A Pilot Prospective Study." *Digestion*85, no. 1 (2012): 1-8. doi:10.1159/000332079.

Lahiff, Conor, and Adam S. Cheifetz. "The Holistic Effects of Cannabis in Crohn's Disease." *Clinical Gastroenterology and Hepatology*12, no. 5 (2014): 898. doi:10.1016/j.cgh.2013.11.013.

Lake, Stephanie, Thomas Kerr, and Julio Montaner. "Prescribing Medical Cannabis in Canada: Are We Being Too Cautious?" *Can J Public Health*106, no. 5 (2015). doi:10.17269/cjph.106.4926.

Lamas, Gervasio A., Christine Goertz, Robin Boineau, Daniel B. Mark, Theodore Rozema, Richard L. Nahin, Lauren Lindblad, Eldrin F. Lewis, Jeanne Drisko, Kerry L. Lee, and For The Tact Investigators. "Effect of Disodium EDTA Chelation Regimen on Cardiovascular Events in Patients with Previous Myocardial Infarction." *Jama*309, no. 12 (2013): 1241. doi:10.1001/jama.2013.2107.

Lau, Nicholas, Paloma Sales, Sheigla Averill, Fiona Murphy, Sye-Ok Sato, and Sheigla Murphy. "A Safer Alternative: Cannabis Substitution as Harm Reduction." *Drug and Alcohol Review*34, no. 6 (2015): 654-59. doi:10.1111/dar.12275.

Lavie, Lena. "Oxidative stress in obstructive sleep apnea and intermittent hypoxia – Revisited – The bad ugly and good: Implications to the heart and brain." *Sleep Medicine Reviews*20 (2015): 27-45. doi:10.1016/j.smrv.2014.07.003.

Law, Meng, Amit M. Saindane, Yulin Ge, James S. Babb, Glyn Johnson, Lois J. Mannon, Joseph Herbert, and Robert I. Grossman. "Microvascular Abnormality in Relapsing-Remitting Multiple Sclerosis: Perfusion MR Imaging Findings in Normal-appearing White Matter." *Radiology*231, no. 3 (2004): 645-52. doi:10.1148/radiol.2313030996.

Lea, Rod, Natalie Colson, Sharon Quinlan, John Macmillan, and Lyn Griffiths. "The effects of vitamin supplementation and MTHFR (C677T) genotype on homocysteine-lowering and migraine disability." *Pharmacogenetics and Genomics*19, no. 6 (2009): 422-28. doi:10.1097/fpc.0b013e32832af5a3.

Lee, M. "Juicing Raw Cannabis." O'Shaugnessy's. beyondthc.com.

Lengfeld, Justin, Tyler Cutforth, and Dritan Agalliu. "The Role of Angiogenesis in the Pathology of Multiple Sclerosis." *Vascular Cell*6, no. 1 (2014). doi:10.1186/s13221-014-0023-6.

Levine, Steven M. "Is There an Increased Risk for Ischemic Stroke in Patients with Multiple Sclerosis, and If So, Should Preventive Treatment Be Considered?" *Frontiers in Neurology*7 (2016). doi:10.3389/fneur.2016.00128.

Leweke, F. M., D. Piomelli, F. Pahlisch, D. Muhl, C. W. Gerth, C. Hoyer, J. Klosterkötter, M. Hellmich, and D. Koethe. "Cannabidiol Enhances Anandamide Signaling and Alleviates Psychotic Symptoms of Schizophrenia." *Translational Psychiatry*2, no. 3 (2012). doi:10.1038/tp.2012.15.

Lewy Body Disease by Edna and Daniel DeJong. Accessed April 30, 2018. http://rxmarijuana.com/lewy.htm.

Liebert, Ann D., Roberta T. Chow, Brian T. Bicknell, and Euahna Varigos. "Neuroprotective Effects against POCD by Photobiomodulation: Evidence from Assembly/Disassembly of the Cytoskeleton." *Journal of Experimental Neuroscience*10 (2016). doi:10.4137/jen.s33444.

Liu, Zhong-Wu, Geliang Gan, Shigetomo Suyama, and Xiao-Bing Gao. "Intracellular Energy Status Regulates Activity in Hypocretin/orexin Neurones: A Link between Energy and Behavioural States." *The Journal of Physiology*589, no. 17 (2011): 4157-166. doi:10.1113/jphysiol.2011.212514.

Logsdon, Aric F., Michelle A. Erickson, Elizabeth M. Rhea, Therese S. Salameh, and William A. Banks. "Gut reactions: How the blood–brain barrier connects the microbiome and the brain." *Experimental Biology and Medicine*243, no. 2 (2017): 159-65. doi:10.1177/1535370217743766.

Long, Ying, Jiewen Tan, Yulin Nie, Yu Lu, Xiufang Mei, and Chaoqun Tu. "Hyperbaric oxygen therapy is safe and effective for the treatment of sleep disorders in children with cerebral palsy." *Neurological Research*39, no. 3 (2017): 239-47. doi:10.1080/01616412.2016.1275454.

Loprinzi, Paul D., Christy D. Wolfe, and Jerome F. Walker. "Exercise Facilitates Smoking Cessation Indirectly via Improvements in Smoking-specific Self-efficacy: Prospective Cohort Study among a National Sample of Young Smokers." *Preventive Medicine*81 (2015): 63-66. doi:10.1016/j.ypmed.2015.08.011.

Loprinzi, Paul D., Skyla M. Herod, Bradley J. Cardinal, and Timothy D. Noakes. "Physical Activity and the Brain: A Review of This Dynamic, Bi-directional Relationship." *Brain Research*1539 (2013): 95-104. doi:10.1016/j.brainres.2013.10.004.

Lotan, Itay, Therese A. Treves, Yaniv Roditi, and Ruth Djaldetti. "Cannabis (Medical Marijuana) Treatment for Motor and Non–Motor Symptoms of Parkinson Disease." *Clinical Neuropharmacology*37, no. 2 (2014): 41-44. doi:10.1097/wnf.0000000000000016.

Louveau, Antoine, Igor Smirnov, Timothy J. Keyes, Jacob D. Eccles, Sherin J. Rouhani, J. David Peske, Noel C. Derecki, David Castle, James W. Mandell, Kevin S. Lee, Tajie H. Harris, and Jonathan Kipnis. "Structural and Functional Features of Central Nervous System Lymphatic Vessels." *Nature*523, no. 7560 (2015): 337-41. doi:10.1038/nature14432.

Lucas, Philippe. "Cannabis as an Adjunct to or Substitute for Opiates in the Treatment of Chronic Pain." *Journal of Psychoactive Drugs*44, no. 2 (2012): 125-33. doi:10.1080/02791072.2012.684624.

Lunetta, Christian, Andrea Lizio, Eleonora Maestri, Valeria Ada Sansone, Gabriele Mora, Robert G. Miller, Stanley H. Appel, and Adriano Chiò. "Serum C-Reactive Protein as a Prognostic Biomarker in Amyotrophic Lateral Sclerosis." *JAMA Neurology*74, no. 6 (2017): 660. doi:10.1001/jamaneurol.2016.6179.

Lương, Khanh Vinh Quốc. "The Role of Thiamine in Schizophrenia." *American Journal of Psychiatry and Neuroscience*1, no. 3 (2013): 38. doi:10.11648/j.ajpn.20130103.11.

Maa, Edward, and Paige Figi. "The Case for Medical Marijuana in Epilepsy." *Epilepsia*55, no. 6 (2014): 783-86. doi:10.1111/epi.12610.

Maccallum, Caroline A., and Ethan B. Russo. "Practical Considerations in Medical Cannabis Administration and Dosing." *European Journal of Internal Medicine*49 (2018): 12-19. doi:10.1016/j.ejim.2018.01.004.

Maccallum, Caroline A., and Ethan B. Russo. "Practical Considerations in Medical Cannabis Administration and Dosing." *European Journal of Internal Medicine*49 (2018): 12-19. doi:10.1016/j.ejim.2018.01.004.

Mahad, Don H., Bruce D. Trapp, and Hans Lassmann. "Pathological Mechanisms in Progressive Multiple Sclerosis." *The Lancet Neurology*14, no. 2 (2015): 183-93. doi:10.1016/s1474-4422(14)70256-x.

Maksimovich, Ivan V. "Dementia and Cognitive Impairment Reduction after Laser Transcatheter Treatment of Alzheimer's Disease." *World Journal of Neuroscience*05, no. 03 (2015): 189-203. doi:10.4236/wjns.2015.53021.

Mander, Palwinder, Vilma Borutaite, Salvador Moncada, and Guy C. Brown. "Nitric oxide from inflammatory-activated glia synergizes with hypoxia to induce neuronal death." *Journal of Neuroscience Research*79, no. 1-2 (2004): 208-15. doi:10.1002/jnr.20285.

Mandolesi, S. "C1-C2 X-Ray assessment of misalignment parameters in patients with Chronic Cerebra-spinal Venous Insufficiency and Multiple Sclerosis versus patients with other pathologies." *Ann Ital Chir*86, no. 4 (2015): 293-300.

Marco, Eva M., Silvana Y. Romero-Zerbo, María-Paz Viveros, and Francisco J. Bermudez-Silva. "The Role of the Endocannabinoid System in Eating Disorders." *Behavioural Pharmacology*23, no. 5 and 6 (2012): 526-36. doi:10.1097/fbp.0b013e328356c3c9.

Marijuana and the Brain, Part II: The Tolerance Factor. Accessed April 30, 2018. http://www.marijuanalibrary.org/brain2.html.

Marrie, R. A., R. Rudick, R. Horwitz, G. Cutter, T. Tyry, D. Campagnolo, and T. Vollmer. "Vascular comorbidity is associated with more rapid disability progression in multiple sclerosis." *Neurology*74, no. 13 (2010): 1041-047. doi:10.1212/wnl.0b013e3181d6b125.

Mate, Gabor. *In the Realm of Hungry Ghosts: Close Encounters with Addiction.* Toronto: Random House, 2013.

Matthay, Michael A. "Saving Lives with High-Flow Nasal Oxygen." *New England Journal of Medicine*372, no. 23 (2015): 2225-226. doi:10.1056/nejme1504852.

May, A., M. Leone, J. Áfra, M. Linde, P. S. Sándor, S. Evers, and P. J. Goadsby. "EFNS Guidelines on the Treatment of Cluster Headache and Other Trigeminal-autonomic Cephalalgias." *European Journal of Neurology*13, no. 10 (2006): 1066-077. doi:10.1111/j.1468-1331.2006.01566.x.

Mcsherry, J. W., C. B. Carroll, J. Zajicek, L. Teare, and P. Bain. "Cannabis for dyskinesia in Parkinson disease: A randomized double-blind crossover study." *Neurology*64, no. 6 (2005): 1100. doi:10.1212/wnl.64.6.1100.

Mech, Arnold W., and Andrew Farah. "Correlation of Clinical Response with Homocysteine Reduction During Therapy with Reduced B Vitamins in Patients with MDD Who Are Positive for MTHFR C677T or A1298C Polymorphism." *The Journal of Clinical Psychiatry*, 2016, 668-71. doi:10.4088/jcp.15m10166.

Mechoulam, R. "Cannabinoids and Brain Injury: Therapeutic Implications." *Trends in Molecular Medicine*8, no. 2 (2002): 58-61. doi:10.1016/s1471-4914(02)02276-1.

Mehta, Vanita, Tajender S. Vasu, Barbara Phillips, and Frances Chung. "Obstructive Sleep Apnea and Oxygen Therapy: A Systematic Review of the Literature and Meta-Analysis." *Journal of Clinical Sleep Medicine*, 2013. doi:10.5664/jcsm.2500.

Meier, M. H., A. Caspi, A. Ambler, H. Harrington, R. Houts, R. S. E. Keefe, K. Mcdonald, A. Ward, R. Poulton, and T. E. Moffitt. "Persistent Cannabis Users Show Neuropsychological Decline from Childhood to Midlife." *Proceedings of the National Academy of Sciences*109, no. 40 (2012). doi:10.1073/pnas.1206820109.

Meirovithz, Elhanan, Judith Sonn, and Avraham Mayevsky. "Effect of hyperbaric oxygenation on brain hemodynamics, hemoglobin oxygenation and mitochondrial NADH" *Brain Research Reviews*54, no. 2 (2007): 294-304. doi:10.1016/j.brainresrev.2007.04.004.

Menni, Cristina, Chihung Lin, Marina Cecelja, Massimo Mangino, Maria Luisa Matey-Hernandez, Louise Keehn, Robert P. Mohney, Claire J. Steves, Tim D. Spector, Chang-Fu Kuo, Phil Chowienczyk, and Ana M. Valdes. "Gut Microbial Diversity Is Associated with Lower Arterial Stiffness in Women." *European Heart Journal*, May 2018. doi:10.1093/eurheartj/ehy226.

Mercola, Joseph. *Fat for Fuel: A Revolutionary Diet to Combat Cancer, Boost Brain Power, and Increase Your Energy*. Carlsbad, CA: Hay House, 2017.

Meschia, James F., Cheryl Bushnell, Bernadette Boden-Albala, Lynne T. Braun, Dawn M. Bravata, Seemant Chaturvedi, Mark A. Creager, Robert H. Eckel, Mitchell S.v. Elkind, Myriam Fornage, Larry B. Goldstein, Steven M. Greenberg, Susanna E. Horvath, Costantino Iadecola, Edward C. Jauch, Wesley S. Moore, and John A. Wilson. "Guidelines for the Primary Prevention of Stroke." *Stroke*45, no. 12 (2014): 3754-832. doi:10.1161/str.0000000000000046.

Mesnage, Robin, George Renney, Gilles-Eric Séralini, Malcolm Ward, and Michael N. Antoniou. "Multiomics reveal non-alcoholic fatty liver disease in rats following chronic exposure to an ultra-low dose of Roundup herbicide." *Scientific Reports*7 (2017): 39328. doi:10.1038/srep39328.

Metz, Luanne, and Stacey Page. "Oral cannabinoids for spasticity in multiple sclerosis: will attitude continue to limit use?" *The Lancet*362, no. 9395 (2003): 1513. doi:10.1016/s0140-6736(03)14776-9.

Micronutrient Information Center. Linus Pauling Institute. October 21, 2016. Accessed May 15, 2018. http://lpi.oregonstate.edu/mic.

Migraine Headache. Physiopedia. Accessed July 23, 2017. https://www.physio-pedia.com/Migraine_Headache.

Mikuriya, Tod H. "Cannabis as a Substitute for Alcohol: A Harm-Reduction Approach." *Journal of Cannabis Therapeutics*4, no. 1 (2004): 79-93. doi:10.1300/j175v04n01_04.

Milham, Samuel. "Historical Evidence That Electrification Caused the 20th Century Epidemic of 'diseases of Civilization.'" *Medical Hypotheses*74, no. 2 (2010): 337-45. doi:10.1016/j.mehy.2009.08.032.

Montagne, Axel, Angeliki M. Nikolakopoulou, Zhen Zhao, Abhay P. Sagare, Gabriel Si, Divna Lazic, Samuel R. Barnes, Madelaine Daianu, Anita Ramanathan, Ariel Go, Erica J. Lawson, Yaoming Wang, William J. Mack, Paul M. Thompson, Julie A. Schneider, Jobin Varkey, Ralf Langen, Eric Mullins, Russell E. Jacobs, and Berislav V. Zlokovic. "Pericyte Degeneration Causes White Matter Dysfunction in the Mouse Central Nervous System." *Nature Medicine*24, no. 3 (2018): 326-37. doi:10.1038/nm.4482.

More, Sandeep Vasant, and Dong-Kug Choi. "Promising cannabinoid-based therapies for Parkinson's disease: motor symptoms to neuroprotection." *Molecular Neurodegeneration*10, no. 1 (2015). doi:10.1186/s13024-015-0012-0.

Moss, Mark C., A. B. Scholey, and Keith Wesnes. "Oxygen Administration Selectively Enhances Cognitive Performance in Healthy Young Adults: A Placebo-controlled Double-blind Crossover Study." *Psychopharmacology*138, no. 1 (1998): 27-33. doi:10.1007/s002130050641.

Mullin, Gerard E. *Integrative gastroenterology*. New York: Oxford University Press, 2011.

Mullin, Gerard E. *The gut balance revolution: boost your metabolism, restore your inner ecology, and lose the weight for good!* New York, NY: Rodale, 2017.

Mullin, Gerard E., and Kathie Madonna. Swift. *The inside tract: your good gut guide to great digestive health*. New York, NY: Rodale, 2011.

Naeser, Margaret A., and Michael R. Hamblin. "Traumatic Brain Injury: A Major Medical Problem That Could Be Treated Using Transcranial, Red/

Near-Infrared LED Photobiomodulation." *Photomedicine and Laser Surgery*33, no. 9 (2015): 443-46. doi:10.1089/pho.2015.3986.

Naeser, Margaret A., Anita Saltmarche, Maxine H. Krengel, Michael R. Hamblin, and Jeffrey A. Knight. "Improved Cognitive Function After Transcranial, Light-Emitting Diode Treatments in Chronic, Traumatic Brain Injury: Two Case Reports." *Photomedicine and Laser Surgery*29, no. 5 (2011): 351-58. doi:10.1089/pho.2010.2814.

Naeser, Margaret A., Paula I. Martin, Kristine Lundgren, Reva Klein, Jerome Kaplan, Ethan Treglia, Michael Ho, Marjorie Nicholas, Miguel Alonso, and Alvaro Pascual-Leone. "Improved Language in a Chronic Nonfluent Aphasia Patient After Treatment with CPAP and TMS." *Cognitive and Behavioral Neurology*23, no. 1 (2010): 29-38. doi:10.1097/wnn.0b013e3181bf2d20.

Naeser, Margaret A., Ross Zafonte, Maxine H. Krengel, Paula I. Martin, Judith Frazier, Michael R. Hamblin, Jeffrey A. Knight, William P. Meehan, and Errol H. Baker. "Significant Improvements in Cognitive Performance Post-Transcranial, Red/Near-Infrared Light-Emitting Diode Treatments in Chronic, Mild Traumatic Brain Injury: Open-Protocol Study." *Journal of Neurotrauma*31, no. 11 (2014): 1008-017. doi:10.1089/neu.2013.3244.

Naftali, Timna, Lihi Bar-Lev Schleider, Iris Dotan, Ephraim Philip Lansky, Fabiana Sklerovsky Benjaminov, and Fred Meir Konikoff. "Cannabis Induces a Clinical Response in Patients With Crohns Disease: A Prospective Placebo-Controlled Study." *Clinical Gastroenterology and Hepatology*11, no. 10 (2013). doi:10.1016/j.cgh.2013.04.034.

Naftali, Timna, Lihi Bar-Lev Schleider, Iris Dotan, Ephraim Philip Lansky, Fabiana Sklerovsky Benjaminov, and Fred Meir Konikoff. "Cannabis Induces a Clinical Response in Patients With Crohns Disease: A Prospective Placebo-Controlled Study." *Clinical Gastroenterology and Hepatology*11, no. 10 (2013). doi:10.1016/j.cgh.2013.04.034.

Narayana, Ponnada A. "Magnetic Resonance Spectroscopy in the Monitoring of Multiple Sclerosis." *Journal of Neuroimaging*15 (2005). doi:10.1177/1051228405284200.

Neretin, V. Ya., M. A. Lobov, S. V. Kotov, G. F. Cheskidova, G. S. Molchanova, and O. G. Safronova. "Hyperbaric Oxygenation in Comprehensive Treatment of Parkinsonism." *Neuroscience and Behavioral Physiology*20, no. 6 (1990): 490-92. doi:10.1007/bf01237273.

Neumeister, A., M. D. Normandin, R. H. Pietrzak, D. Piomelli, M. Q. Zheng, A. Gujarro-Anton, M. N. Potenza, C. R. Bailey, S. F. Lin, S. Najafzadeh, J. Ropchan, S. Henry, S. Corsi-Travali, R. E. Carson, and Y. Huang. "Elevated Brain Cannabinoid CB1 Receptor Availability in Post-traumatic Stress Disorder: A Positron Emission Tomography Study." *Molecular Psychiatry*18, no. 9 (2013): 1034-040. doi:10.1038/mp.2013.61.

Nguyen, B. M., D. Kim, S. Bricker, F. Bongard, A. Neville, B. Putnam, J. Smith, and D. Plurad. "Effect of Marijuana Use on Outcomes in Traumatic Brain Injury." Advances in Pediatrics. October 2014. Accessed May 13, 2018. https://www.ncbi.nlm.nih.gov/pubmed/25264643.

Nieves, Jeri W., Chris Gennings, Pam Factor-Litvak, Jonathan Hupf, Jessica Singleton, Valerie Sharf, Björn Oskarsson, J. Americo M. Fernandes Filho, Eric J. Sorenson, Emanuele D'Amico, Ray Goetz, and Hiroshi Mitsumoto. "Association Between Dietary Intake and Function in Amyotrophic Lateral Sclerosis." *JAMA Neurology*73, no. 12 (2016): 1425. doi:10.1001/jamaneurol.2016.3401.

Nozari, Ala, Ergin Dilekoz, Inna Sukhotinsky, Thor Stein, Katharina Eikermann-Haerter, Christina Liu, Yumei Wang, Matthew P. Frosch, Christian Waeber, Cenk Ayata, and Michael A. Moskowitz. "Microemboli May Link Spreading Depression, Migraine Aura, and Patent Foramen Ovale." *Annals of Neurology*67, no. 2 (2010): 221-29. doi:10.1002/ana.21871.

Nugent, Shannon M., Benjamin J. Morasco, Maya E. Oneil, Michele Freeman, Allison Low, Karli Kondo, Camille Elven, Bernadette Zakher, Makalapua Motuapuaka, Robin Paynter, and Devan Kansagara. "The Effects of Cannabis Among Adults with Chronic Pain and an Overview of General Harms." *Annals of Internal Medicine*167, no. 5 (2017): 319. doi:10.7326/m17-0155.

Omalu, Bennet I., Steven T. Dekosky, Ryan L. Minster, M. Ilyas Kamboh, Ronald L. Hamilton, and Cyril H. Wecht. "Chronic Traumatic Encephalopathy in a National Football League Player." *Neurosurgery*57, no. 1 (2005): 128-34. doi:10.1227/01.neu.0000163407.92769.ed.

Omalu, Bennet I., Steven T. Dekosky, Ryan L. Minster, M. Ilyas Kamboh, Ronald L. Hamilton, and Cyril H. Wecht. "Chronic Traumatic Encephalopathy in a National Football League Player." *Neurosurgery*59, no. 5 (2006): 1086-092. doi:10.1097/00006123-200605000-00036.

Oneil, Maya E., Shannon M. Nugent, Benjamin J. Morasco, Michele Freeman, Allison Low, Karli Kondo, Bernadette Zakher, Camille Elven, Makalapua

Motuapuaka, Robin Paynter, and Devan Kansagara. "Benefits and Harms of Plant-Based Cannabis for Posttraumatic Stress Disorder." *Annals of Internal Medicine*167, no. 5 (2017): 332. doi:10.7326/m17-0477.

Orlander, Philip R., and George T. Griffing. "Hypothyroidism Clinical Presentation." Hypothyroidism Clinical Presentation: History, Physical Examination. March 06, 2018. Accessed July 24, 2017. https://emedicine.medscape.com/article/122393-clinical.

Ornish, D., S. E. Brown, J. H. Billings, L. W. Scherwitz, W. T. Armstrong, T. A. Ports, S. M. Mclanahan, R. L. Kirkeeide, K. L. Gould, and R. J. Brand. "Can Lifestyle Changes Reverse Coronary Heart Disease?" *The Lancet*336, no. 8708 (1990): 129-33. doi:10.1016/0140-6736(90)91656-u.

Oron, Amir, Uri Oron, Jieli Chen, Anda Eilam, Chunling Zhang, Menachem Sadeh, Yair Lampl, Jackson Streeter, Luis Detaboada, and Michael Chopp. "Low-Level Laser Therapy Applied Transcranially to Rats After Induction of Stroke Significantly Reduces Long-Term Neurological Deficits." *Stroke*37, no. 10 (2006): 2620-624. doi:10.1161/01.str.0000242775.14642.b8.

Owens, R. L. "Supplemental Oxygen Needs During Sleep. Who Benefits?" *Respiratory Care*58, no. 1 (2012): 32-47. doi:10.4187/respcare.01988.

Özdemir, F., M. Birtane, and S. Kokino. "The Clinical Efficacy of Low-Power Laser Therapy on Pain and Function in Cervical Osteoarthritis." *Clinical Rheumatology*20, no. 3 (2001): 181-84. doi:10.1007/s100670170061.

Panda, Suchita, Francisco Guarner, and Chaysavanh Manichanh. "Structure and Functions of the Gut Microbiome." *Endocrine, Metabolic & Immune Disorders-Drug Targets*14, no. 4 (2014): 290-99. doi:10.2174/1871530314666140714120744.

Passos, Giselle Soares, Dalva Poyares, Marcos Gonçalves Santana, Carolina Vicaria Rodrigues D'Aurea, Shawn D. Youngstedt, Sergio Tufik, and Marco Túlio De Mello. "Effects of Moderate Aerobic Exercise Training on Chronic Primary Insomnia." *Sleep Medicine*12, no. 10 (2011): 1018-027. doi:10.1016/j.sleep.2011.02.007.

Penn Study Finds Hyperbaric Oxygen Treatments Mobilize Stem Cells. ScienceDaily. December 28, 2005. Accessed July 23, 2016. https://www.sciencedaily.com/releases/2005/12/051228175511.htm.

Perlmutter, David. *Brain Maker: The Power of Gut Microbes to Heal and Protect Your Brain-for Life*. Little, Brown and Company, 2015.

Pertwee, R. G. "The Diverse CB1and CB2receptor Pharmacology of Three Plant Cannabinoids: Δ9-tetrahydrocannabinol, Cannabidiol and Δ9-tetrahydrocannabivarin." *British Journal of Pharmacology*153, no. 2 (2008): 199-215. doi:10.1038/sj.bjp.0707442.

Petersen, Anja S., Mads Cj Barloese, Nunu Lt Lund, and Rigmor H. Jensen. "Oxygen Therapy for Cluster Headache. A Mask Comparison Trial. A Single-blinded, Placebo-controlled, Crossover Study." *Cephalalgia*37, no. 3 (2016): 214-24. doi:10.1177/0333102416637817.

Petrov, Ivo, Lachezar Grozdinski, Svetlin Tsonev, Mariana Iloska, and Iveta Tasheva. "Hypercapnia and Hypoxaemia Due to Impaired Venous Blood Draining and Significant Improvement after Endovascular Treatment in Patients with Chronic Cerebrospinal Venous Insufficiency." *Phlebological Review*1 (2016): 20-24. doi:10.5114/pr.2016.61534.

Piepmeier, Aaron T., and Jennifer L. Etnier. "Brain-derived Neurotrophic Factor (BDNF) as a Potential Mechanism of the Effects of Acute Exercise on Cognitive Performance." *Journal of Sport and Health Science*4, no. 1 (2015): 14-23. doi:10.1016/j.jshs.2014.11.001.

Pisa, Diana, Ruth Alonso, Ana M. Fernández-Fernández, Alberto Rábano, and Luis Carrasco. "Polymicrobial Infections In Brain Tissue From Alzheimer's Disease Patients." *Scientific Reports*7, no. 1 (2017). doi:10.1038/s41598-017-05903-y.

Pokorski, M., and U. Jernajczyk. "Nocturnal Oxygen Enrichment in Sleep Apnoea." *Journal of International Medical Research*28, no. 1 (2000): 1-8. doi:10.1177/147323000002800101.

Pollan, Michael. *The Omnivores Dilemma a Natural History of Four Meals*. New York, NY: Penguin Books, 2016.

Popper, Charles W. "Single-Micronutrient and Broad-Spectrum Micronutrient Approaches for Treating Mood Disorders in Youth and Adults." *Child and Adolescent Psychiatric Clinics of North America*23, no. 3 (2014): 591-672. doi:10.1016/j.chc.2014.04.001.

Pröbstel, Anne-Katrin, and Sergio E. Baranzini. "The Role of the Gut Microbiome in Multiple Sclerosis Risk and Progression: Towards Characterization of the 'MS Microbiome.'" *Neurotherapeutics*15, no. 1 (2017): 126-34. doi:10.1007/s13311-017-0587-y.

Pryce, Gareth, and David Baker. "Potential Control of Multiple Sclerosis by Cannabis and the Endocannabinoid System." *CNS & Neurological Disorders - Drug Targets*11, no. 5 (2012): 624-41. doi:10.2174/187152712801661310.

Purandare, Nitin, Alistair Burns, Kevin J. Daly, Jayne Hardicre, Julie Morris, Gary Macfarlane, and Charles Mccollum. "Cerebral emboli as a potential cause of Alzheimers disease and vascular dementia: casecontrol study." *Bmj*332, no. 7550 (2006): 1119-124. doi:10.1136/bmj.38814.696493.ae.

Raby, Wilfrid Noel, Kenneth M. Carpenter, Jami Rothenberg, Adam C. Brooks, Huiping Jiang, Maria Sullivan, Adam Bisaga, Sandra Comer, and Edward V. Nunes. "Intermittent Marijuana Use Is Associated with Improved Retention in Naltrexone Treatment for Opiate-Dependence." *American Journal on Addictions*18, no. 4 (2009): 301-08. doi:10.1080/10550490902927785.

Rain, Alesandra, Andrea Crocker, and Bill Code. *Point of Return: Your Personal Guide to Taper off Anti-anxiety & Anti-depressant Drugs*. Label Me Sane, 2006.

Rain, Alesandra. *Deeds of Trust: A True Story*. Malibu, CA: Label Me Sane, 2005.

Ramirez, B. G. "Prevention of Alzheimers Disease Pathology by Cannabinoids: Neuroprotection Mediated by Blockade of Microglial Activation." *Journal of Neuroscience*25, no. 8 (2005): 1904-913. doi:10.1523/jneurosci.4540-04.2005.

Reddy, P. Hemachandra. "Mitochondrial Medicine for Aging and Neurodegenerative Diseases." *NeuroMolecular Medicine*10, no. 4 (2008): 291-315. doi:10.1007/s12017-008-8044-z.

Reiman, Amanda, Mark Welty, and Perry Solomon. "Cannabis as a Substitute for Opioid-Based Pain Medication: Patient Self-Report." *Cannabis and Cannabinoid Research*2, no. 1 (2017): 160-66. doi:10.1089/can.2017.0012.

Reisman, Mark, Ryan D. Christofferson, Jill Jesurum, John V. Olsen, Merrill P. Spencer, Kimberly A. Krabill, Lance Diehl, Sheena Aurora, and William A. Gray. "Migraine Headache Relief after Transcatheter Closure of Patent Foramen Ovale." *Journal of the American College of Cardiology*45, no. 4 (2005): 493-95. doi:10.1016/j.jacc.2004.10.055.

Rhyne, Danielle N., Sarah L. Anderson, Margaret Gedde, and Laura M. Borgelt. "Effects of Medical Marijuana on Migraine Headache Frequency in an Adult Population." *Pharmacotherapy: The Journal of Human Pharmacology and Drug Therapy*36, no. 5 (2016): 505-10. doi:10.1002/phar.1673.

Roberts, Emmert, Vanessa Delgado Nunes, Sara Buckner, Susan Latchem, Margaret Constanti, Paul Miller, Michael Doherty, Weiya Zhang, Fraser Birrell, Mark Porcheret, Krysia Dziedzic, Ian Bernstein, Elspeth Wise, and Philip G. Conaghan. "Paracetamol: not as safe as we thought? A systematic literature review of observational studies." *Annals of the Rheumatic Diseases*75, no. 3 (2015): 552-59. doi:10.1136/annrheumdis-2014-206914.

Rogers, Sherry A. *Detoxify or Die*. Sarasota, FL: Sand Key Company, 2002.

Rosenberg, Gary A. "Neurological Diseases in Relation to the Blood–Brain Barrier." *Journal of Cerebral Blood Flow & Metabolism*32, no. 7 (2012): 1139-151. doi:10.1038/jcbfm.2011.197.

Rossi, Silvia, Caterina Motta, Valeria Studer, Giulia Macchiarulo, Elisabetta Volpe, Francesca Barbieri, Gabriella Ruocco, Fabio Buttari, Annamaria Finardi, Raffaele Mancino, Sagit Weiss, Luca Battistini, Gianvito Martino, Roberto Furlan, Jelena Drulovic, and Diego Centonze. "Interleukin-1β Causes Excitotoxic Neurodegeneration and Multiple Sclerosis Disease Progression by Activating the Apoptotic Protein P53." *Molecular Neurodegeneration*9, no. 1 (2014): 56. doi:10.1186/1750-1326-9-56.

Rossignol, Daniel A. "Hyperbaric oxygen treatment for inflammatory bowel disease: a systematic review and analysis." *Medical Gas Research*2, no. 1 (2012): 6. doi:10.1186/2045-9912-2-6.

Round, June L., and Sarkis K. Mazmanian. "The gut microbiota shapes intestinal immune responses during health and disease." *Nature Reviews Immunology*9, no. 5 (2009): 313-23. doi:10.1038/nri2515.

Rubin, Clinton, Stefan Judex, and Yi-Xian Qin. "Low-level mechanical signals and their potential as a non-pharmacological intervention for osteoporosis." *Age and Ageing*35, no. Suppl_2 (2006): Ii32-i36. doi:10.1093/ageing/afl082.

Rundshagen, Ingrid. "Postoperative Cognitive Dysfunction." *Deutsches Aerzteblatt Online*, 2014. doi:10.3238/arztebl.2014.0119.

Russell, James. "RESONANCE—BEINGS OF FREQUENCY." Vimeo. 2013. https://vimeo.com/54189727.

Russo, Ethan B. "Cannabidiol Claims and Misconceptions." *Trends in Pharmacological Sciences*38, no. 3 (2017): 198-201. doi:10.1016/j.tips.2016.12.004.

Russo, Ethan B. "Clinical Endocannabinoid Deficiency Reconsidered: Current Research Supports the Theory in Migraine, Fibromyalgia, Irritable Bowel, and

Other Treatment-Resistant Syndromes." *Cannabis and Cannabinoid Research*1, no. 1 (2016): 154-65. doi:10.1089/can.2016.0009.

Russo, Ethan B. "Current Therapeutic Cannabis Controversies and Clinical Trial Design Issues." *Frontiers in Pharmacology*7 (2016). doi:10.3389/fphar.2016.00309.

Russo, Ethan B. "Taming THC: Potential Cannabis Synergy and Phytocannabinoid-terpenoid Entourage Effects." *British Journal of Pharmacology*163, no. 7 (2011): 1344-364. doi:10.1111/j.1476-5381.2011.01238.x.

Russo, Ethan B., and Jahan Marcu. "Cannabis Pharmacology: The Usual Suspects and a Few Promising Leads." *Cannabinoid Pharmacology Advances in Pharmacology*, 2017, 67-134. doi:10.1016/bs.apha.2017.03.004.

Russo, Ethan. "Cannabis for Migraine Treatment: The Once and Future Prescription? An Historical and Scientific Review." *Pain*76, no. 1 (1998): 3-8. doi:10.1016/s0304-3959(98)00033-5.

Ryu, Jae Kyu, Mark A. Petersen, Sara G. Murray, Kim M. Baeten, Anke Meyer-Franke, Justin P. Chan, Eirini Vagena, Catherine Bedard, Michael R. Machado, Pamela E. Rios Coronado, Thomas Prodhomme, Israel F. Charo, Hans Lassmann, Jay L. Degen, Scott S. Zamvil, and Katerina Akassoglou. "Blood Coagulation Protein Fibrinogen Promotes Autoimmunity and Demyelination via Chemokine Release and Antigen Presentation." *Nature Communications*6, no. 1 (2015). doi:10.1038/ncomms9164.

Ryz, Natasha R., David J. Remillard, and Ethan B. Russo. "Cannabis Roots: A Traditional Therapy with Future Potential for Treating Inflammation and Pain." *Cannabis and Cannabinoid Research*2, no. 1 (2017): 210-16. doi:10.1089/can.2017.0028.

Sadrzadeh, S.m. Hossein, and Yasi Saffari. "Iron and Brain Disorders." *Pathology Patterns Reviews*121, no. Suppl_1 (2004). doi:10.1309/ew0121lg9n3n1yl4.

Sakurai, Takeshi. "The Neural Circuit of Orexin (hypocretin): Maintaining Sleep and Wakefulness." *Nature Reviews Neuroscience*8, no. 3 (2007): 171-81. doi:10.1038/nrn2092.

Salatin, Joel. *Everything I Want to Do Is Illegal.* Swoope, VA: Polyface, 2007.

Salgado, Afonso S. I., Renato A. Zângaro, Rodolfo B. Parreira, and Ivo I. Kerppers. "The effects of transcranial LED therapy (TCLT) on cerebral blood flow in the elderly women." *Lasers in Medical Science*30, no. 1 (2014): 339-46. doi:10.1007/s10103-014-1669-2.

Sampson, Timothy R., Justine W. Debelius, Taren Thron, Stefan Janssen, Gauri G. Shastri, Zehra Esra Ilhan, Collin Challis, Catherine E. Schretter, Sandra Rocha, Viviana Gradinaru, Marie-Francoise Chesselet, Ali Keshavarzian, Kathleen M. Shannon, Rosa Krajmalnik-Brown, Pernilla Wittung-Stafshede, Rob Knight, and Sarkis K. Mazmanian. "Gut Microbiota Regulate Motor Deficits and Neuroinflammation in a Model of Parkinson's Disease." *Cell*167, no. 6 (2016). doi:10.1016/j.cell.2016.11.018.

Samsel, Anthony, and Stephanie Seneff. "Glyphosate, pathways to modern diseases II: Celiac sprue and gluten intolerance." *Interdisciplinary Toxicology*6, no. 4 (2013). doi:10.2478/intox-2013-0026.

Sandler, Richard H., Sydney M. Finegold, Ellen R. Bolte, Cathleen P. Buchanan, Anne P. Maxwell, Marja-Liisa Väisänen, Michael N. Nelson, and Hannah M. Wexler. "Short-Term Benefit From Oral Vancomycin Treatment of Regressive-Onset Autism." *Journal of Child Neurology*15, no. 7 (2000): 429-35. doi:10.1177/088307380001500701.

Sarchielli, Paola, Luigi Alberto Pini, Francesca Coppola, Cristiana Rossi, Antonio Baldi, Maria Luisa Mancini, and Paolo Calabresi. "Endocannabinoids in Chronic Migraine: CSF Findings Suggest a System Failure." *Neuropsychopharmacology*32, no. 6 (2007): 1432. doi:10.1038/sj.npp.1301320.

Saresella, Marina, Laura Mendozzi, Valentina Rossi, Franca Mazzali, Federica Piancone, Francesca Larosa, Ivana Marventano, Domenico Caputo, Giovanna E. Felis, and Mario Clerici. "Immunological and Clinical Effect of Diet Modulation of the Gut Microbiome in Multiple Sclerosis Patients: A Pilot Study." *Frontiers in Immunology*8 (2017). doi:10.3389/fimmu.2017.01391.

Sathasivam, Sivarani, and Sivakumar Sathasivam. "Patent Foramen Ovale and Migraine: What Is the Relationship between the Two?" *Journal of Cardiology*61, no. 4 (2013): 256-59. doi:10.1016/j.jjcc.2012.12.005.

Savage, Judith. "Oxygen Therapy for Cluster Headaches." Accessed July 17, 2017. https://www.uhb.nhs.uk/Downloads/pdf/PiOxygenTherapyCluster-Headaches.pdf.

Scavone, J.l., R.c. Sterling, and E.j. Van Bockstaele. "Cannabinoid and Opioid Interactions: Implications for Opiate Dependence and Withdrawal." *Neuroscience*248 (2013): 637-54. doi:10.1016/j.neuroscience.2013.04.034.

Schalinske, Kevin L., and Anne L. Smazal. "Homocysteine Imbalance: A Pathological Metabolic Marker." *Advances in Nutrition*3, no. 6 (2012): 755-62. doi:10.3945/an.112.002758.

Schelling, F. "Multiple Sclerosis." Multiple Sclerosis. Accessed May 15, 2018. http://www.ms-info.net/evo/msmanu/984.htm.

Scheperjans, Filip, Velma Aho, Pedro A. B. Pereira, Kaisa Koskinen, Lars Paulin, Eero Pekkonen, Elena Haapaniemi, Seppo Kaakkola, Johanna Eerola-Rautio, Marjatta Pohja, Esko Kinnunen, Kari Murros, and Petri Auvinen. "Gut Microbiota Are Related to Parkinsons Disease and Clinical Phenotype." *Movement Disorders*30, no. 3 (2014): 350-58. doi:10.1002/mds.26069.

Schicho, Rudolf, and Martin Storr. "Patients with IBD Find Symptom Relief in the Cannabis Field." *Nature Reviews Gastroenterology & Hepatology*11, no. 3 (2013): 142-43. doi:10.1038/nrgastro.2013.245.

Schiffer, Fredric, Andrea L. Johnston, Caitlin Ravichandran, Ann Polcari, Martin H. Teicher, Robert H. Webb, and Michael R. Hamblin. "Psychological benefits 2 and 4 weeks after a single treatment with near infrared light to the forehead: a pilot study of 10 patients with major depression and anxiety." *Behavioral and Brain Functions*5, no. 1 (2009): 46. doi:10.1186/1744-9081-5-46.

Scholey, Andrew B., Mark C. Moss, Nick Neave, and Keith Wesnes. "Cognitive Performance, Hyperoxia, and Heart Rate Following Oxygen Administration in Healthy Young Adults." *Physiology & Behavior*67, no. 5 (1999): 783-89. doi:10.1016/s0031-9384(99)00183-3.

Schuhfried, Othmar, Christian Mittermaier, Tatjana Jovanovic, Karin Pieber, and Tatjana Paternostro-Sluga. "Effects of whole-body vibration in patients with multiple sclerosis: a pilot study." *Clinical Rehabilitation*19, no. 8 (2005): 834-42. doi:10.1191/0269215505cr919oa.

Schwarcz, Glenn, Basawaraj Karajgi, and Richard Mccarthy. "Synthetic Δ-9-Tetrahydrocannabinol (Dronabinol) Can Improve the Symptoms of Schizophrenia." *Journal of Clinical Psychopharmacology*29, no. 3 (2009): 255-58. doi:10.1097/jcp.0b013e3181a6bc3b.

Semenza, Gregg L., MD, PhD. "Oxygen Sensing, Homeostasis, and Disease." *New England Journal of Medicine*365, no. 19 (2011): 1845-846. doi:10.1056/nejmc1110602.

Seneff, Stephanie, Glyn Wainwright, and Luca Mascitelli. "Nutrition and Alzheimers Disease: The Detrimental Role of a High Carbohydrate Diet." *European Journal of Internal Medicine*22, no. 2 (2011): 134-40. doi:10.1016/j.ejim.2010.12.017.

Sepe, Vincenzo, Gabriella Adamo, Maria Grazia Giuliano, Carmelo Libetta, and Antonio Dal Canton. "Folic acid for stroke prevention." *The Lancet*370, no. 9588 (2007): 651. doi:10.1016/s0140-6736(07)61328-2.

Shahripour, Reza Bavarsad, et al. "N-Acetylcysteine (NAC) in Neurological Disorders: Mechanisms of Action and Therapeutic Opportunities." *Brain and Behavior*, vol. 4, no. 2, 2014, pp. 108–122., doi:10.1002/brb3.208.

Shalev, Arieh, Israel Liberzon, and Charles Marmar. "Post-Traumatic Stress Disorder." *New England Journal of Medicine*376, no. 25 (2017): 2459-469. doi:10.1056/nejmra1612499.

Shaw, William, and Bernard Rimland. *Biological Treatments for Autism & PDD:*. Lenexa, Kan.: Great Plains Laboratory, 2008.

Shaw, William, Kurt Woeller, Daniel Rossignol, Lenny Gonzalez, Denise Tarasuk, and Doris Rapp. *Autism: Beyond the Basics: Treating Autism Spectrum Disorders*. Lenexa, Kan.: W. Shaw, 2009.

Shaw, William. "Evidence That Increased Acetaminophen Use in Genetically Vulnerable Children Appears to Be a Major Cause of the Epidemics of Autism, Attention Deficit with Hyperactivity, and Asthma." *Journal of Restorative Medicine*2, no. 1 (2013): 14-29. doi:10.14200/jrm.2013.2.0101.

Shaw, William. "Increased urinary excretion of a 3-(3-hydroxyphenyl)-3-hydroxypropionic acid (HPHPA), an abnormal phenylalanine metabolite of Clostridia spp in the gastrointestinal tract, in urine samples from patients with autism and schizophrenia." *Nutritional Neuroscience*13, no. 3 (2010): 135-43. doi:10.1179/147683010x12611460763968.

Shaw, William. "The Unique Vulnerability of the Human Brain to Toxic Chemical Exposure and the Importance of Toxic Chemical Evaluation and Treatment in Orthomolecular Psychiatry." *Journal of Orthomolecular Medicine*25, no. 3 (2010): 125-34. http://www.isom.ca/wp-content/uploads/2013/01/The-Unique-Vulnerability-of-the-Human-Brain-to-Toxic-Chemical-Exposure-and-the-Importance-of-Toxic-Chemical-Evaluation-and-Treatment-in-Orthomolecular-Psychiatry-25.3.pdf.

Shehata, Awad A., Wieland Schrödl, Alaa. A. Aldin, Hafez M. Hafez, and Monika Krüger. "The Effect of Glyphosate on Potential Pathogens and Beneficial Members of Poultry Microbiota In Vitro." *Current Microbiology*66, no. 4 (2012): 350-58. doi:10.1007/s00284-012-0277-2.

Shoenfeld, Y. "Are You Developing an Autoimmune Disease Years Before Symptoms." The Gluten Summit. 2013. Accessed May 15, 2018. http://theglutensummit.com/.

Shohami, Esther, Ayelet Cohen-Yeshurun, Lital Magid, Merav Algali, and Raphael Mechoulam. "Endocannabinoids and Traumatic Brain Injury." *British Journal of Pharmacology*163, no. 7 (2011): 1402-410. doi:10.1111/j.1476-5381.2011.01343.x.

Shungu, Dikoma C., Nora Weiduschat, James W. Murrough, Xiangling Mao, Sarah Pillemer, Jonathan P. Dyke, Marvin S. Medow, Benjamin H. Natelson, Julian M. Stewart, and Sanjay J. Mathew. "Increased Ventricular Lactate in Chronic Fatigue Syndrome. III. Relationships to Cortical Glutathione and Clinical Symptoms Implicate Oxidative Stress in Disorder Pathophysiology." *NMR in Biomedicine*25, no. 9 (2012): 1073-087. doi:10.1002/nbm.2772.

Simpson, R. "FAQ about RSO." FAQ about RSO « Phoenix Tears | Rick Simpson. Accessed May 12, 2018. http://phoenixtears.ca/faq-about-rso/.

Siri-Tarino, Patty W., Qi Sun, Frank B. Hu, and Ronald M. Krauss. "Saturated fat, carbohydrate, and cardiovascular disease." *The American Journal of Clinical Nutrition*91, no. 3 (2010): 502-09. doi:10.3945/ajcn.2008.26285.

Sjösten, Noora, and Sirkka-Liisa Kivelä. "The Effects of Physical Exercise on Depressive Symptoms among the Aged: A Systematic Review." *International Journal of Geriatric Psychiatry*21, no. 5 (2006): 410-18. doi:10.1002/gps.1494.

Slesserev, M., and J. Fisher. "Oxygen Administration in the Emergency Department: Choosing the Appropriate Dosage and the Technology." *Israeli Journal of Emergency Medicine*6, no. 1 (January 2006): 10-21.

Smith, Fran. "The Science of Addiction." National Geographic. September 2017. Accessed May 12, 2018. https://www.nationalgeographic.com/magazine/2017/09/science-of-addiction/.

Socías, M. Eugenia, Thomas Kerr, Evan Wood, Huiru Dong, Stephanie Lake, Kanna Hayashi, Kora Debeck, Didier Jutras-Aswad, Julio Montaner, and M-J Milloy. "Intentional Cannabis Use to Reduce Crack Cocaine Use in a Canadian Setting: A Longitudinal Analysis." *Addictive Behaviors*72 (2017): 138-43. doi:10.1016/j.addbeh.2017.04.006.

Somers, Emily C., Sara L. Thomas, Liam Smeeth, and Andrew J. Hall. "Auto-immune Diseases Co-occurring Within Individuals and Within Families." *Epidemiology*17, no. 2 (2006): 202-17. doi:10.1097/01.ede.0000193605.93416.df.

Sommer, Isolde, Ursula Griebler, Christina Kien, Stefanie Auer, Irma Kler-ings, Renate Hammer, Peter Holzer, and Gerald Gartlehner. "Vitamin D Deficiency as a Risk Factor for Dementia: A Systematic Review and Meta-analysis." *BMC Geriatrics*17, no. 1 (2017). doi:10.1186/s12877-016-0405-0.

Sparling, P. B., A. Giuffrida, D. Piomelli, L. Rosskopf, and A. Dietrich. "Exer-cise Activates the Endocannabinoid System." *NeuroReport*14, no. 17 (2003): 2209-211. doi:10.1097/00001756-200312020-00015.

Stankiewicz, James M., Mohit Neema, and Antonia Cecca-relli. "Iron and multiple sclerosis." *Neurobiology of Aging*35 (2014). doi:10.1016/j.neurobiolaging.2014.03.039.

Stoller, Kenneth P. "All the right moves: the need for the timely use of . . ." 2015. Accessed June 6, 2017. https://link.springer.com/content/pdf/10.1186%2Fs13618-015-0028-0.pdf.

Stoller, Kenneth P. "All the Right Moves: The Need for the Timely Use of Hyperbaric Oxygen Therapy for Treating TBI/CTE/PTSD." *Medical Gas Research*5, no. 1 (2015). doi:10.1186/s13618-015-0028-0.

Strause, Tyler. "Supporting Your Endocannabinoid System: - Randy's Club - Medium." Medium. June 28, 2016. Accessed May 13, 2018. https://medium.com/randy-s-club/supporting-your-endocannabinoid-system-5db4c35d6037.

Sullan, Molly J., Breton M. Asken, Michael S. Jaffee, Steven T. Dekosky, and Russell M. Bauer. "Glymphatic System Disruption as a Mediator of Brain Trauma and Chronic Traumatic Encephalopathy." *Neuroscience & Biobehav-ioral Reviews*84 (2018): 316-24. doi:10.1016/j.neubiorev.2017.08.016.

Svensson, Elisabeth, Reimar W. Thomsen, Jens Christian Djurhuus, Lars Pedersen, Per Borghammer, and Henrik Toft Sørensen. "Vagotomy and Subse-quent Risk of Parkinson's Disease." FEBS Letters. July 17, 2015. Accessed May 16, 2018. https://febs.onlinelibrary.wiley.com/doi/10.1002/ana.24448.

Swank, R. L. "Subcutaneous Hemorrhages in Multiple Sclerosis." *Neurology*8, no. 6 (1958): 497. doi:10.1212/wnl.8.6.497.

Swash, Michael. "Dietary Factors and Amyotrophic Lateral Sclerosis." *JAMA Neurology*73, no. 12 (2016): 1398. doi:10.1001/jamaneurol.2016.3905.

Taboada, Luis De, Jin Yu, Salim El-Amouri, Sebastiano Gattoni-Celli, Steve Richieri, Thomas Mccarthy, Jackson Streeter, and Mark S. Kindy. "Transcranial Laser Therapy Attenuates Amyloid-β Peptide Neuropathology in Amyloid-β Protein Precursor Transgenic Mice." *Journal of Alzheimer's Disease*23, no. 3 (2011): 521-35. doi:10.3233/jad-2010-100894.

Takahashi, Kazuhiro, Zenei Arihara, Takashi Suzuki, Masahiko Sone, Kumi Kikuchi, Hironobu Sasano, Osamu Murakami, and Kazuhito Totsune. "Expression of orexin-A and orexin receptors in the kidney and the presence of orexin-A-like immunoreactivity in human urine." *Peptides*27, no. 4 (2006): 871-77. doi:10.1016/j.peptides.2005.08.008.

Talbert, David G. "Raised venous pressure as a factor in multiple sclerosis." *Medical Hypotheses*70, no. 6 (2008): 1112-117. doi:10.1016/j.mehy.2007.10.009.

Tam, Joseph, Jie Liu, Bani Mukhopadhyay, Resat Cinar, Grzegorz Godlewski, and George Kunos. "Endocannabinoids in Liver Disease." *Hepatology*53, no. 1 (2011): 346-55. doi:10.1002/hep.24077.

Tarnopolsky, M. A. "The Mitochondrial Cocktail: Rationale for Combined Nutraceutical Therapy in Mitochondrial Cytopathies." *Advanced Drug Delivery Reviews*60, no. 13-14 (2008): 1561-567. doi:10.1016/j.addr.2008.05.001.

Taylor, Enid. *Kefir—Nature's Little Miracle?* Letchworth Garden City: Taymount Clinic, 2016.

Teller, Edward, PhD. "On Hyperbaric Oxygenation." *Journal of American Physicians and Surgeons*8, no. 4 (2003): 97.

Tergau, Frithjof, Ute Naumann, Walter Paulus, and Bernhard J. Steinhoff. "Low-frequency Repetitive Transcranial Magnetic Stimulation Improves Intractable Epilepsy." *The Lancet*353, no. 9171 (1999): 2209. doi:10.1016/s0140-6736(99)01301-x.

The World of Cannabinoid Acids Like THCa and CBDa Will Make You Re-Think Cannabis. Green Flower Media. Accessed May 13, 2018. https://www.learngreenflower.com/articles/539/the-world-of-cannabinoid-acids-like-thca-and-cbda-will-make-you-re-think-cannabis.

Thom, Stephen R. "Hyperbaric Oxygen: Its Mechanisms and Efficacy." *Plastic and Reconstructive Surgery*127 (2011). doi:10.1097/prs.0b013e3181fbe2bf.

Thom, Stephen R., Ming Yang, Veena M. Bhopale, Tatyana N. Milovanova, Marina Bogush, and Donald G. Buerk. "Intramicroparticle nitrogen dioxide is a bubble nucleation site leading to decompression-induced neutrophil activation and vascular injury." *Journal of Applied Physiology*114, no. 5 (2013): 550-58. doi:10.1152/japplphysiol.01386.2012.

Thom, Stephen R., Veena M. Bhopale, Omaida C. Velazquez, Lee J. Goldstein, Lynne H. Thom, and Donald G. Buerk. "Stem Cell Mobilization by Hyperbaric Oxygen." *American Journal of Physiology-Heart and Circulatory Physiology*290, no. 4 (2006). doi:10.1152/ajpheart.00888.2005.

Tomassini, Valentina, Heidi Johansen-Berg, Saad Jbabdi, Richard G. Wise, Carlo Pozzilli, Jacqueline Palace, and Paul M. Matthews. "Relating Brain Damage to Brain Plasticity in Patients with Multiple Sclerosis." *Neurorehabilitation and Neural Repair*26, no. 6 (2012): 581-93. doi:10.1177/1545968311433208.

Tunez, Isaac. "Gut Microbiota and Central Nervous System Condemned to Understand Each Other: Their Role in Multiple Sclerosis." *MOJ Cell Science & Report*1, no. 2 (2014). doi:10.15406/mojcsr.2014.01.00005.

Tyler, Mitchell E., Kurt A. Kaczmarek, Kathy L. Rust, Alla M. Subbotin, Kimberly L. Skinner, and Yuri P. Danilov. "Non-invasive neuromodulation to improve gait in chronic multiple sclerosis: a randomized double blind controlled pilot trial." *Journal of NeuroEngineering and Rehabilitation*11, no. 1 (2014): 79. doi:10.1186/1743-0003-11-79.

Uttara, Bayani, Ajay Singh, Paolo Zamboni, and R. Mahajan. "Oxidative Stress and Neurodegenerative Diseases: A Review of Upstream and Downstream Antioxidant Therapeutic Options." *Current Neuropharmacology*7, no. 1 (2009): 65-74. doi:10.2174/157015909787602823.

Valdeolivas, Sara, Carmen Navarrete, Irene Cantarero, María L. Bellido, Eduardo Muñoz, and Onintza Sagredo. "Neuroprotective Properties of Cannabigerol in Huntington's Disease: Studies in R6/2 Mice and 3-Nitropropionate-lesioned Mice." *Neurotherapeutics*12, no. 1 (2014): 185-99. doi:10.1007/s13311-014-0304-z.

Vanga, Rohini, and Daniel A. Leffler. "Gluten Sensitivity: Not Celiac and Not Certain." *Gastroenterology*145, no. 2 (2013): 276-79. doi:10.1053/j.gastro.2013.06.027.

Velarde, Michael C. "Mitochondrial and Sex Steroid Hormone Crosstalk during Aging." *Longevity & Healthspan*3, no. 1 (2014): 2. doi:10.1186/2046-2395-3-2.

Venderová, Kateřina, Evžen Růžička, Viktor Voříšek, and Peter Višňovský. "Survey on Cannabis Use in Parkinsons Disease: Subjective Improvement of Motor Symptoms." *Movement Disorders*19, no. 9 (2004): 1102-106. doi:10.1002/mds.20111.

Verhoeckx, Kitty C.m., Henrie A.a.j. Korthout, A.p. Van Meeteren-Kreikamp, Karl A. Ehlert, Mei Wang, Jan Van Der Greef, Richard J.t. Rodenburg, and Renger F. Witkamp. "Unheated Cannabis Sativa Extracts and Its Major Compound THC-acid Have Potential Immuno-modulating Properties Not Mediated by CB1 and CB2 Receptor Coupled Pathways." *International Immunopharmacology*6, no. 4 (2006): 656-65. doi:10.1016/j.intimp.2005.10.002.

Vojdani, A., T. Obryan, J. A. Green, J. Mccandless, K. N. Woeller, E. Vojdani, A. A. Nourian, and E. L. Cooper. "Immune Response to Dietary Proteins, Gliadin and Cerebellar Peptides in Children with Autism." *Nutritional Neuroscience*7, no. 3 (2004): 151-61. doi:10.1080/10284150400004155.

Vojdani, Aristo. "The Characterization of the Repertoire of Wheat Antigens and Peptides Involved in the Humoral Immune Responses in Patients with Gluten Sensitivity and Crohns Disease." *ISRN Allergy*2011 (2011): 1-12. doi:10.5402/2011/950104.

Volek, Jeff S., Maria Luz Fernandez, Richard D. Feinman, and Stephen D. Phinney. "Dietary carbohydrate restriction induces a unique metabolic state positively affecting atherogenic dyslipidemia, fatty acid partitioning, and metabolic syndrome." *Progress in Lipid Research*47, no. 5 (2008): 307-18. doi:10.1016/j.plipres.2008.02.003.

Vu, Michelle P., Gil Y. Melmed, and Stephan R. Targan. "Weeding Out the Facts: The Reality About Cannabis and Crohns Disease." *Clinical Gastroenterology and Hepatology*12, no. 5 (2014): 898-99. doi:10.1016/j.cgh.2013.11.016.

Wahls, Terry L. *Minding My Mitochondria: How I Overcame Secondary Progressive Multiple Sclerosis (MS) and Got out of My Wheelchair: Includes over 100 Recipes for a Healthy Brain!: A Practical Guide to Understanding Mitochondrial Health and the Steps You Can Take to Improve Your Brains Function and Health.* IA City, IA, U.S.A.: TZ Press, 2010.

Wahls, Terry L., and Eve Adamson. *The Wahls Protocol: A Radical New Way to Treat All Chronic Autoimmune Conditions Using Paleo Principles.* New York: Avery, 2015.

Walker, J. M., and A. G. Hohmann. "Cannabinoid Mechanisms of Pain Suppression." *Handbook of Experimental Pharmacology Cannabinoids*, 2005, 509-54. doi:10.1007/3-540-26573-2_17.

Walsh, Zach, Raul Gonzalez, Kim Crosby, Michelle S. Thiessen, Chris Carroll, and Marcel O. Bonn-Miller. "Medical cannabis and mental health: A guided systematic review." *Clinical Psychology Review*51 (2017): 15-29. doi:10.1016/j.cpr.2016.10.002.

Wang, Xiaobin, Xianhui Qin, Hakan Demirtas, Jianping Li, Guangyun Mao, Yong Huo, Ningling Sun, Lisheng Liu, and Xiping Xu. "Efficacy of folic acid supplementation in stroke prevention: a meta-analysis." *The Lancet*369, no. 9576 (2007): 1876-882. doi:10.1016/s0140-6736(07)60854-x.

Wang, Yan, and Lloyd H. Kasper. "The Role of Microbiome in Central Nervous System Disorders." *Brain, Behavior, and Immunity*38 (2014): 1-12. doi:10.1016/j.bbi.2013.12.015.

Walsh, William. *Nutrient Power: Heal Your Biochemistry and Heal Your Brain.* Skyhorse Publishing, 2014.

Ward, Roberta J., David T. Dexter, and Robert R. Crichton. "Neurodegenerative Diseases and Therapeutic Strategies Using Iron Chelators." *Journal of Trace Elements in Medicine and Biology*31 (2015): 267-73. doi:10.1016/j.jtemb.2014.12.012.

Ware, Mark A., Crystal R. Doyle, Ryan Woods, Mary E. Lynch, and Alexander J. Clark. "Cannabis Use for Chronic Non-cancer Pain: Results of a Prospective Survey." *Pain*102, no. 1 (2003): 211-16. doi:10.1016/s0304-3959(02)00400-1.

Wei, L., J. Wang, Y. Cao, Q. Ren, L. Zhao, X. Li, and J. Wang. "Hyperbaric oxygenation promotes neural stem cell proliferation and protects the learning and memory ability in neonatal hypoxic-ischemic brain damage." *International Journal of Clinical and Experimental Pathology*8, no. 2 (2015): 1752-759.

West, J. B. "A strategy for reducing neonatal mortality at high altitude using oxygen conditioning." *Journal of Perinatology*35, no. 11 (2015): 900-02. doi:10.1038/jp.2015.108.

West, J. B., and O. Mathieu-Costello. "Stress Failure of Pulmonary Capillaries: Role in Lung and Heart Disease." *The Lancet*340, no. 8822 (1992): 762-67. doi:10.1016/0140-6736(92)92301-u.

West, John B. "Oxygen Conditioning: A New Technique for Improving Living and Working at High Altitude." *Physiology*31, no. 3 (2016): 216-22. doi:10.1152/physiol.00057.2015.

West, John B. "Oxygen enrichment of room air to relieve the hypoxia of high altitude." *Respiration Physiology*99, no. 2 (1995): 225-32. doi:10.1016/0034-5687(94)00094-g.

West, John B. "Physiological Effects of Chronic Hypoxia." *New England Journal of Medicine*376, no. 20 (2017): 1965-1971. doi:10.1056/nejmra1612008.

Wheeler, Mark. "UCLA Study Suggests Iron Is at Core of Alzheimer's Disease." UCLA Newsroom. August 20, 2013. Accessed May 13, 2018. http://newsroom.ucla.edu/releases/ucla-study-suggests-that-iron-247864.

Whiting, Penny F., Robert F. Wolff, Sohan Deshpande, Marcello Di Nisio, Steven Duffy, Adrian V. Hernandez, J. Christiaan Keurentjes, Shona Lang, Kate Misso, Steve Ryder, Simone Schmidlkofer, Marie Westwood, and Jos Kleijnen. "Cannabinoids for Medical Use." *Jama*313, no. 24 (2015): 2456. doi:10.1001/jama.2015.6358.

Whitmarsh, Thomas E. "Homeopathy in Multiple Sclerosis." *Complementary Therapies in Nursing and Midwifery*9, no. 1 (2003): 5-9. doi:10.1016/s1353-6117(02)00105-1.

Wilcox, Anna. Multiple Sclerosis: Here's Why Cannabis Is So Effective Against MS. March 22, 2018. Accessed April 09, 2018. https://herb.co/marijuana/news/marijuana-and-ms.

Wilmshurst, P. T., J. C. Byrne, and M. M. Webb-Peploe. "Relation Between Interatrial Shunts And Decompression Sickness In Divers." *The Lancet*334, no. 8675 (1989): 1302-306. doi:10.1016/s0140-6736(89)91911-9.

Wilson, Mark H., Christopher H. E. Imray, and Alan R. Hargens. "The Headache of High Altitude and Microgravity—Similarities with Clinical Syndromes of Cerebral Venous Hypertension." *High Altitude Medicine & Biology*12, no. 4 (2011): 379-86. doi:10.1089/ham.2011.1026.

Wilson, R. I. "Endocannabinoid Signaling in the Brain." *Science*296, no. 5568 (2002): 678-82. doi:10.1126/science.1063545.

Witte, Maarten E., Jeroen J. G. Geurts, Helga E. De Vries, Paul Van Der Valk, and Jack Van Horssen. "Mitochondrial Dysfunction: A Potential Link between

Neuroinflammation and Neurodegeneration?" *Mitochondrion*10, no. 5 (2010): 411-18. doi:10.1016/j.mito.2010.05.014.

Woeller, Kurt N. *Autism - the Road to Recovery (Dr. Kurt N. Woellers Autism Action Plan): An Autism Recovery Guide for Parents and Physicians.* (Lexington, KY): Dr. Kurt N. Woeller, 2012.

Woodfield, H. Charles, D. Gordon Hasick, Werner J. Becker, Marianne S. Rose, and James N. Scott. "Effect of Atlas Vertebrae Realignment in Subjects with Migraine: An Observational Pilot Study." *BioMed Research International*2015 (2015): 1-18. doi:10.1155/2015/630472.

Xie, L., H. Kang, Q. Xu, M. J. Chen, Y. Liao, M. Thiyagarajan, J. Odonnell, D. J. Christensen, C. Nicholson, J. J. Iliff, T. Takano, R. Deane, and M. Nedergaard. "Sleep Drives Metabolite Clearance from the Adult Brain." *Science*342, no. 6156 (2013): 373-77. doi:10.1126/science.1241224.

Yang, Jingke, Qi Zhang, Peiyu Li, Tingting Dong, and Mei X. Wu. "Low-level light treatment ameliorates immune thrombocytopenia." *Scientific Reports*6, no. 1 (2016). doi:10.1038/srep38238.

Yeshurun, Moshe, Ofer Shpilberg, Corina Herscovici, Liat Shargian, Juliet Dreyer, Anat Peck, Moshe Israeli, Maly Levy-Assaraf, Tsipora Gruenewald, Raphael Mechoulam, Pia Raanani, and Ron Ram. "Cannabidiol for the Prevention of Graft-versus-Host-Disease after Allogeneic Hematopoietic Cell Transplantation: Results Of a Phase II Study." *Biology of Blood and Marrow Transplantation*21, no. 10 (2015): 1770-775. doi:10.1016/j.bbmt.2015.05.018.

Younger, Jarred, Luke Parkitny, and David Mclain. "The Use of Low-dose Naltrexone (LDN) as a Novel Anti-inflammatory Treatment for Chronic Pain." *Clinical Rheumatology*33, no. 4 (2014): 451-59. doi:10.1007/s10067-014-2517-2.

Yu, Yigang, Long Zhou, Jinhuang Lin, Junming Lin, Guoju Kui, and Jianhua Zhang. "Neuroprotective Effects of Vagus Nerve Stimulation on Traumatic Brain Injury." *Neural Regeneration Research*9, no. 17 (2014): 1585. doi:10.4103/1673-5374.141783.

Yucel, M., E. Bora, D. I. Lubman, N. Solowij, W. J. Brewer, S. M. Cotton, P. Conus, M. J. Takagi, A. Fornito, S. J. Wood, P. D. Mcgorry, and C. Pantelis. "The Impact of Cannabis Use on Cognitive Functioning in Patients With Schizophrenia: A Meta-analysis of Existing Findings and New Data in a First-Episode Sample." *Schizophrenia Bulletin*38, no. 2 (2010): 316-30. doi:10.1093/schbul/sbq079.

Zajicek, John, Patrick Fox, Hilary Sanders, David Wright, Jane Vickery, Andrew Nunn, and Alan Thompson. "Cannabinoids for treatment of spasticity and other symptoms related to multiple sclerosis (CAMS study): multicentre randomised placebo-controlled trial." *The Lancet*362, no. 9395 (2003): 1517-526. doi:10.1016/s0140-6736(03)14738-1.

Zamboni, P., V. Tisato, E. Menegatti, F. Mascoli, S. Gianesini, F. Salvi, and P. Secchiero. "Ultrastructure of internal jugular vein defective valves." *Phlebology: The Journal of Venous Disease*30, no. 9 (2014): 644-47. doi:10.1177/0268355514541980.

Zhang, Rongzhen, Robert G. Miller, Ron Gascon, Stacey Champion, Jonathan Katz, Mariselle Lancero, Amy Narvaez, Ronald Honrada, David Ruvalcaba, and Michael S. Mcgrath. "Circulating Endotoxin and Systemic Immune Activation in Sporadic Amyotrophic Lateral Sclerosis (sALS)." *Journal of Neuroimmunology*206, no. 1-2 (2009): 121-24. doi:10.1016/j.jneuroim.2008.09.017.

Zhang, Yonghua, Aasheeta Parikh, and Shuo Qian. "Migraine and Stroke." *Stroke and Vascular Neurology*2, no. 3 (2017): 160-67. doi:10.1136/svn-2017-000077.

Zivadinov, Robert, Bianca Weinstock-Guttman, and Istvan Pirko. "Iron deposition and inflammation in multiple sclerosis. Which one comes first?" *BMC Neuroscience*12, no. 1 (2011): 60. doi:10.1186/1471-2202-12-60.

Zivadinov, Robert, Deepa P. Ramasamy, Ralph R. H. Benedict, Paul Polak, Jesper Hagemeier, Christopher Magnano, Michael G. Dwyer, Niels Bergsland, Nicola Bertolino, Bianca Weinstock-Guttman, Channa Kolb, David Hojnacki, David Utriainen, E. Mark Haacke, and Ferdinand Schweser. "Cerebral Microbleeds in Multiple Sclerosis Evaluated on Susceptibility-weighted Images and Quantitative Susceptibility Maps: A Case-Control Study." *Radiology*281, no. 3 (2016): 884-95. doi:10.1148/radiol.2016160060.

Zivadinov, Robert, Stefano Bastianello, Michael D. Dake, Hector Ferral, E. Mark Haacke, Ziv J. Haskal, David Hubbard, Nikolaos Liasis, Kenneth Mandato, Salvatore Sclafani, Adnan H. Siddiqui, Marian Simka, and Paolo Zamboni. "Recommendations for Multimodal Noninvasive and Invasive Screening for Detection of Extracranial Venous Abnormalities Indicative of Chronic Cerebrospinal Venous Insufficiency: A Position Statement of the International Society for Neurovascular Disease." *Journal of Vascular and Interventional Radiology*25, no. 11 (2014). doi:10.1016/j.jvir.2014.07.024.

Zlokovic, Berislav V. "The Blood-Brain Barrier in Health and Chronic Neurodegenerative Disorders." *Neuron*57, no. 2 (2008): 178-201. doi:10.1016/j.neuron.2008.01.003.

Zoladz, J. A., and A. Pilc. "The Effect of Physical Activity on the Brain Derived Neurotrophic Factor: From Animal to Human Studies." *J Physiol Pharmacol*61, no. 5 (2010): 533-41.

Zonis, Svetlana, Robert N. Pechnick, Vladimir A. Ljubimov, Michael Mahgerefteh, Kolja Wawrowsky, Kathrin S. Michelsen, and Vera Chesnokova. "Chronic Intestinal Inflammation Alters Hippocampal Neurogenesis." *Journal of Neuroinflammation*12, no. 1 (2015). doi:10.1186/s12974-015-0281-0.

Acknowledgements

I am grateful for the support of family, friends and colleagues in this major life endeavor. Many of these are listed within the book so are not repeated here. However, a large number of individuals are sincerely thanked for their efforts, input and wisdom. I sincerely appreciate the contributions from the various authors. As experts in their fields, their work added significantly to this important topic of brain health. For all others, if you had any input, whether a comment a query, or a reference, I thank you for this.

A special thank you to Andrew Paterson for his computer and bibliography expertise. His daughter, MacKenzie was a great assist in this. Special thanks are also extended to Elaine O'Rourke, Candace Appleby, Mary Cook, Brian Code and Denise Code for the many hours they spent helping to complete this book.

Editing, artwork, and proofreading were well done by FriesenPress.

Index

Please note that the italicized letter "*n*" after a page number refers to a footnote and the italicized "*f*" refers to a figure.

C

E

I

MRI. *See* magnetic resonance imaging (MRI)

MRSA. *See* methicillin-resistant staph infection (MRSA)

MRV. *See* magnetic resonance venography (MRV)

MS. *See* multiple sclerosis or microvascular syndrome (MS)

MSH. *See* alpha melanocyte-stimulating hormone (MSH)

MTHFR. *See* methylenetetrahydrofolate reductase (MTHFR)

O

R

T

V

W

Yu, Yigang, 140

Printed in Canada